Moyamoya Disease Update

Byung-Kyu Cho · Teiji Tominaga
Editors

Moyamoya Disease Update

Springer

Editors

Byung-Kyu Cho M.D., Ph.D.
Professor
Department of Neurosurgery
Seoul National University College of Medicine
Seoul National University Children's Hospital
101 Daehangno, Jongno-gu
Seoul 110-744
Republic of Korea
bkcho@snu.ac.kr

Teiji Tominaga M.D., Ph.D.
Professor, Chairman
Department of Neurosurgery
Tohoku University Graduate School of Medicine
1-1 Seiryo-machi, Aoba-ku
Sendai 980-8578
Japan
tomi@nsg.med.tohoku.ac.jp

ISBN 978-4-431-54649-8 ISBN 978-4-431-99703-0 (eBook)
DOI 10.1007/978-4-431-99703-0
Springer Tokyo Berlin Heidelberg New York

Printed on acid-free paper

Springer is part of Springer Science+Business Media (www.springer.com)

Foreword

The emblem of Seoul National University bears the apothegm *Veritas lux mea*, "The truth enlightens me." The phrase may serve as a source of pride for new students as well as a creed for life kept deeply in the hearts of graduates of Seoul National University. Although every scholar seeks after the truth for various reasons, it is hard to live up to the sincere purpose of abandoning all greed in life. I think Professor Byung-Kyu Cho lived such a life.

Back in 1979, Professor Cho had just become a member of the faculty of the Department of Neurosurgery at Seoul National University College of Medicine. I vividly remember his enthusiasm at that time, as it was also the first year of my training course in neurosurgery. As time surely flies as fast as an arrow, he is about to finish his respectable period of three decades as a neurosurgeon in his alma mater. He has never neglected his duty as a scholar throughout his career. He never missed a conference, listened very carefully to the end, always put forth proper questions, and gave kind advice based on his vast experience and profound knowledge. "Meticulousness" is the best word to characterize his attitude in clinical and academic activities.

This book about moyamoya disease is like a reflection of his characteristics. Since Professor Jiro Suzuki introduced the new disease category of moyamoya disease in 1969, it has been found to have a geographical preponderance in the East Asia, and many important investigations have been carried out in Japan and Korea. However, moyamoya disease is still a medical syndrome for which the pathophysiology remains to be discovered. Systematic compilation of scattered current knowledge may be the starting point for a new step toward complete comprehension of the disease. This book scrupulously covers a diversity of topics from the evidence provided by basic research to the clinical investigations on moyamoya disease. It consists of 13 sections with 52 chapters written by 74 authors, and each subject begins with an overview and goes on to specific details, with "special consideration" sections to provide readers with practical information. Professor Teiji Tominaga of Tohoku University, Japan, took part in preparing the book as a co-editor, and his perceptive insight was invaluable.

The publication of this monograph on moyamoya disease is well timed to provide inspirational guidance for future directions. The book is especially meaningful for Professor Byung-Kyu Cho, as it not only deals with the field of his special interest but also includes the integration of achievements by him and his colleagues. I am convinced that this work will inspire coming generations with great ideas and motivation.

Dong Gyu Kim, MD, PhD
Professor and Chairman
Department of Neurosurgery
Seoul National University College of Medicine
Seoul, Republic of Korea

Preface

It has been half a century since Takeuchi K. and Shimizu K. first reported a new entity of vascular disease in 1957 that they called "hypogenesis of bilateral internal carotid arteries." The name "moyamoya disease" (MMD) was coined by Suzuki J. and Takaku A. in 1969, after the characteristic angiographic finding that showed abnormal vascular networks around the occluded distal internal carotid artery looking like a puff of smoke (*moyamoya* in Japanese). The first monograph on moyamoya disease was published in 1986 by Professor Jiro Suzuki of Tohoku University, Japan. In 2001, Ikezaki K. and Loftus CM published the second monograph on moyamoya disease. Since then, a large amount of clinical as well as basic research data on MMD has been gathered.

The purpose of this monograph is to present a summary of the accumulated information to help readers understand the current status of MMD in clinical practice and basic research.

For this reason we have tried to include all the important issues involved both in current development and in controversy. The chapters of the book provide readers with the current concepts and future directions of study. Genetics, computational analysis of hemodynamic shear stress, new imaging techniques including magnetic resonance angiography and magnetoencephalography, and endovascular treatment of MMD are those focused on in the book. In addition, "special consideration" sections deal with practical topics in the chapters on very young children with MMD, adult hemorrhagic MMD, post-direct bypass hyperperfusion syndrome, moyamoya syndrome, pregnancy and delivery-related problems, and asymptomatic MMD, as well as the future direction of the management of cerebral ischemia with enhancers of revascularization, and gene and stem cell therapies. We hope this information will lead to more efficient and predictive management of MMD in the near future.

We greatly appreciate the contributors of all the chapters as well as our colleagues who devoted their time and effort to make this book meaningful. We also give special thanks to the publisher, Springer Japan, for their generous assistance and superb work in producing this monograph on MMD. Above all, we send our thanks and love to our patients and their families, without whom this volume could not have come into existence.

Editors
Byung-Kyu Cho, MD, PhD
Teiji Tominaga, MD, PhD

Contents

Contributors

Jong-Hee Chae MD, PhD
Department of Pediatrics, Pediatric Clinical Neuroscience Center,
Seoul National University Children's Hospital, Research Center for Rare Disease
Seoul National University College of Medicine, Seoul, Republic of Korea

Jung-Eun Cheon MD
Department of Radiology, Seoul National University Hospital, Seoul National University
College of Medicine, Seoul, Republic of Korea

Hae Il Cheong MD, PhD
Department of Pediatrics, Seoul National University Children's Hospital,
Kidney Research Institute, Medical Research Center, Research Center for Rare Disease
Seoul National University College of Medicine, Seoul, Republic of Korea

Byung-Kyu Cho MD, PhD
Division of Pediatric Neurosurgery, Pediatric Clinical Neuroscience Center,
Seoul National University Children's Hospital, Seoul National University
College of Medicine, Seoul, Republic of Korea

Joong-Uhn Choi MD, PhD
Department of Neurosurgery, CHA Bundang Medical Center, CHA University,
Gyeonggi-do, Republic of Korea

Yong Choi MD, PhD
Department of Pediatrics,
Seoul National University Children's Hospital, Kidney Research Institute, Medical Research
Center, Seoul National University College of Medicine, Seoul, Republic of Korea

Isao Date MD, PhD
Department of Neurological Surgery, Okayama University Graduate School of Medicine,
Dentistry and Pharmaceutical Sciences, Okayama, Japan

Kent Doi MD, PhD
Department of Neurosurgery, Kyoto University Graduate School of Medicine, Kyoto, Japan

Javier Fandino MD
Department of Neurosurgery, Kantonsspital Aarau, Aarau, Switzerland

Yukihiko Fujii MD, PhD
Department of Neurosurgery, Brain Research Institute, University of Niigata, Niigata, Japan

Miki Fujimura MD, PhD
Department of Neurosurgery, Kohnan Hospital, Sendai, Japan

Masayuki Fujioka MD
Department of Neurosurgery, Kantonsspital Aarau, Aarau, Switzerland
University of Zürich, Zürich, Switzerland

Raphael Guzman MD
Department of Neurosurgery, Stanford Stroke Center, Stanford Institute for Neuro-Innovation and Translational Neurosciences, Stanford University School of Medicine, Stanford, CA, USA

Kentaro Hayashi MD, PhD
Department of Neurosurgery, Nagasaki University School of Medicine, Nagasaki, Japan

Seok Ho Hong MD
Department of Neurosurgery, Asan Medical Center, University of Ulsan College of Medicine, Seoul, Republic of Korea

Haruhiko Hoshino MD, PhD
Preventive Medicine for Cerebrovascular Disease, Department of Neurology, Keio University School of Medicine, Tokyo, Japan

Kiyohiro Houkin MD, DMSc
Department of Neurosurgery, Sapporo Medical University, Sapporo, Japan

Martina Hug MD
Children's Hospital of Zürich, University Clinic, Zürich, Switzerland

Gyojun Hwang MD
Division of Cerebrovascular Surgery, Department of Neurosurgery, Seoul National University Bundang Hospital, Seoul National University College of Medicine, Gyeonggi-do, Republic of Korea

Yong-Seung Hwang MD, PhD
Department of Pediatrics, Pediatric Clinical Neuroscience Center Seoul National University Children's Hospital, Seoul National University College of Medicine, Seoul, Republic of Korea

Satoshi Iihoshi MD, PhD
Department of Neurosurgery, Sapporo Medical University, Sapporo, Japan

So-Hyang Im MD
Department of Neurosurgery, Thomas Jefferson University, Philadelphia, Pennsylvania, USA

Hyun-Seung Kang MD, PhD
Department of Neurosurgery, Seoul National University Hospital, Seoul National University College of Medicine, Seoul, Republic of Korea

Akitake Kanno PhD
MEG Laboratory Kohnan Hospital, Sendai, Japan

Masatou Kawashima MD, PhD
Department of Neurosurgery, Faculty of Medicine, Saga University, Saga, Japan

Nadia Khan MD
Department of Neurosurgery, Stanford Stroke Center, Stanford Institute for Neuro-Innovation and Translational Neurosciences, Stanford University School of Medicine, Stanford, CA, USA

Ken-ichiro Kikuta MD, PhD
Division of Neurosurgery, Department of Sensory and Locomotor Medicine, Faculty of Medical Sciences, University of Fukui, Fukui, Japan

Byong Cheol Kim MD, PhD
Department of Neurosurgery, Seoul National University Bundang Hospital, Seoul National University College of Medicine, Seoul, Republic of Korea

Chae-Yong Kim MD, PhD
Department of Neurosurgery, Seoul National University Bundang Hospital, Seoul National University College of Medicine, Seoul, Republic of Korea

Dal-Soo Kim MD, PhD
Stroke Center, Department of Neurosurgery, Myong-Ji St. Mary's Hospital, Seoul, Republic of Korea

Hee-Soo Kim MD, PhD
Division of Pediatric Anesthesiology and Pain Medicine, Seoul National University Children's Hospital, Seoul National University College of Medicine, Seoul, Republic of Korea

In-One Kim MD, PhD
Department of Radiology, Seoul National University Hospital, Seoul National University College of Medicine, Seoul, Republic of Korea

Jeong Chul Kim PhD
Institute of Medical and Biological Engineering, Medical Research Center, Seoul National University College of Medicine, Seoul, Republic of Korea,

Jin Hyun Kim PhD
Clinical Research Institute, Gyeongsang National University Hospital, Gyeongnam-do, Republic of Korea

Jeong Eun Kim MD, PhD
Department of Neurosurgery, Seoul National University Hospital, Seoul National University College of Medicine, Seoul, Republic of Korea

Ki Joong Kim MD, PhD
Department of Pediatrics, Pediatric Clinical Neuroscience Center, Seoul National University Children's Hopital, Seoul Notional University College of Medicine, Seoul, Republic of Korea

Seong Hyun Kim MD
Department of Radiology, Clinical Neuroscience Center, Seoul National University Bundang Hospital, Seoul National University College of Medicine, Gyeonggi-do, Republic of Korea

Seung-Ki Kim MD, PhD
Division of Pediatric Neurosurgery, Pediatric Clinical Neuroscience Center, Seoul National University Children's Hospital, Research Center for Rare Disease, Seoul National University College of Medicine, Seoul, Republic of Korea

Shigeo Kure MD, PhD
Department of Pediatrics, Tohoku University School of Medicine, Sendai, Japan

Satoshi Kuroda MD, PhD
Department of Neurosurgery, Hokkaido University Graduate School of Medicine, Sapporo, Japan

O-Ki Kwon MD, PhD
Division of Cerebrovascular Surgery, Department of Neurosurgery, Seoul National University Bundang Hospital, Seoul National University College of Medicine, Gyeonggi-do, Republic of Korea

Dong Soo Lee MD, PhD
Department of Nuclear Medicine, and Department of Molecular Medicine and Biopharmaceutical Sciences, Seoul National University, Seoul, Republic of Korea

Jianmin Liu MD
Department of Neurosurgery, Changhai Hospital, Shanghai, China

Jun Masuoka MD, PhD
Department of Neurosurgery, Faculty of Medicine, Saga University, Saga, Japan

Toshio Matsushima MD, PhD
Department of Neurosurgery, Faculty of Medicine, Saga University, Saga, Japan

Takeshi Mikami MD, PhD
Department of Neurosurgery, Sapporo Medical University, Sapporo, Japan

Susumu Miyamoto MD, PhD
Department of Neurosurgery, Kyoto University, Kyoto, Japan

Izumi Nagata MD, PhD
Department of Neurosurgery, Nagasaki University School of Medicine, Nagasaki, Japan

Jyoji Nakagawara MD
Department of Neurosurgery, Nakamura Memorial Hospital, Sapporo, Japan

Nobukazu Nakasato MD, PhD
MEG Laboratory and Department of Neurosurgery, Kohnan Hospital, Sendai, Japan

Tadashi Nariai MD, PhD
Department of Neurosurgery, Tokyo Medical and Dental University, Tokyo, Japan

Kazuhiko Nishino MD
Department of Neurosurgery, Brain Research Institute, University of Niigata, Niigata, Japan

Shigeru Nogawa MD, PhD
Department of Neurology, Tokyo Dental College Ichikawa General Hospital, Ichikawa, Japan

Chang-Wan Oh MD, PhD
Division of Cerebrovascular Surgery, Department of Neurosurgery, Seoul National Univeristy Bundang Hospital, Seoul National University College of Medicine, Gyeonggi-do, Republic of Korea

Koichi Oki MD
Department of Neurology, Keio University School of Medicine, Tokyo, Japan

Jin Chul Paeng MD
Department of Nuclear Medicine, Seoul National University Hospital, Seoul National University College of Medicine, Seoul, Republic of Korea

Myoung Hee Park MD, PhD
Department of Laboratory Medicine, Seoul National University Hospital, Seoul National University College of Medicine, Seoul, Republic of Korea

Ji Hoon Phi MD
Division of Pediatric Neurosurgery, Pediatric Clinical Neuroscience Center, Seoul National University Children's Hospital, Seoul National University College of Medicine, Seoul, Republic of Korea

R. Michael Scott MD
Department of Neurosurgery, Children's Hospital, Harvard Medical School, Boston, Massachusetts, USA

Ho Jun Seol MD, PhD
Department of Neurosurgery, Kangwon National University Hospital, Kangwon-do, Republic of Korea

Eun Bo Shim PhD
Department of Mechanical and Biomedical Engineering, Kangwon National University, Kangwon-do, Republic of Korea

Reizo Shirane MD, PhD
Department of Neurosurgery, Miyagi Children's Hospital, Sendai, Japan

Edward R. Smith MD
Department of Neurosurgery, Children's Hospital, Harvard Medical School, Boston, Massachusetts, USA

Takatoshi Sorimachi MD, PhD
Department of Neurosurgery, Brain Research Institute, University of Niigata, Niigata, Japan

Gary K. Steinberg MD, PhD
Department of Neurosurgery, Stanford Stroke Center, Stanford Institute for Neuro-Innovation and Translational Neurosciences, Stanford University School of Medicine, Stanford, CA, USA

Norihiro Suzuki MD, PhD
Department of Neurology, Keio University School of Medicine, Tokyo, Japan

Yasushi Takagi MD, PhD
Department of Neurosurgery, Kyoto University Graduate School of Medicine, Kyoto, Japan

Jun C. Takahashi MD, PhD
Department of Neurosurgery, Kyoto University, Kyoto, Japan

Koji Tokunaga MD, PhD
Department of Neurological Surgery, Okayama University Graduate School of Medicine, Dentistry and Pharmaceutical Sciences, Okayama, Japan

Teiji Tominaga MD, PhD
Department of Neurosurgery, Tohoku University Graduate School of Medicine, Sendai, Japan

Kyu-Chang Wang MD, PhD
Division of Pediatric Neurosurgery, Pediatric Clinical Neuroscience Center, Seoul National University Children's Hospital, Seoul National University College of Medicine, Seoul, Republic of Korea

Weimin Wang MD
Department of Neurosurgery, Guangzhou General Hospital of Guangzhou Military Area Command, Guangzhou, China

Markus Wiesli MD
Klinik im Park, Zürich, Switzerland

Wenyuan Zhao MD, PhD
Department of Neurosurgery, Changhai Hospital, Shanghai, China

Yasuhiro Yonekawa MD
University of Zürich, Zürich, Switzerland
Department of Neurosurgery, Kantonsspital Aarau, Aarau, Switzerland
Children's Hospital of Zürich, University Clinic, Zürich, Switzerland
Klinik im Park, Zürich, Switzerland

Part I
Introduction

Overview

Teiji Tominaga

Introduction

Moyamoya disease is a unique cerebrovascular disease with steno-occlusive changes at the terminal portion of the internal carotid artery and fine vascular network, the so-called "moyamoya" vessels [1]. This vascular network forms a collateral pathway and compensates reduced cerebral blood flow due to steno-occlusive changes of the trunk arteries. The characteristics of moyamoya disease can be summarized as follows. Moyamoya disease shows racial difference in incidence and predominantly occurs in the Eastern Asia among a worldwide distribution. Clinical manifestation includes ischemia and hemorrhage, epilepsy, headache, etc., and young patients usually present with ischemia and adult patients with either ischemia or hemorrhage [2]. Evidence indicates that revascularization surgery can prevent an ischemic event, although its effect on prevention of hemorrhagic events is yet to be determined [2–6]. Since the familial occurrence reaches 12%, an intense effort has been focused on genetic analysis during the past decade which has found that several genetic loci associate with this disease [7, 8]. Nevertheless, the conclusive pathogenesis of this disease still remains unknown. In this chapter, the author seeks to focus on the diagnostic criteria, the definition, and the history of this disease.

Definition and Diagnostic Criteria

The first English report of moyamoya disease described its clinical features including steno-occlusive changes of the carotid fork with abnormal vascular network (moyamoya vessels) in the base of the brain [1]. In addition, these vascular changes have features of bilateral location and progression. The pathogenesis is unknown. In 1977, the research committee supported by the Japanese Ministry of Health and Welfare started basic and clinical research on this disease, and in 1995 (in English, 1997), this committee proposed guidelines for diagnosis and treatment of moyamoya disease [9].

T. Tominaga (✉)
Department of Neurosurgery, Tohoku University Graduate School of Medicine, 1-1 Seiryo-machi, Aoba-ku, Sendai, 980-8574, Japan
e-mail: tomi@nsg.med.tohoku.ac.jp

B.-K. Cho and T. Tominaga (eds.), *Moyamoya Disease Update*,
DOI 10.1007/978-4-431-99703-0_1, © Springer 2010

The diagnostic criteria of these guidelines are summarized in Table 1. Since the characteristic vascular changes have been confirmed by conventional angiography, this examination has been essential for the diagnosis of this disease (Fig. 1). However, recent

Table 1 Diagnostic criteria of moyamoya disease

1. Vascular changes		
	Angiography	MRI/MRA
(1)	Stenosis or occlusion at the terminal portion of the internal carotid artery w/wo that at the proximal portion of the anterior and/or middle cerebral arteries	MRA: Stenosis or occlusion at the terminal portion of the internal carotid artery w/wo that at the proximal portion of the anterior and/or middle cerebral arteries
(2)	Abnormal vascular network in the vicinity of the occlusive or stenotic lesions in the arterial	MRA: Abnormal vascular network in the vicinity of the occlusive or stenotic lesions MRI: Two or more than two flow voids in the basal ganglia in the same side
(3)	(1) and (2) present bilaterally	
2. Etiology and exclusion c riteria		
Etiology is unknown, and vascular changes associated with following diseases or conditions should be excluded; atherosclerosis, autoimmune diseases, meningitis, brain tumors, Down syndrome, Recklinghausen's disease, traumatic brain injury, irradiation, and others.		

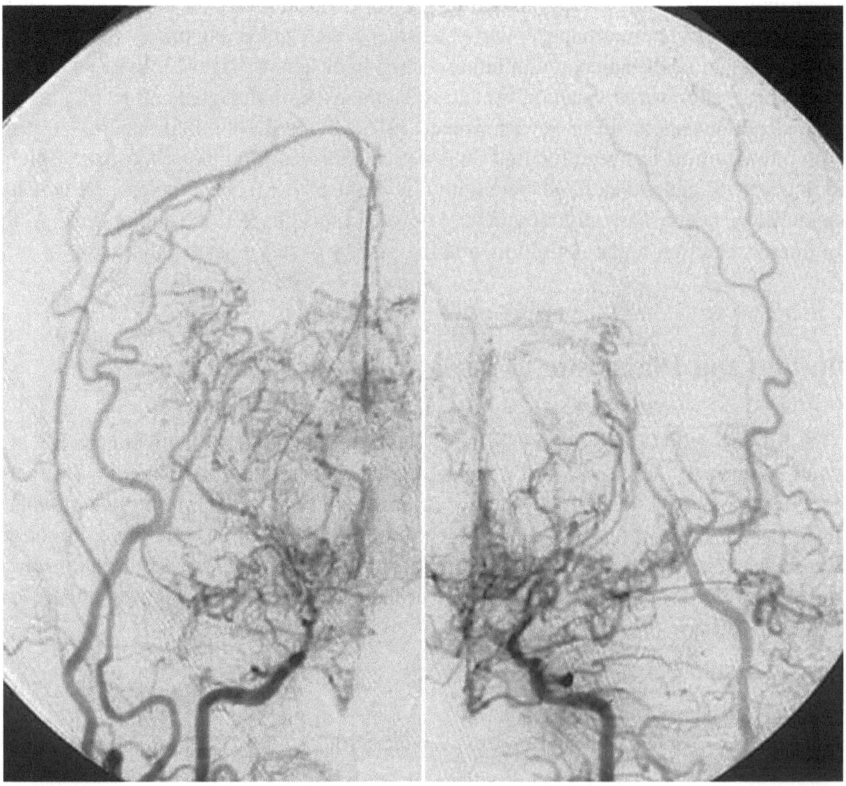

Fig. 1 Carotid angiogram of moyamoya disease. Note stenosis at the terminal portion of the internal carotid artery and disappearance of the main trunks of the anterior and middle cerebral arteries in both sides. Moyamoya vessels are seen bilaterally and transdural anastomoses are well developed

advances and widespread use of magnetic resonance imaging and angiography (MRI/MRA) has provided information adequate for identifying vascular changes characteristic of moyamoya disease. The MRI/MRA makes the evaluation more convenient and safer, particularly in pediatric patients and in out-patient screening of this disease. Therefore, the research committee introduced MRI/MRA as a diagnostic means in addition to conventional angiography. It is noted that the existence of flow voids in the basal ganglia (two or more, unilateral side) can be considered as the finding corresponding to moyamoya vessels on angiography (Fig. 2).

Unknown etiology consists of the definition of this disease. When a risk factor or condition which may cause vascular changes presents, the diagnosis should be moyamoya syndrome, instead of moyamoya disease. The research committee indicated the disorders or conditions to exclude moyamoya disease as follows:

1. Arteriosclerosis
2. Autoimmune disease
3. Meningitis
4. Brain neoplasm
5. Down syndrome
6. Recklinghausen's disease
7. Head trauma
8. Irradiation to the head
9. Others

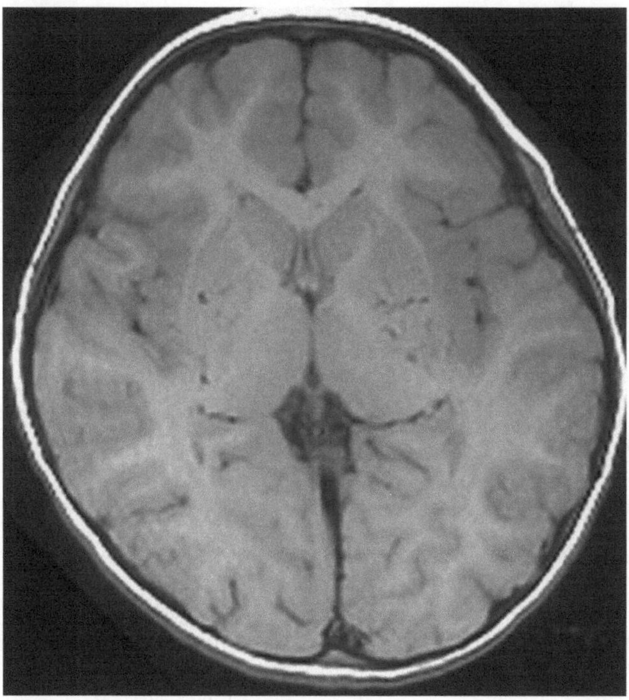

Fig. 2 MRI of moyamoya disease. Note several flow voids in the basal ganglia on both sides. These flow voids correspond to moyamoya vessels on angiography [9]

In addition to those diagnostic criteria, pathological findings suggestive of moyamoya disease are as follows [9]:

1) Stenosis or occlusion of the inner lumen of the terminal portion of the internal carotid artery due to hyperplasia or thickening of the intimal layer is usually seen on both sides. Deposition of lipid is occasionally seen within the thickened intimal layer.
2) In the arteries consisting of the circle of Willis, such as the anterior, middle, or posterior cerebral artery, stenotic change in various degrees or occlusion is often observed with fibrous hyperplasia of the intimal layer, a waving of the internal elastic lamina, and thinning of the medial layer.
3) There are a number of fine vessels (perforators and anastomotic vascular channels) mainly at the site of or surrounding the circle of Willis.
4) Frequent observation of rete-like small vessels congregated in the pia mater.

These diagnostic criteria do not differ from the original description of this disease. However, the progressive nature of moyamoya disease was highlighted in the original report and included in the important features of this disease. As shown in Fig. 3 and Table 2, angiographic progression has been classified into the six stages based on its appearance, development, diminishment, and disappearance of moyamoya vessels [1].

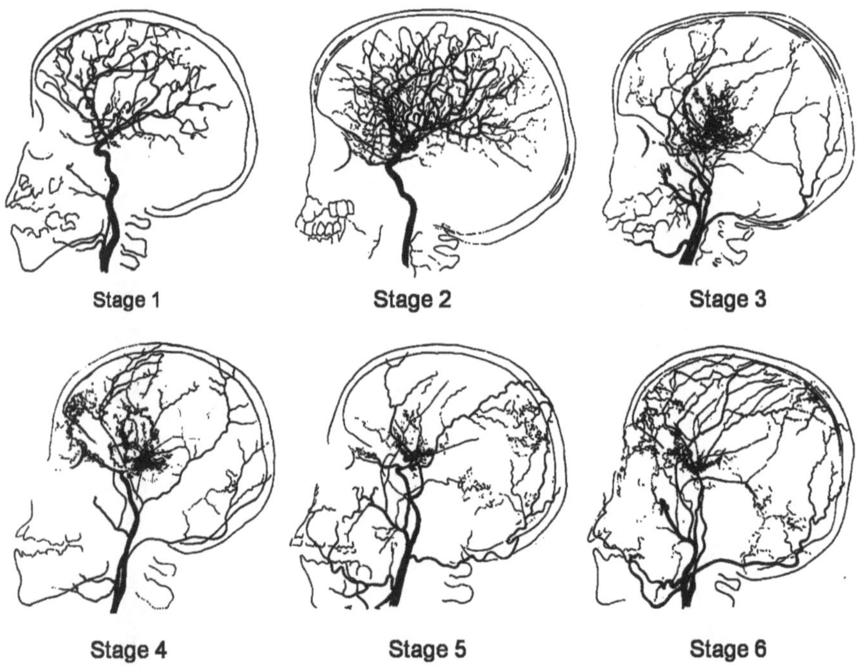

Fig. 3 Angiographic stages of moyamoya disease [1]

Table 2 Angiographic stages and its feature

Stage 1: Narrowing of the carotid fork
Stage 2: Initiation of moyamoya vessels
Stage 3: Intensification of moyamoya vessels
Stage 4: Minimization of moyamoya vessels
Stage 5: Reduction of moyamoya vessels
Stage 6: Disappearance of moyamoya vessels

Diagnosis

Diagnosis of moyamoya disease depends on the peculiar vascular changes, cause of disease, age of patient, and unilateral or bilateral location of vascular changes. Definitive moyamoya disease, probable or unilateral moyamoya disease, and moyamoya syndrome include the following factors, respectively. Figure 4 shows a flow chart for practical diagnosis of moyamoya-associated entities.

1. *Definitive moyamoya disease:*
   Adult: steno-occlusive change of the carotid fork and moyamoya vessels, bilateral, unknown cause
   Child: above findings, either bilateral or unilateral
2. *Probable or unilateral moyamoya disease:*
   Adult: steno-occlusive change of the carotid fork and moyamoya vessels, unilateral, unknown cause
   Child: (-)
   Recent evidence indicated that about 36% of patients with unilateral moyamoya disease progressed to bilateral lesions (moyamoya disease) during 5 years after the onset [10]. Another report indicated that 30% of patients with unilateral moyamoya syndrome who underwent revascularization showed progression to bilateral lesions with a more rapid progression rate in younger ages at the diagnosis [11]. These are suggestive that unilateral moyamoya disease has a pathogenesis similar to that of moyamoya disease. Indeed, a recent study reported that unilateral moyamoya disease has a genetic background similar to that of definitive moyamoya disease [12].
3. *Moyamoya syndrome (quasi-moyamoya disease):*
   Adult/child: steno-occlusive change of the carotid fork and moyamoya vessels, unilateral or bilateral, presence of associated disease or condition (a possible risk associated with the occurrence of such vascular changes)
   A variety of clinical conditions or systemic disorders have been reported in conjunction with moyamoya syndrome as indicated in Table 3 [4, 13]. Across those congenital,

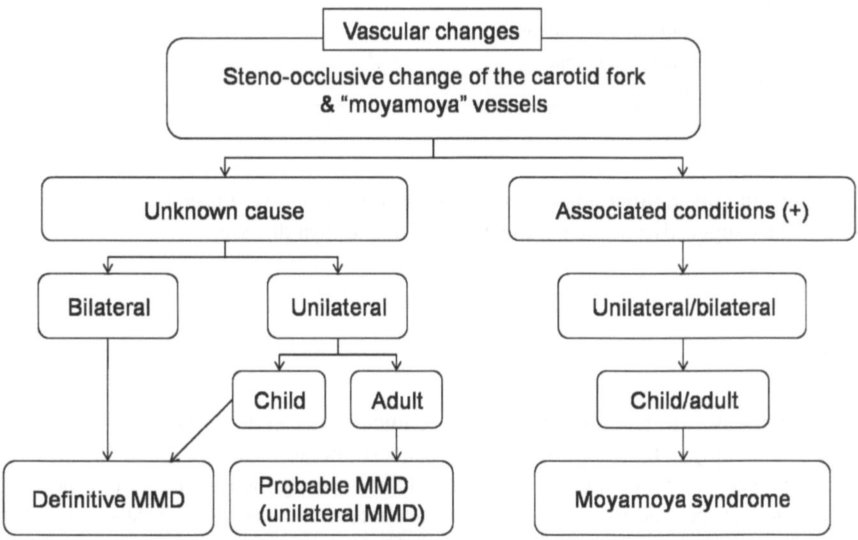

Fig. 4 A flow chart for diagnosis of moyamoya disease

Table 3 Moyamoya syndrome and associated disorders and conditions (Ikezaki et al. [13], modified)

Congenital disorder	Acquired disorders
Hematological disorders	*Autoimmune diseases*
Anaplastic anemia	Systemic lupus erythematosis
Fanconi's anemia	Anti-phospholipid antibody syndrome
Sickle cell anemia	Thrombotic thrombocytopenic purpura
Thalassemia	Periarteritis nodusa
Spherocytosis	Sjögren syndrome
Protein C deficiency	Hyperthyroidism
Protein S deficiency	*Neoplasm*
Plasminogen deficiency	Parasellar tumor
Congenital anomalies	*Infectious diseases*
Down syndrome	Leptospirosis
NF type I	Tuberculosis
Tuberous sclerosis	Meningitis
Marfan syndrome	*Others*
Coarctation of aorta	Traumatic brain injury
Fibromuscular dysplasia	Cranial irradiation
Osteogenesis imperfect	Oral contraceptive
Turner's syndrome	Drug abuse (cocaine etc.)
Hirschsprung disease	
Wilms' tumor	Unclassified disorders
Polycystic kidney	*Vascular disorders*
Prader Willi syndrome	Cerebral aneurysm
Apert's syndrome	Arteriovenous malformation
Allagille syndrome	Venous angioma
Williams syndrome	Cavernous angioma
Noonan syndrome	Athersclerotic disease
Metabolic disorders	Renovascular hypertension
Hyperlipoproteinemia (type 2A)	
Glycogen storage disease	
Lipohyalinosis	
NADH-CoQ reductase activity	
Pyruvate kinase deficiency	
Homocystinuria	

acquired, and unclassified disorders and conditions, it is very difficult to discover consistent factors suggestive of the pathogenesis of moyamoya disease.

History

Moyamoya disease was recognized as a single clinical entity in the early 1960s in Japan. The name of "moyamoya" first appeared in the Japanese literature in 1965, and in the English literature in 1969 [1]. Since those reports, there have been a growing number of reports from America and Europe, and moyamoya disease has become a worldwide disease, while it was initially thought to be the regional disease of the Eastern Asia.

In 1955, the first patient with this disease was reported at the 14th Annual Meeting of the Japan Neurosurgical Society by Shimizu and Takeuchi. The title was "Hypoplasia of the bilateral internal carotid arteries," and they published this case in the Japanese journal *Brain Nerve* in 1957 [14]. In the same year, Kudo published a case report entitled "a case of hypoplasia of the circle of Willis" in the same journal [15]. Thereafter, patients with angiographic vascular changes characteristic of moyamoya disease have been reported sporadically in Japan. At that time, occlusion of bilateral carotid arteries and the formation of net-like vessels (moyamoya vessels) have been considered as congenital anomalies, like hypoplasia or vascular tumor.

In 1963, Suzuki et al. reported six cases of moyamoya disease at the 22nd Annual Meeting of the Japan Neurosurgical Society. They proposed that net-like vessels at the base of the brain serve as collateral channels which were necessitated by acquired and gradual stenosis of the internal carotid arteries. In addition, more importantly, these findings on the cerebral angiogram consist of a single clinical entity.

In the United States and Europe, patients with moyamoya disease seem to appear in 1965 [16–18]. Weidner et al. reported angiographic findings of four patients with cerebrovascular disease focusing on the leptomeningeal and rete mirabile (meningeal to pial) anastomoses [16]. Among the four patients, a 31-year-old Japanese-American woman who presented with intracranial bleeding showed angiographic findings typical of moyamoya disease. In the same year, Krayenbuhl and Yasargil also described one case of cerebral angiogram characteristic of moyamoya disease in their textbook, and mentioned it as an extremely rare anomaly, namely "Kapillareiffuse cerebrale angioectasie" [17]. Also in 1965, Leeds and Abbott reported two such cases [18], and thereafter, a growing number of patients have been reported in the English language literature.

In 1969, the name of "moyamoya" first appeared in the English literature. In this original report, the main arterial trunk lesions included stenosis or occlusion of the terminal portion of the internal carotid artery [1]. They say, "in some cases, there is a defect or an abnormality observed in the middle or anterior cerebral artery." They also stressed that this disease or angiographic change is progressive. It is surprising that they proposed the six stages of angiographic findings along the progress of this disease, based on only 20 cases that they experienced (Fig. 3 and Table 2).

Before the name of "moyamoya" disease appeared, a variety of names were proposed for this pathological condition; cerebral juxta-basal teleangiectasia, hemangiomatous malformation of the bilateral internal carotid arteries at the base of the brain, cerebral arterial rete, and Nishimoto (or Nishimoto-Takeuchi-Kudo) disease [19], etc. The name of "Spontaneous occlusion of the circle of Willis" was reported in 1968 [20] and used particularly in Japan, while the more evocative name "moyamoya" has spread widely and has been recognized as the name specific to this condition.

Why "Moyamoya" (Fig. 5)

The Japanese word "moyamoya" means something hazy such as a puff of cigarette smoke drifting in the air, and indicates the appearance of the network of fine vessels formed as collateral circulation on the angiogram of patients with this disease. First, Suzuki and Takaku submitted a manuscript entitled "A disease showing abnormal net-like vessels at the base of the brain" with a subtitle of "moyamoya disease". The editor of the journal *Archives of Neurology*, who received this manuscript, exchanged the main title and subtitle, which

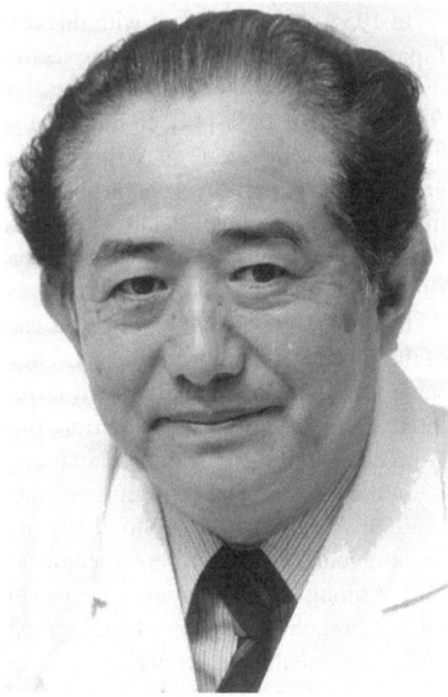

Fig. 5 Professor Jiro Suzuki (1924–1990)

led to the name of "moyamoya" disease becoming popular and spread all over the world [21]. Along the progression of this disease, moyamoya vessels first become evident and dense, and then diminish and disappear from the angiogram. This process again resembles cigarette smoke in the air. Because of the nuance of vague, mysterious, and unsolved in Japanese, the word "moyamoya" also fits the unknown etiology of disease. In future, when the etiology of this disease is fully elucidated, the name "moyamoya" will become somewhat ill-fitting.

Evolution of Research and Lessons from Moyamoya Disease

During the past half century since the first report of this disease, efforts have been concentrated on clinical and basic research to understand and conquer this mysterious disease. Major topics on this disease are thoroughly covered in the later chapters. For instance, genetic analysis indicated close association to several foci, molecular biology allowed us to clarify the involvement of growth factors in this disease, advances in neuroimaging have provided safer and more informative evaluation, and accumulating evidence indicates the significant effect of surgical treatment for prevention of ischemic stroke. It is noteworthy that guidelines for treatment have been recently proposed in both the United States and Japan. (Evidence-based recommendation for the prevention of ischemic stroke in infants and children caused by moyamoya disease, by the American Heart Association Stroke Council 2008 [3]; the guidelines for the diagnosis and treatment of moyamoya disease, by the research committee on moymoya disease supported by the Japanese ministry, 2009.)

In the process of this research and management of patients, we have learned valuable lessons concerning moyamoya disease: how the human brain is resistant to chronic ischemia and how the brain vessels are elaborative and, sometimes, fragile. Investigations on various aspects of this disease have substantially contributed to a better understanding of the pathophysiology of brain ischemia and angiogenesis, etc. Further, requirements for the prevention of ischemic stroke have led to the refinement of surgical intervention such as direct bypass techniques and indirect vascularization.

References

1. Suzuki J, Takaku A (1969) Cerebrovascular "Moaymoya" disease. Disease showing abnormal net-like vessels in base of brain. Arch Neurol 20:288–299
2. Kuroda S, Houkin K (2008) Moyamoya disease: current concepts and future perspectives. Lancet Neurol 7:1056–1066
3. Roach ES, Colomb MR, Adam R et al (2008) Management of stroke in infants and children. A scientific statement from a special writing group of the American heart association stroke council and the council on cardiovascular disease in the young. Stroke 39:2644–2691
4. Scott RM, Smith ER (2009) Moyamoya disease and moyamoya syndrome. N Eng J Med 360: 1226–1237
5. Hallemeier CL, Rich KM, Grubb RL et al (2006) Clinical features and outcome in North American adults with moyamoya phenomenon. Stroke 37:1490–1496
6. Mesiwala AH, Sviri G, Fatemi N et al (2008) Long-term outcome of superficial temporal artery-middle cerebral artery bypass for patients with moyamoya disease in the U.S. Neurosurg Focus. doi: 10.3171/FOC/2008/24/2/E15
7. Kuriyama S, Kusaka Y, Fujimura M et al (2008) Prevalence and clinicoepidemiological features of moyamoya disease in Japan. Findings from a nationwide epidemiological surgery. Stroke 39:42–47
8. Achrol AD, Guzman R, Lee M et al (2009) Pathophysiology and genetic factors in moyamoya disease. Neurosurg Focus. doi: 10.3171.2009.1.FOCUS08302
9. Fukui M, Members of the Research Committee on Spontaneous Occlusion of the Circle of Willis (Moyamoya Disease) of the Ministry of Health and Welfare, Japan (1997) Guideline for the diagnosis and treatment of spontaneous occlusion of the circle of Willis ('Moyamoya' disease). Clin Neurol Neurosurg 99:S238–S240
10. Kuroda S, Hashimoto N, Yoshimoto T et al (2007) Radiological findings, clinical course, and outcome in asymptomatic moyamoya disease: results of multicenter survey in Japan. Stroke 38:1430–1435
11. Smith ER, Scott RM (2008) Progression of disease in unilateral moyamoya syndrome. Neurosurg Focus doi: 10.3171/FOC/2008/24/2/E17
12. Mineharu Y, Liu W, Inoue K, et al (2008) Autosomal dominant moyamoya disease maps to chromosome 17q25.3. Neurology 70:2357–2363
13. Ikezaki K, Loftus CM (2001) Quasi-moyamoya disease: definition, classification, and therapy. In Moyamoya disease, Ikezaki K, Loftus CM (eds) AANS, USA, pp 23–41
14. Takeuchi K, Shimizu K (1957) Hypoplasia of the bilateral internal carotid arteries. Brain Nerve (Tokyo) 9:37–43
15. Kudo T, Takayama R, Mikawakuchi K, et al. (1957) Occlusion of internal carotid artery. Brain Nerve (Tokyo) 9:757
16. Weidner W, Hanafee W, Markham CH (1965) Intracranial collateral circulation via leptomeningeal and rete mirabile anastomoses. Neurology 15:39–48
17. Kraynbuhl HA, Yasargil MG (1965) Cerebral angiography. Butterworth, London
18. Leeds NE, Abott KH (1965) Collateral circulation in cerebrovascular disease in childhood via rete mirabile and perforating branches of anterior choroidal and posterior cerebral arteries. Radiology 85:628–634
19. Nishimoto A, Takeuchi T (1968) Abnormal cerebrovascular network related to the internal carotid arteries. J Neurosurg 29:255–260
20. Kudo T (1968) Spontaneous occlusion of the circle of Willis: a disease apparently confined to Japanese. Neurology 18:485–496
21. Suzuki J (1983) Moyamoya disease. Springer, Tokyo, preface VII–VIII

Pathology of Moyamoya Disease

Kent Doi and Ken-ichiro Kikuta

Abbreviations

APAS	Antiphospholipid antibody syndromes
EMS	Encephalo-myo-synangiosis
EPC	Endothelial progenitor cell
MB	Microbleed
MCA	Middle cerebral artery
MMD	Moyamoya disease
MR	Magnetic resonance
mRNA	Messenger ribonucleic acid

Introduction: Pathology of Moyamoya Disease

Moyamoya disease (MMD) is a cerebrovascular occlusive disease first reported by Japanese surgeons in 1957 as hypoplasia of the bilateral internal carotid arteries [1]. The entity is characterized by steno-occlusive changes at the terminal portion of the bilateral internal carotid arteries and by development of an abnormal vascular network near the arterial occlusion [2, 3].

In the criteria prepared by the Research Committee in Japan [4], instructive pathological findings are as follows: (1) intimal thickening and the resulting stenosis or occlusion of the lumen is observed in and around the terminal portion of the internal carotid artery, usually on both sides; lipid deposits are occasionally seen in the proliferating intima; (2) arteries

K. Doi
Department of Neurosurgery, Kyoto University Graduate School of Medicine, Yoshida-Konoe-cho, Sakyo-ku, Kyoto 606-8501, Japan

K. Kikuta (✉)
Division of Neurosurgery, Department of Sensory and Locomotor Medicine, Faculty of Medical Sciences, University of Fukui, 23-3 Matsuokashimoaizuki, Eiheiji-cho, Yoshida-gun, Fukui 910-1193, Japan
e-mail: kikuta@u-fukui.ac.jp

B.-K. Cho and T. Tominaga (eds.), *Moyamoya Disease Update*,
DOI 10.1007/978-4-431-99703-0_2, © Springer 2010

constituting the circle of Willis, such as the anterior and the middle cerebral and the posterior communicating arteries, often show stenosis of various degrees or occlusion associated with fibrocellular thickening of the intima, waving of the internal elastic lamina, and attenuation of the media; (3) numerous small vascular channels (perforators and anastomotic branches) are observed around the circle of Willis; and (4) reticular conglomerates of small vessels are often seen in the pia mater.

Although MMD was first reported more than half a century ago, its pathophysiology remains unknown. In this chapter, we present the current knowledge of MMD from the perspective of pathology.

Histological Findings in Moyamoya Disease

Intraoperative observations have shown that the outer diameters of the relevant carotid artery terminations are markedly diminished in MMD [5]. Similarly, autopsy studies of adult patients have shown that the external diameter and lumens of the arteries of the circle of Willis are narrowed or occluded by a thickening of the intima [3, 6].

Histopathological findings in the carotid terminations and the middle cerebral artery (MCA) have shown fibrocellular thickening of the intima, irregular undulation ("waving") of the internal elastic lamina, and attenuation of the media [5]. The thickened intima contains an increased number of smooth muscle cells, which are considered to be synthetic-type smooth muscle cells migrating from the media [3, 7, 8]. Disruption of the internal elastic lamina and inflammatory cell infiltration are generally absent, and deposits of lipid are rare [3]. Mural thrombi are frequently seen in the stenotic lesions, and the organization of repeated mural thrombi is suspected by some authors to be responsible for multilayered eccentric intimal thickening [3, 9–11].

Leptomeningeal Vessels

In 1990, Kono et al. [12] investigated the leptomeningeal vessels of six autopsied patients with MMD. They found that the vessels were histologically characterized by the dilation of preexisting arteries and veins, and were accompanied by intimal thickening and alterations of the internal elastic lamina as the clinical period lengthened. These dilated leptomeningeal vessels may participate in collateral circulations at the cerebral surface (Fig. 1a, b).

Vessels with Encephalo-myo-synangiosis

Kono et al. identified collateral vessels formed by encephalo-myo-synangiosis in a 67-year-old man who had undergone surgery 10 years before the study [13].

Thick fibrous tissue containing atrophic striated muscles was seen adjacent to the underlying cortex. Several arteries with thickened walls and multilaminated internal elastic lamina were scattered in the muscular flap, along with some veins with fibroelastosis. The largest artery in the muscular flap extended into the subarachnoid space, and two of its small branches were traced to their entry into the cerebral parenchyma. There was no infarction or gliosis around those intraparenchymal vessels.

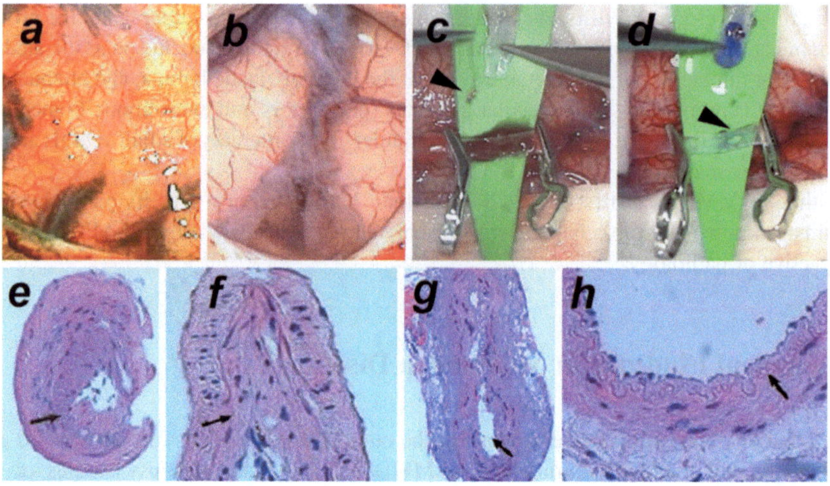

Fig. 1 Macroscopic and microscopic findings of middle cerebral arteries in MMD. Intraoperative photographs of the brain surface at bypass surgery in patients with MMD (**a**) and eit non-MMD patients (**b**). Pial arteries develop extensively and dilated on the brain surface of MMD. Surgical specimens of the middle cerebral artery were obtained at arteriotomy in a round shape at bypass surgery (**c**, **d**: *arrow head*). Specimens taken from patients with MMD showed intimal hyperplasia (**e**) and thin media (**f**) compared with specimens from control subjects (**g**, **h**) (*arrows* in **e**–**h** indicating internal elastic lamina) [27]

Perforators

Moyamoya vessels are dilated perforating arteries exhibiting various histopathological changes, including fibrin deposits in the walls, fragmented elastic lamina, attenuated media, and the formation of microaneurysms. Collapse of the arterial lumen and subsequent thrombosis can also be seen in moyamoya vessels [5]. These histopathological changes might therefore be closely associated with the onset of ischemic and hemorrhagic stroke [5].

The perforating arteries in the basal ganglia, thalamus, and internal capsule are dilated with either relatively thin walls or stenotic thin walls [3, 7]. A histological survey and morphometry of cerebral arteries in 22 patients with MMD indicated the prevalence of severe stenotic lesions in older patients and dilatation and attenuation of the media in younger patients [7]. This is consistent with the angiographic progression and attenuation of moyamoya vessels in the long clinical course of the disease [3, 7, 14].

Hemorrhage from Perforators

In 1980, Mauro et al. [15] found two types of vascular lesions in the perforators of a patient with hemorrhagic events: microaneurysms and lipohyalinosis of the vascular wall. The microaneurysms (100–2,500 μm) were located within the thalamic hemorrhage foci and showed apparent disruption of the wall. Lipohyalinosis was identified among the small perforating arteries (100–500 μm in diameter) with focal disintegration of elastic lamina, marked hyalinization of the vascular wall, and accumulation of foam cells.

In 1983, Yamashita et al. [7] studied 22 patients and suggested that the initial vascular lesions of small perforating arteries that could contribute to wall rupture might comprise fibrosis and attenuation of tunica media in association with luminal dilatation.

Focal fibrin deposits and a true microaneurysm were considered further advanced lesions predisposed to rupture. Their materials provided no evidence for lipohyalinosis of the vascular wall.

Their findings indicate that rupturing of vessels in MMD could occur in the absence of microaneurysms or fibrinoid necrosis, which are often found in hypertensives.

Increased blood supply would lead to hemodynamic stress on these moyamoya vessels as a collateral pathway. In addition, the progressive stenoses of moyamoya vessels, in both severity and distribution, might induce further stress on the remaining vessels, leading to eventual disruption of the wall. The disrupted and organized small arteries within the old hemorrhagic foci indicate that the rupture of moyamoya vessels might even occur repeatedly.

These vascular abnormalities resulted in cerebral hypoperfusion and subsequent ischemic or hemorrhagic stroke. Over the past few decades, numerous studies have been conducted on the genes or proteins (mostly growth factors or angiogenic factors) that expressed highly in the vascular walls, dura mater, or cerebrospinal fluid [16–24]. However, the etiology remains unclear.

Molecular Analysis with Intracranial Vessels

Several histological findings regarding extracranial vessels have been reported [25, 26], and the expression of some genes was found in specimens from the superficial temporal artery or in cultured vascular smooth muscle cells from these extracranial arteries [16, 17, 20–22]. However, few studies on intracranial arteries were made with patients with MMD, and most of these studies were based on only a small number of autopsy specimens [23, 24].

Takagi et al. [27] analyzed 35 specimens of the MCAs from patients with MMD; these specimens were obtained during bypass surgery and were freshly fixed with formalin. They found intimal hyperplasia and medial thinness in the M4 portion of MCA, as was found in the internal cerebral artery from the previous autopsy studies. In addition, Takagi et al. analyzed the incidence of the abnormal elastic lamina and the thickness of the intima and media (Fig. 1c–h). They speculated that intimal hyperplasia and medial thinness occur even in young patients with MMD, and that abnormality of the internal elastic lamina might occur as a secondary effect.

Since their samples were fresh, they found it easy to collect the messenger ribonucleic acid from these samples. They also investigated the molecular mechanisms of MMD using these specimens [18, 19].

Microbleeds in Moyamoya Disease

Recent progress in neuroimaging could offer a key to understanding the pathology of MMD. Microbleeds (MBs) detected by T2*-weighted magnetic resonance (MR) imaging are considered a general marker of vascular vulnerability in cerebral angiopathy with a tendency to bleeding. Asymptomatic MBs are significantly more common in patients with MMD, and multiple MBs have been reported as a possible predictor of subsequent hemorrhage [28, 29].

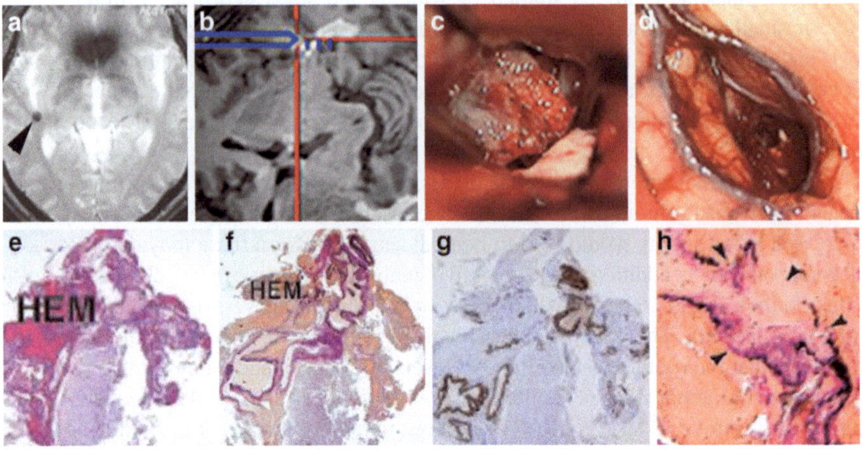

Fig. 2 Histology of a microbleeds in patient with MMD. A specimen of the microbleed in the right temporal operculum in patient with MMD (**a**) was removed by using neuronavigation system (**b**). Photomicrographs of the microbleed revealed encapsulized hematoma (HEM) with small vessels (**e**: hematoxilin-eosin stain, ×20) and many small vessels within the deposition of erythrocytes and clearly visualized internal elastic lamina (**f**: elastica-van Gieson stain, ×30). Immunostaining with antibody against human alpha-smooth muscle actin (**g**: ×25) showed thick smooth muscle layers in those vessels indicating arteries, and some arterioles with disrupted internal elastic lamina (*arrow heads*) (**h**: elastica-van Gieson stain, ×200) [30]

Histological analysis of an MB following surgical resection in a patient with MMD revealed an encapsulated hematoma containing small vessels. Many small vessels were located within the deposition of erythrocytes, and these had smooth muscle layers indicating arteries. Some of the vessels exhibited disrupted internal elastic lamina (Fig. 2a–h) [30].

An enlarged MB with perifocal edema resulting in a fatal intracerebral hemorrhage was also reported [29]. Although MBs are usually located in both the basal ganglia and subcortical regions in patients with small vessel diseases [31, 32], MBs in patients with MMD are located mainly in the periventricular white matter. Development and dilatation of the arteries situated in the periventricular white matter, such as choroidal arteries and branches of posterior communicating arteries, have been reported as risk factors for hemorrhage in MMD [33, 34]. MBs might be related to these risk factors [29].

Epidemiology

MMD is found mostly in Asia, especially in Japan and Republic of Korea. The clinical background of MMD in Republic of Korea is similar to that in Japan [35–37]. However, MMD as it occurs in people of European ethnicity differs from that occurring in Asians in the later timing of the onset of vasculopathy and in the lower rate of hemorrhages [38–41]. Gaining an awareness of both the similarities and difference between these two groups could provide new insights into the etiology of MMD.

Kraemer et al. [38] performed a biopsy during revascularization surgery. Their histological examination of two of the six cerebral blood vessel specimens obtained from ethno-Europeans patients with MMD revealed a thickened internal elastic lamina and intima, which are characteristic findings for MMD. In their speculation, the difference in presentation between Asian and ethno-Europeans patients is related to the later onset of vaso-occlusive vasculopathy in the ethno-European group [38]. Further research on MMD among ethno-Europeans could clarify the underlying mechanism of racial differences related to MMD.

Comparison with Moyamoya Syndrome

Radiographic changes similar to those found in MMD can also be found in certain infections, head trauma, brain neoplasms, autoimmune diseases, and hematologic, metabolic, genetic, and chromosomal disorders [4, 5, 42]. Because the etiology of MMD is unknown, we should distinguish MMD from cerebrovascular diseases arising from these underlying diseases and conditions [4, 42]. These changes are sometimes referred to as "moyamoya syndrome." Some vessels affected in moyamoya syndrome have been analyzed for comparison with those affected by MMD.

von Recklinghausen Disease

Histopathological observation of a case with von Recklinghausen disease revealed that the vascular changes in this case differ from those exhibited in MMD [11]. Namely, those in von Recklinghausen disease include the interruption of internal elastic lamina and mild to moderate infiltration of macrophages and lymphocytes, neither of which is fundamentally observed in MMD. These results indicate that clinical or angiographical manifestations similar to MMD could be due to different pathogenesis, and that diagnosis of MMD should be done from a clinical viewpoint as well as using a pathomorphological approach [11].

Neurofibromin, the protein product of the *NF1* gene, is expressed in endothelial and smooth muscle cells of blood vessels and is likely to be involved in pathogenesis [43, 44]. It has been hypothesized that the loss of neurofibromin expression in endothelial cells may somehow trigger the proliferation of vascular smooth muscle cells. It has also been suggested that neurofibromin helps maintain the integrity of the endothelial cell layer, and that if this integrity is lost because of aberrant neurofibromin, vascular smooth muscle cells could proliferate [43, 44].

Irradiation

Radiation-induced occlusive vasculopathy of the large cerebral arteries is an important delayed complication of radiation therapy, usually evolving slowly to produce ischemic effects years or even decades after irradiation. Patients who receive radiation therapy at a younger age were found to have an increased risk for moyamoya syndrome [45, 46].

Several case studies and experimental radiation damage studies [47–49] have typically shown subintimal collections of foam cells with myointimal proliferation, which has been broadly characterized as premature or accelerated arteriosclerosis. A prominent thickened wall with an increased outer diameter was demonstrated in some studies [48, 49]. On the other hand, in idiopathic (primary) MMD, the outer diameter of occluded and stenotic arteries is decreased [50, 51].

Contrast-enhanced MR imaging has revealed arterial wall thickening and enhancement in patients with radiation-induced large-vessel vasculopathy. These findings are similar to those frequently observed in patients with aortitis syndrome and atherosclerosis [46]. However, the arteries of patients with idiopathic MMD showed no prominent enhancement of the arterial wall. These results suggest that these two conditions have different pathophysiologies [46].

Down Syndrome

Patients with Down syndrome are at increased risk for cerebral infarction. In the majority of cases, the strokes are secondary to cerebral embolism, originating from atrioventricular canal defects, right-to-left shunting, myocardial dysmotility, or cardiac valvular abnormalities.

Moreover, they sometimes present clinical and radiological features similar to those of primary MMD [52–55]. The autopsy of a 4 year old with Down syndrome and ischemic stroke showed intimal thickening with collagen deposition in the affected cerebral vessels [54]. Patients with Down syndrome are also known to have a predisposition for vascular disease, such as abnormal nail-bed capillary morphology, abnormalities of retinal vessels, and primary intimal fibroplasia. Genes on chromosome 21 are suspected to be the causes of these features [55].

Postinfection

Vascular events are a known complication of bacterial meningitis, and the formation of moyamoya vessels has been found in some cases [56–59]. The pathogenesis of this type of postinfectious vasculopathy is unknown, although an infection could trigger an autoimmune process in the cerebral blood vessels. For example, streptococcal infections are associated with a variety of autoimmune diseases, including glomerulonephritis, chorea, myocarditis, arthritis, tics, and obsessive-compulsive disorder. Triggering of antiphospholipid antibody syndromes (APAS) has also been reported following infections, and antibodies to β2-GP 1 are associated with postinfectious autoimmune APAS. The autopsy of a patient with MMD revealed the absence of inflammation of the cerebral vessels, which implies that the patient either responded to the aggressive immunomodulatory therapy or that the autoimmune process spontaneously ceased [57].

Endothelial Progenitor Cells in MMD

Recently, some groups have shown that endothelial progenitor cells (EPCs) play a role in MMD [60–62]. EPCs are bone-marrow-derived somatic stem cells and work for angiogenesis and endothelial repair [63, 64]. The number of EPCs was reportedly related to cardiac and cerebrovascular functions or outcomes [64–70]. For example, an increase in circulating EPCs following acute ischemic stroke is associated with a good outcome [69]. Although EPC research requires further development and its significance in MMD is unclear, it could contribute to new insights into the pathogenesis of MMD.

Genetic Analysis

In accordance with the advance of the worldwide genomic research, several genetic analyses for familial MMD have been reported. These reports have suggested the disease is probably inherited in a polygenic or autosomal dominant mode with a low penetrance [71]. Microsatellite linkage analysis has identified genetic loci associated with MMD on chromosomes 3, 6, 8, and 17 [72–77]. However, the relevant genes remain to be investigated.

Summary and Conclusion

Histological findings observed in major vascular lesions of MMD include fibrocellular thickening of the intima, waving of the internal elastic lamina, and attenuation of the media. The pathology-inducing cerebral ischemia or hemorrhage requires further investigation. Clues to understanding the disease could be revealed from a study of racial differences between Asians and ethno-Europeans and from a comparison with moyamoya syndrome. Multidimensional research with further histological, neuroimaging, molecular-biological, and genetic approaches could clarify the etiology of MMD.

References

1. Takeuchi K, Shimizu K (1957): Hypoplasia of the bilateral internal carotid arteries (in Japanese). No to Shinkei 9:37–43
2. Suzuki J, Takaku A (1969): Cerebrovascular 'Moyamoya disease': A disease showing abnormal net-like vessels in base of brain. Arch Neurol 20:288–299
3. Fukui M, Kono S, Sueishi K et al. (2000): Moyamoya disease. Neuropathology 20:S61–S64
4. Fukui M, Members of the Research Committee on Spontaneous Occlusion of the circle of Willis (Moyamoya disease) of the Ministry of Health and Welfare, Japan (1997): Guidelines for the diagnosis and treatment for spontaneous occlusion of the circle of Willis ('moyamoya' disease). Clin Neurol Neurosurg 99(S2):S238–S240
5. Kuroda S, Houkin K (2008): Moyamoya disease: current concepts and future perspectives. Lancet Neurol 7:1056–1066
6. Takekawa Y, Umezawa T, Ueno Y et al. (2004): Pathological and immunohistochemical findings of an autopsy case of adult moyamoya disease. Neuropathology 24:236–242
7. Yamashita M, Oka K, Tanaka K (1983): Histopathology of the brain vascular networks in moyamoya disease. Stroke 14:50–58
8. Masuda J, Ogata J, Yutani C (1993): Smooth muscle cell proliferation and localization of macrophage and T cells in the occlusive intracranial major arteries in moyamoya disease. Stroke 24:1960–1967
9. Yamashita M, Oka K, Tanaka K (1984): Cervico-cephalic arterial thrombi and thromboemboli in moyamoya disease, possible correlation with progressive intimal thickening in the intracranial major arteries. Stroke 15:264–270

10. Ikeda E, Hosoda Y (1993): Disruption of the thrombotic lesions in the cerebral arteries in spontaneous occlusion of the circle of Willis: cerebrovascular moyamoya disease. Clin Neuropathol 12:44–48
11. Hosoda Y, Ikeda E, Hirose S (1997): Histopathological studies on spontaneous occlusion of the circle of Willis (cerebrovascular moyamoya disease). Clin Neurol Neurosurg 99(S2):S203–S208
12. Kono S, Oka K, Sueishi K (1990): Histopathologic and morphometric studies of leptomeningeal vessels in moyamoya disease. Stroke 21:1044–1050
13. Kono S, Oka K, Sueishi K et al. (1997): Histopathological studies on spontaneous vault Moyamoya and revascularized collaterals formed by encephalomyosynangiosis. Clin Neurol Neurosurg 99(S2):S209–S212
14. Takebayashi S, Matsuo K, Kaneko M (1984): Ultrastructural studies of cerebral arteries and collateral vessels in moyamoya disease. Stroke 15(4):728–732
15. Mauro AJ, Johnson ES, Chikos PM et al. (1980): Lipohyalinosis and military microaneurysms causing cerebral hemorrhage in a patient with moyamoya. A clinicopathological study. Stroke 11:405–412
16. Hojo M, Hoshimaru M, Miyamoto S et al. (1998): Role of transforming growth factor-beta1 in the pathogenesis of moyamoya disease. J Neurosurg 89:623–629
17. Hoshimaru M, Takahashi JA, Kikuchi H et al. (1991): Possible roles of basic fibroblast growth factor in the pathogenesis of moyamoya disease. J Neurosurg 75:267–270
18. Takagi Y, Kikuta K, Nozaki K et al. (2007): Expression of hypoxia-inducing factor-1 alpha and endoglin in intimal hyperplasia of the middle cerebral artery of patients with moyamoya disease. Neurosurgery 60:338–345
19. Takagi Y, Kikuta K, Sadamasa N et al. (2006): Caspase-3-dependent apoptosis in middle cerebral arteries in patients with moyamoya disease. Neurosurgery 59:894–901
20. Yamamoto M, Aoyagi M, Tajima S et al. (1997): Increase in elastin gene expression and protein synthesis in arterial smooth muscle cells derived from patients with moyamoya disease. Stroke 28:1733–1738
21. Aoyagi M, Fukai N, Matsushima Y et al. (1993): Kinetics of 125I-PDGF binding and down-regulation of PDGF receptor in arterial smooth muscle cells derived from patients with moyamoya disease. J Cell Physiol 154:281–288
22. Yamamoto M, Aoyagi M, Fukai N (1999): Increase in prostaglandin E2 production by interleukin-1beta in arterial smooth muscle cells derived from patients with moyamoya disease. Circ Res 85:912–918
23. Houkin K, Yoshimoto T, Abe H et al. (1998): Role of basic fibroblast growth factor in the pathogenesis of moyamoya disease. Neurosurg Focus 5:e2
24. Nanba R, Kuroda S, Ishikawa T et al. (2004): Increased expression of hepatocyte growth factor in cerebrospinal fluid and intracranial artery in moyamoya disease. Stroke 34:2385–2841
25. Aoyagi M, Fukai N, Yamamoto M et al. (1996): Early development of intimal thickening in superficial temporal arteries in patients with moyamoya disease. Stroke 27:1750–1754
26. Aoyagi M, Fukai N, Yamamoto M et al. (1997): Development of intimal thickening in superficial temporal arteries in patients with moyamoya disease. Clin Neurol Neurosurg 99(S2):S213–S217
27. Takagi Y, Kikuta K, Nozaki K et al. (2007): Histological features of middle cerebral arteries from patients treated for moyamoya disease. Neurol Med Chir (Tokyo) 47:1–4
28. Kikuta K, Takagi Y, Nozaki K et al. (2005): Asymptomatic microbleeds in moyamoya disease: T2*-weighted gradient-echo magnetic resonance imaging study. J Neurosurg 102:470–475
29. Kikuta K, Takagi Y, Nozaki K et al. (2008): The presence of multiple microbleeds as a predictor of subsequent cerebral hemorrhage in patients with moyamoya disease. Neurosurgery 62:104–112
30. Kikuta K, Takagi Y, Nozaki K et al. (2007): Histological analysis of microbleed after surgical resection in a patient with moyamoya disease. Neurol Med Chir 47:564–567
31. Koennecke HC (2006): Cerebral microbleeds on MRI: prevalence, associations, and potential clinical implications. Neurology 66:165–171
32. Viswanathan A, Chabriat H (2006): Cerebral microhemorrhage. Stroke 37:550–557
33. Irikura K, Miyasaka Y, Kurata A et al. (1996): A source of haemorrhage in adult patients with moyamoya disease: the significance of tributaries from the choroidal artery. Acta Neurochir (Wien) 138:1282–1286
34. Morioka M, Hamada J, Kawano T et al. (2003): Angiographic dilatation and branch extension of the anterior choroidal and posterior communicating arteries are predictors of hemorrhage in adult moyamoya patients. Stroke 34:90–95
35. Ikezaki K, Han DH, Kawano T et al. (1997): A clinical comparison of definite moyamoya disease between South Korea and Japan. Stroke 28:2513–2517

36. Han DH, Kwon OK, Byun BJ et al., The Korean Society for Cerebrovascular Disease, Seoul, Korea (2000): A co-operative study: clinical characteristics of 334 Korean patients with moyamoya disease treated at neurosurgical institutes (1976–1994). Acta Neurochir (Wien) 142:1263–1274
37. Kuriyama S, Kusaka Y, Fujimura M (2008): Prevalence and clinicoepidemiological features of moyamoya disease in Japan: findings from a nationwide epidemiological survey. Stroke 39:42–47
38. Kraemer M, Heinenbrok W, Berlit P (2008): Moyamoya disease in Europeans. Stroke 39:3193–3200
39. Hallemeier CL, Rich KM, Grubb RL et al. (2006): Clinical features and outcome in North American adults with moyamoya phenomenon. Stroke 37:1490–1496
40. Chui D, Shedden P, Bratina P et al. (1998): Clinical features of moyamoya disease in the United States. Stroke 29:1347–1351
41. Khan N, Yonekawa Y (2005): Moyamoya angiopathy in Europe. Acta Neurochir Suppl 94:149–152
42. Achrol AS, Guzman R, Lee M et al (2009): Pathophysiology and genetic factors in moyamoya disease. Neurosurg Focus 26(4):E4
43. Norton KK, Xu J, Gutmann DH (1995): Expression of the neurofibromatosis 1 gene product, neurofibromin, in blood vessel endothelial cells and smooth muscle. Neurobiol Dis 2:13–21
44. Rosser TL, Vezina G, Packer RJ (2005): Cerebrovascular abnormalities in a population of children with neurofibromatosis type 1. Neurology 64:553–555
45. Desai SS, Paulino AC, Mai WY et al. (2006): Radiation-induced moyamoya syndrome. Int J Radiation Oncol Biol Phys 65(4):1222–1227
46. Aoki S, Hayashi N, Abe O et al. (2002): Radiation-induced arteritis: thickened wall with prominent enhancement on cranial MR images – report of five cases and comparison with 18 cases of moyamoya disease. Radiology 223:683–688
47. Bitzer M, Topka H (1995): Progressive cerebral occlusive disease after radiation therapy. Stroke 26:131–136
48. Brant-Zawadzki M, Anderson M, DeArmond SJ et al. (1980): Radiation-induced large intracranial vessel occlusive vasculopathy. AJR Am J Roentgenol 134:51–55
49. Kamiryo T, Lopes MBS, Berr SS et al. (1996): Occlusion of the anterior cerebral artery after gamma knife irradiation in a rat. Acta Neurochir 138:983–991
50. Hosoda Y (1984): Pathology of so-called "spontaneous occlusion of the circle of Willis." Pathol Ann 19(pt 2):221–244
51. Haltia M, Iivanainen M, Majuri H et al. (1982): Spontaneous occlusion of the circle of Willis (moyamoya syndrome). Clin Neuropathol 1:11–22
52. Dai AI, Shaikh ZA, Cohen ME (2000): Early-onset moyamoya syndrome in a patient with Down syndrome: case report and review of the literature. J Child Neurol 15:696–699
53. Fukuyama Y, Osawa M, Kanai N (1992): Moyamoya disease (syndrome) and the Down syndrome. Brain Dev 14:254–256
54. Mito T, Becker LE (1992): Vascular dysplasia in Down syndrome: a possible relationship to moyamoya disease. Brain Dev 14:248–251
55. Cramer SC, Robertson RL, Dooling EC et al. (1996): Moyamoya and Down syndrome, clinical and radiological features. Stroke 27:2131–2135
56. Palacio S, Hart RG, Vollmer DG et al. (2003): Late-developing cerebral arteriopathy after pyogenic meningitis. Arch Neurol 60:431–433
57. Czartoski T, Hallam D, Lacy JM et al. (2005): Postinfectious vasculopathy with evolution to moyamoya syndrome. J Neurol Neurosurg Psychiatry 76:256–259
58. Weststrate W, Hijdra A, deGans J (1996): Brain infarcts in adults with bacterial meningitis. Lancet 347:399
59. Pfister HW, Barasio GD, Dirnagl U et al. (1992): Cerebrovascular complications of bacterial meningitis in adults. Neurology 42:1497–1504
60. Yoshihara T, Taguchi A, Matsuyama T et al. (2008): Increase in circulating CD34-positive cells in patients with angiographic evidence of moyamoya-like vessels. J Cereb Blood Flow Metab 28(6):1086–1089
61. Jung KH, Chu K, Lee ST et al. (2008): Circulating endothelial progenitor cells as a pathogenic marker of moyamoya disease. J Cereb Blood Flow Metab 28(11):1795–1803
62. Rafat N, Beck GCh, Peña-Tapia PG et al. (2009): Increased levels of circulating endothelial progenitor cells in patients with moyamoya disease. Stroke 40(2):432–438
63. Asahara T, Murohara T, Sullivan A et al. (1997): Isolation of putative progenitor endothelial cells for angiogenesis. Science 275:964–967

64. Rouhl RP, van Oostenbrugge RJ, Damoiseaux J et al. (2008): Endothelial progenitor cell research in stroke: a potential shift in pathophysiological and therapeutical concepts. Stroke 39(7):2158–2165
65. Hill JM, Zalos G, Halcox JP et al. (2003): Circulating endothelial progenitor cells, vascular function, and cardiovascular risk. N Engl J Med 348:593–600
66. Werner N, Kosiol S, Schiegl T et al. (2005): Circulating endothelial progenitor cells and cardiovascular outcomes. N Engl J Med 353:999–1007
67. Schmidt-Lucke C, Rossig L, Fichtlscherer S et al. (2005): Reduced number of circulating endothelial progenitor cells predicts future cardiovascular events: proof of concept for the clinical importance of endogenous vascular repair. Circulation 111:2981–2987
68. Ghani U, Shuaib A, Salam A et al. (2005): Endothelial progenitor cells during cerebrovascular disease. Stroke 36:151–153
69. Sobrino T, Hurtado O, Moro MA et al. (2007): The increase of circulating endothelial progenitor cells after acute ischemic stroke is associated with good outcome. Stroke 38:2759–2764
70. Taguchi A, Matsuyama T, Moriwaki H et al. (2004): Circulating cd34-positive cells provide an index of cerebrovascular function. Circulation 109:2972–2975
71. Mineharu Y, Takenaka K, Yamakawa H et al. (2006): Inheritance pattern of familial moyamoya disease: autosomal dominant mode and genomic imprinting. J Neurol Neurosurg Psychiatry 77:1025–1029
72. Ikeda H, Sasaki T, Yoshimoto T et al. (1999): Mapping of a familial moyamoya disease gene to chromosome 3p24.2–p26. Am J Hum Genet 64:533–537
73. Inoue TK, Ikezaki K, Sasazuki T et al. (2000): Linkage analysis of moyamoya disease on chromosome 6. J Child Neurol 15:179–182
74. Yamauchi T, Tada M, Houkin K et al. (2000): Linkage of familial moyamoya disease (spontaneous occlusion of the circle of Willis) to chromosome 17q25. Stroke 31:930–935
75. Sakurai K, Horiuchi Y, Ikeda H et al. (2004): A novel susceptibility locus for moyamoya disease on chromosome 8q23. J Hum Genet 49:278–281
76. Nanba R, Tada M, Kuroda S et al. (2005): Sequence analysis and bioinformatics analysis of chromosome 17q25 in familial moyamoya disease. Childs Nerv Syst 21:62–68
77. Mineharu Y, Liu W, Inoue K Y et al. (2008): Autosomal dominant moyamoya disease maps to chromosome 17q25. Neurology 70:2353–2363

Unilateral Moyamoya Disease

Chang-Wan Oh and Gyojun Hwang

Introduction

The Research Committee on Spontaneous Occlusion of the Circle of Willis of the Ministry of Health and Welfare, Japan, defines typical moyamoya disease as specific angiographic findings of diffuse stenotic or occlusive lesions of the bilateral carotid fork and unique collateral vessels at the base of the brain. However, there are some atypical cases of moyamoya disease that show unilateral lesions on angiography and a normal terminal portion of contralateral internal carotid artery or proximal middle cerebral artery. These patients are categorized as having 'unilateral' moyamoya disease. Kelly et al. reported that patients with angiographically unilateral lesions comprised up to 18% of patients with moyamoya disease who were treated surgically [1]. Recently, however, asymptomatic moyamoya diseases detected by MRI have been increasing, so that the real incidence is thought to be higher than expected. Also, until now, the natural history of unilateral moyamoya disease has been unclear, and whether it is an early form of moyamoya disease remains controversial.

Here, although there have been only a small number of reports related to this topic, we will review the clinical features and progression of disease in unilateral moyamoya disease.

Clinical Features of Unilateral Moyamoya Disease

Many authors have reported chronic ischemia (transient ischemic attack or completed stroke), hemorrhage, seizure, and intractable headache in order as the initial presenting symptoms [1–4]. There seem to be no differences from typical moyamoya disease in presenting symptoms, but their features are somewhat different, especially in chronic ischemic symptoms.

Interestingly, Ogata et al. found that both rCBF at rest and after acetazolamide injection in unilateral moyamoya disease was higher than in typical moyamoya disease. They explained

C.-W. Oh and G. Hwang (✉)
Division of Cerebrovascular Surgery, Department of Neurosurgery, Seoul National Univeristy Bundang Hospital, Seoul National University College of Medicine, 300 Gummi-dong, Bundang-gu, Seongnam-si, Gyeonggi-do 463-707, Republic of Korea
e-mail: wanoh@snu.ac.kr

B.-K. Cho and T. Tominaga (eds.), *Moyamoya Disease Update*,
DOI 10.1007/978-4-431-99703-0_3, © Springer 2010

that the result was due to easier development of the collateral network from the unaffected side [2]. Hallemeier et al. reported that patients presenting with unilateral moyamoya disease had a better functional outcome than those with bilateral moyamoya disease, although they did not analyze the relationship between rCBF and outcome. However, this result is also likely to be related to increased rCBF.

Concerning the hemorrhage in adult unilateral moyamoya disease, its incidence is variable. Ikezaki et al. found that 58% of the adult unilateral moyamoya disease patients suffered from hemorrhagic stroke [5]. Other recent reports showed 0–2% incidence of hemorrhage in initial presenting symptoms [1–3]. Because hemorrhage in moyamoya disease is thought to be caused by rupture of friable transmedullary collateral vessels or related aneurysms, the angiographic comparison between unilateral and typical moyamoya disease may be important for the comparison of incidence between the two diseases. Until now, there has been only one report on this topic, in which the author found that there was no significant difference between the two diseases in the basal collateral vessel. Thus, based on this limited reference, we cannot conclude whether the incidence of hemorrhage is higher in unilateral moyamoya.

Progression of Unaffected Hemisphere

There have already been many reports about the progression of the unaffected hemisphere in pediatric unilateral moyamoya disease [6–13]. According to long-term follow-up results with pediatric unilateral moyamoya disease (mean age 6.2–10 years) [3, 6, 7, 14], the average time of progression to bilateral disease was 24.7 months (11–72 months). More recently, Smith et al. reported that a younger age at diagnosis was associated with a more rapid rate of progression [3]. Also, they found that if age was less than 7 years, average time to progression was 0.9 years, and if more than 7 years, average time to progression was 3.1 years.

Of course, such cases have also been reported in adult unilateral moyamoya disease [12, 15–21]. In recent large series, progression of unaffected side occurred in 23.8% of unilateral adult moyamoya disease [4]. These reports warrant careful follow-up of the unaffected side in adult unilateral moyamoya disease.

Other reported risk factors related to bilateral progression were angiographic features, female sex, Asian origin, congenital cardiac anomaly, previous cranial irradiation, and familial moyamoya disease [1, 3]. Interestingly, Kelly et al. found that 75% with equivocal or mild contralateral disease progressed to bilateral MMD, whereas only 10.0% with no initial contralateral disease did so. They concluded that the presence of minor changes in the contralateral ACA, intracranial ICA, and MCA was an important predictor of increased risk of progression, and patients with a completely normal angiogram on the contralateral side had a very low risk of progression [1].

Management Plans

In unilateral moyamoya disease, follow-up imaging studies at shorter intervals should be planned in pediatric patients of younger ages (<7 years) or with any of the risk factors noted. On the other hand, in patients without the risk factors, of older age (especially adults), or with angiographically normal intracranial vasculature on the unaffected side, they can be reassured that the likelihood of disease progression may be low, although they should be cautioned that follow-up is still warranted.

Concerning surgical treatment for the affected side, the same indications and surgical methods can be applied to patients with unilateral moyamoya disease. Preventive treatment for the unaffected side is not necessary, because the natural history of the asymptomatic side is variable.

References

1. Kelly ME, Bell-Stephens TE, Marks MP et al (2006) Progression of unilateral moyamoya disease: a clinical series. Cerebrovasc Dis 22:109–115
2. Ogata T, Yasaka M, Inoue T et al (2008) The clinical features of adult unilateral moyamoya disease: does it have the same clinical characteristics as typical moyamoya disease? Cerebrovasc Dis 26:244–249
3. Smith ER, Scott RM (2008) Progression of disease in unilateral moyamoya syndrome. Neurosurg Focus 24:E17
4. Kuroda S, Ishikawa T, Houkin K et al (2005) Incidence and clinical features of disease progression in adult moyamoya disease. Stroke 36:2148–2153
5. Ikezaki K, Inamura T, Kawano T et al (1997) Clinical features of probable moyamoya disease in Japan. Clin Neurol Neurosurg 99 Suppl 2:S173–177
6. Inoue T, Matsushima T, Nagata S et al (1991) [Two pediatric cases of moyamoya disease with progressive involvement from unilateral to bilateral]. No Shinkei Geka 19:179–183
7. Kawano T, Fukui M, Hashimoto N et al (1994) Follow-up study of patients with "unilateral" moyamoya disease. Neurol Med Chir (Tokyo) 34:744–747
8. Kurose K, Kishi H, Nishijima Y (1991) Moyamoya disease developing from unilateral moyamoya disease--case report. Neurol Med Chir (Tokyo) 31:597–599
9. Matsushima T, Fukui M, Fujii K et al (1990) Two pediatric cases with occlusions of the ipsilateral internal carotid and posterior cerebral arteries associated with moyamoya vessels: "unilateral" moyamoya disease. Surg Neurol 33:276–280
10. Matsushima T, Inoue T, Natori Y et al (1994) Children with unilateral occlusion or stenosis of the ICA associated with surrounding moyamoya vessels – "unilateral" moyamoya disease. Acta Neurochir (Wien) 131:196–202
11. Matsushima T, Take S, Fujii K et al (1988) A case of moyamoya disease with progressive involvement from unilateral to bilateral. Surg Neurol 30:471–475
12. Wanifuchi H, Takeshita M, Aoki N et al (1996) Adult moyamoya disease progressing from unilateral to bilateral involvement. Neurol Med Chir (Tokyo) 36:87–90
13. Yoshida S, Matsumoto S, Ban S et al (1992) Moyamoya disease progressing from unilateral to bilateral involvement – case report. Neurol Med Chir (Tokyo) 32:900–903
14. Hirotsune N, Meguro T, Kawada S et al (1997) Long-term follow-up study of patients with unilateral moyamoya disease. Clin Neurol Neurosurg 99 Suppl 2:S178–181
15. Aoki N, Kagawa M, Wanifuchi H et al (1989) [An adult case of moyamoya disease associated with marked advance of occlusive lesion in the bilateral carotid system]. No Shinkei Geka 17:399–403
16. Fujiwara F, Yamada H, Hayashi S et al (1997) [A case of adult moyamoya disease showing fulminant clinical course associated with progression from unilateral to bilateral involvement]. No Shinkei Geka 25:79–84
17. Kagawa R, Okada Y, Moritake K et al (2004) Magnetic resonance angiography demonstrating adult moyamoya disease progressing from unilateral to bilateral involvement – case report. Neurol Med Chir (Tokyo) 44:183–186
18. Oka Y, Kusunoki K, Nochide I et al (2000) [A case of adult moyamoya disease progressed after vascular reconstructive surgery]. No Shinkei Geka 28:373–378
19. Shirane R, Mikawa S, Ebina T (1999) A case of adult moyamoya disease showing progressive angiopathy on cerebral angiography. Clin Neurol Neurosurg 101:210–214
20. Takeshita I, Tsukamoto H, Yamaguchi T et al (1995) A progressive occlusion of the internal carotid arteries in a case of adult-onset moyamoya disease. Fukuoka Igaku Zasshi 86:367–372
21. Tomida M, Muraki M, Yamasaki K (2000) Angiographically verified progression of moyamoya disease in an adult. Case report. J Neurosurg 93:1055–1057

Part II
Epidemiology

Epidemiology of Moyamoya Disease

Koichi Oki, Haruhiko Hoshino, and Norihiro Suzuki

Introduction

Moyamoya disease has a high incidence in East Asian countries, and many large-scale epidemiological surveys of this disease have been conducted in East-Asian countries such as Japan and Republic of Korea.

In the early 1970s, several surveys first reported the epidemiological features of moyamoya disease in Japan. Since 1977, a research committee on moyamoya disease, established by the Ministry of Health and Welfare, Japan (RCMJ), has studied the epidemiology of this disease, and four nationwide surveys were conducted in Japan in 1984, 1990, 1995, and 2003 [1–5]. In Republic of Korea, a survey of moyamoya disease was first conducted in 1988, and several reports on the epidemiology of this disease in Republic of Korea have been published [6, 7].

In this chapter, we will review the epidemiology of moyamoya disease by investigating data mainly from these two countries.

Prevalence and Incidence (Especially in Japan)

In the latest nationwide survey conducted in Japan in 2003 [5], the total number of patients treated with moyamoya disease was estimated to be 7,700 based on data from selected hospitals. (The total population of Japan in 2003 was about 120 million.) The annual prevalence of moyamoya disease in Japan was estimated to be 6.03/1,00,000 individuals and the incidence was estimated to be 0.54/1,00,000 individuals. This survey revealed a substantial increase in the number of moyamoya patients, based on a comparison with the previous three nationwide surveys (which reported 1,900 affected individuals in 1984, 3,300 individuals in 1990, and 3,900 individuals in 1994, respectively) [1–3, 5] (Fig. 1).

K. Oki (✉) and N. Suzuki
Department of Neurology, Keio University School of Medicine, 35 Shinanomachi, Shinjuku-ku, Tokyo 160-8582, Japan
e-mail: koki-keio@umin.ac.jp

H. Hoshino
Preventive Medicine for Cerebrovascular Disease, Department of Neurology, Keio University School of Medicine, 35 Shinanomachi, Shinjuku-ku, Tokyo 160-8582, Japan

B.-K. Cho and T. Tominaga (eds.), *Moyamoya Disease Update*,
DOI 10.1007/978-4-431-99703-0_4, © Springer 2010

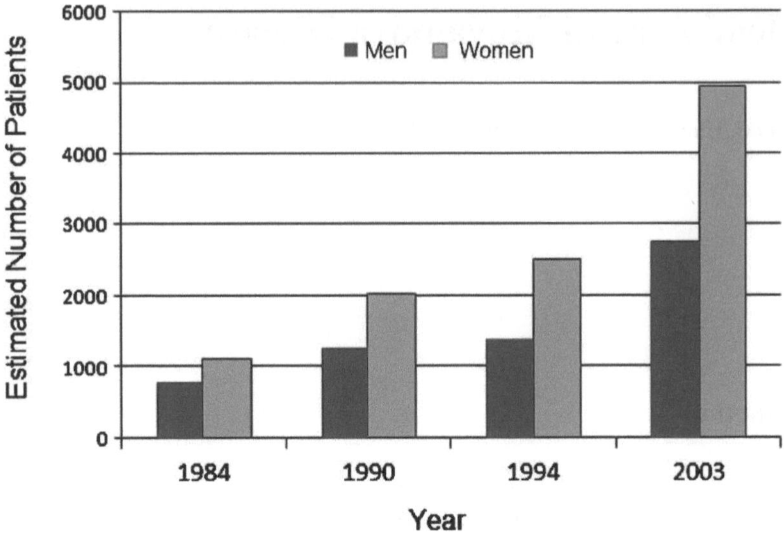

Fig. 1 Increase of estimated number of patients in Japan (based on [1–5])

To avoid a selection bias, an all-inclusive study in a well-delimited area, Hokkaido (the second largest island in Japan), was performed from 2002 to 2006. In this survey, the annual prevalence and incidence of moyamoya disease were estimated to be 10.5/1,00,000 individuals and 0.94/1,00,000 individuals, respectively [8]. The discrepancy between the above two studies was thought to have been caused by differences in the survey methods or survey areas.

The widespread use of noninvasive MRI might increase the detection of asymptomatic people with an occlusion of the circle of Willis. The annual prevalence of moyamoya disease, including this asymptomatic population, was estimated to be 50.7/1,00,000 individuals [9]. Further discussion is needed to determine whether these asymptomatic people with occlusion of the circle of Willis should be regarded as having moyamoya disease. However, there is a possibility that many people who have not been diagnosed as moyamoya disease because of their slight symptoms are potentially present.

Gender Differences

The sex ratio has remained approximately constant throughout recent several surveys. Moyamoya disease occurs much more frequently among women than among men, a sex ratio (women to men) reported in several surveys were 1.6 [3, 4], 1.8 [5], and 2.18 [8].

Familial Occurrence

A family history of moyamoya disease was observed in 10–15% of all the patients [4, 5, 8, 10]. In a study comparing 24 familial cases with 131 sporadic cases, the ratio of women to men was 5.0 among the familial cases but only 1.6 among the sporadic cases. In eight parent–offspring pairs, the parents exhibited their first symptoms at an age of 22–36 years, but their children presented with symptoms at an age of 5–11 years. These results suggest that familial moyamoya disease is strongly associated with genetic anticipation and a female predominance [11].

Age at Onset

The distribution of the age of onset among patients with moyamoya disease is characterized by two peaks. The nationwide survey conducted in Japan in 1997 revealed one peak at an age of less than 5 years and a smaller peak at an age of around 40 years [4]. Similarly, in the RCMJ database for 2003–2007 [10], two peaks in the age of onset distribution were observed, one at 5–9 years and another lower peak at around 40 years (Fig. 2). In contrast, the main peak was shifted towards the adult age group in the all-inclusive study conducted in Hokkaido: the highest peak was observed at 45–49 years, while a smaller peak was observed at 5–9 years [8]. This discrepancy might have been caused by a bias in the sampling of hospitals. The distributions of university hospitals, general hospitals, and small hospitals or clinics specializing in pediatrics may have influenced this shift in the main peak of the age of onset.

Types of Clinical Findings

Two surveys conducted in Japan [8, 10] reported similar percentages of the types of clinical findings and the age of onset distributions according to the types of clinical findings (Fig. 3). The percentage of cases with ischemia (including TIA and stroke) was about 60%. These cases showed two peaks in the age of onset: one at 5–9 years and the other at around 40 years. The percentage of cases with hemorrhage was about 20%, and these cases only exhibited one

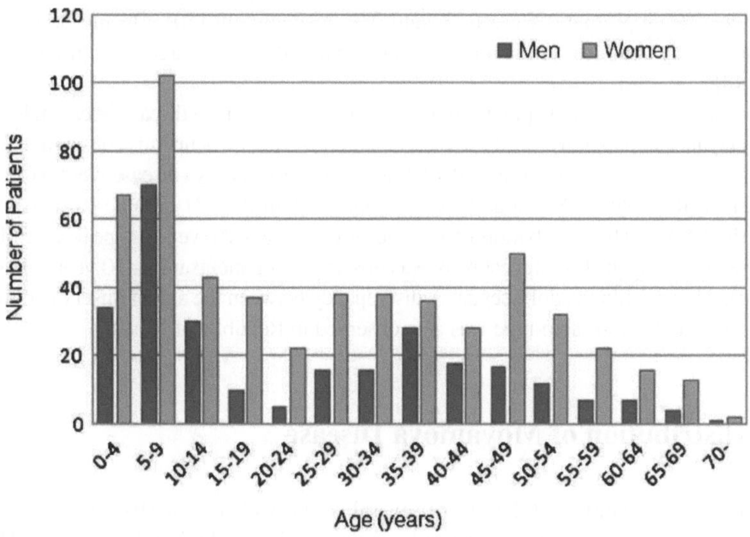

Fig. 2 Age of onset distribution for moyamoya disease (modified from [10])

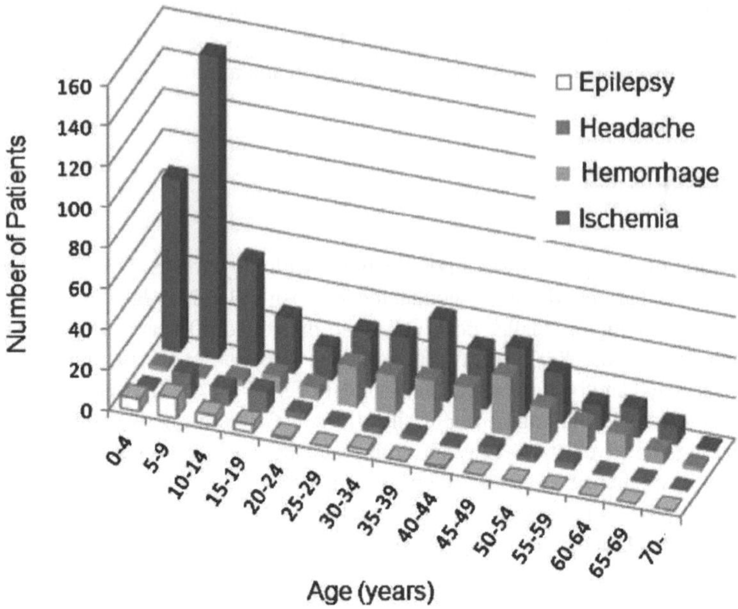

Fig. 3 Age of onset distributions according to clinical types (modified from [10])

peak at around 40 years. The difference in the age distributions for these two clinical types is thought to reflect the fact that ischemic symptoms arising from the occlusion of intracranial arteries can occur in all decades of life, whereas hemorrhagic symptoms are only observed in adulthood because the collateral pathways that gradually develop to compensate for ischemia, known as moyamoya vessels, are very fragile and tend to bleed during adulthood.

The RCMJ database revealed that the percentages of patients with headache, epilepsy, and who were asymptomatic were 6, 3, and 3%, respectively [10]. On the other hand, the all-inclusive study conducted in Hokkaido reported that the percentage of asymptomatic cases was 18% [8].

To compare the clinical and epidemiologic features of moyamoya disease between Republic of Korea and Japan, a collaborative study was organized with Korean neurosurgeons as a main project of the RCMJ in 1995 [7]. In this study, 296 definite case of moyamoya disease were collected from 26 hospitals in Republic of Korea and were compared with the 731 definite cases registered in Japan by the RCMJ. The distribution of the age of onset also showed two peaks, similar to the results observed in Japan. The highest peak was observed for patients under 10 years of age, while the second peak was seen in adolescence. A discrepancy between the age of onset distributions for ischemic-type and hemorrhagic-type was also observed in Republic of Korea.

World Distribution of Moyamoya Disease

An evaluation of the published data from several countries between 1972 and 1989 revealed 1,063 cases of moyamoya disease throughout the world, excluding Japan [12]. The study reported 625 cases in Asia, 201 in Europe, 176 in North and South America, 52 in Africa, and

9 in Oceania. In a survey of 298 cases of moyamoya disease in Washington state and California from 1987 to 1998 [13], the incidence was estimated to be 0.086/1,00,000 individuals, which was lower than that of Japan. However, the ethnicity-specific incidences varied. The highest incidence was observed among Asian Americans (0.28/1,00,000 person-years), followed by African Americans (0.13), whites (0.06), and Hispanics (0.03). This report revealed that genetic, rather than environmental, factors may influence the incidence of moyamoya disease, and that this disease was observed most frequently among people of Asian origin.

Conclusion

Moyamoya disease is an uncommon cerebrovascular disease, and its pathophysiology remains uncertain. Several surveys of the epidemiological features of moyamoya disease have revealed not only its incidence and prevalence, but also a gender difference, the age of onset distribution, and ethnic differences. These epidemiological findings may help to clarify the pathogenesis of moyamoya disease.

Acknowledgment This study was assisted by a research grant from the Research Committee on Spontaneous Occlusion of the Circle of Willis (Moyamoya Disease) in the Ministry of Health, Labor and Welfare, Japan.

References

1. Aoki K, Handa H, Terayama K et al (1986) A nationwide epidemiological survey of intractable diseases in Japan. In: Aoki K (ed) Annual Report of Epidemiology of Intractable Diseases Research Committee. The Research Committee on Epidemiology of Intractable Diseases, Nagoya, Japan, p 9–22
2. Ohno Y, Yonekawa Y, Handa H et al (1987) Clinicoepidemiological features of Spontaneous Occlusion of the Circle of Willis. In: Aoki K (ed) Annual Report of Epidemiology of Intractable Diseases Research Committee. The Research Committee on Epidemiology of Intractable Diseases, Nagoya, Japan, p 29–32
3. Sasaki R, Suzuki S, Tamakoshi A et al (1991) Clinicoepidemiological features of Spontaneous Occlusion of the Circle of Willis from a nationwide epidemiologcal survey. In: Yanagawa H (ed) Annual Report of Epidemiology of Intractable Diseases Research Committee. The Research Committee on Epidemiology of Intractable Diseases, Tochigi, Japan, p 30–32
4. Wakai K, Tamakoshi A, Ikezaki K et al (1997) Epidemiological features of moyamoya disease in Japan: findings from a nationwide survey. Clin Neurol Neurosurg 99 (suppl 2):S1–5
5. Kuriyama S, Kusaka Y, Fujimura M et al (2008) Prevalence and clinicoepidemiological features of moyamoya disease in Japan: findings from a nationwide epidemiological survey. Stroke 39:42–47
6. Choi KS (1988) Moyamoya disease in Korea: a cooperative study. In: Suzuki J (ed) Advances in surgery for cerebral stroke. Springer, Tokyo, Japan, p 107–109
7. Han DH, Kwon OK, Byun BJ et al (2000) A co-operative study: clinical characteristics of 334 Korean patients with moyamoya disease treated at neurosurgical institutes (1976–1994). The Korean Society for Cerebrovascular Disease. Acta Neurochir (Wien) 142:1263–1273; discussion 1273–1274
8. Baba T, Houkin K, Kuroda S (2008) Novel epidemiological features of moyamoya disease. J Neurol Neurosurg Psychiatry 79:900–904
9. Ikeda K, Iwasaki Y, Kashihara H et al (2006) Adult moyamoya disease in the asymptomatic Japanese population. J Clin Neurosci 13:334–338
10. Oki K, Hoshino H, Suzuki N et al (2008) Database count of the Research Committee on Spontaneous Occlusion of the Circle of Willis (moyamoya disease) In: Hashimoto N (ed) A summarized report of

2005–2007 of the Research Committee on Spontaneous Occlusion of the Circle of Willis (Moyamoya Disease). The Research Committee on Spontaneous Occlusion of the Circle of Willis (Moyamoya Disease) Kyoto, Japan, p 15–20

11. Nanba R, Kuroda S, Tada M et al (2006) Clinical features of familial moyamoya disease. Childs Nerv Syst 22:258–262
12. Goto Y, Yonekawa Y (1992) Worldwide distribution of moyamoya disease. Neurol Med Chir (Tokyo) 32:883–886
13. Uchino K, Johnston SC, Becker KJ et al (2005) Moyamoya disease in Washington State and California. Neurology 65:956–958

Familial Moyamoya Disease

Joong-Uhn Choi

Introduction

Moyamoya disease (MMD) is an idiopathic angiopathy characterized progressive stenosis or occlusion of terminal portion of bilateral internal carotid artery and circle of Willis.

Collateral vessels develop at the base of brain to compensate for the progressive stenosis. The slowly developed collaterals appear as puff of smoke in angiography which give name of disease in Japanese.

Definite cases of MMD are diagnosed in patients with bilateral lesion whereas patients with unilateral lesion are diagnosed as probable cases. So-called quasi-MMD or moyamoya syndrome is the same condition combined with a disease such as atherosclerosis, meningitis, brain tumor, head trauma, irradiation to head, neurofibromatosis, or Down's syndrome.

Epidemiology

MMD is predominantly found in East Asian countries like Japan, Republic of Korea, and China. There are general female predominance. Male and female ratio is 1:1.8 in Japan. MMD has two peak ages of onset, initially at 5 years of age (juvenile type) and subsequently at 30–50 years of age (adult type). Peak age in male is 10–14 years and 35–49 years whereas peak in female is 20–24 years and 50–54 years.

Percentage of patients younger than 10 years and over 50 years was about 11.9 and 25.5% respectively. Annual rate of newly diagnosed cases in 2003 was 0.54/1,00,000 population in Japan [1].

Familial occurrence of MMD has been reported to be approximately 6–12% of all reported cases. Approximately 50–70% of cases of MMD among family members occur in siblings, and 24% occur in a parent and offspring [2, 3].

J.-U. Choi (✉)
Department of Neurosurgery, CHA Bundang Medical Center, CHA University, 351 Yatap-dong, Bundang-gu, Seongnam-si, Gyeonggi-do 463-712, Republic of Korea
e-mail: juchoi@yuhs.ac, juchoi@cha.ac.kr

B.-K. Cho and T. Tominaga (eds.), *Moyamoya Disease Update*,
DOI 10.1007/978-4-431-99703-0_5, © Springer 2010

The incidence in siblings of proband with this disease is about 3% which is 42 times higher than that in general population. The incidence of offspring of proband is about 2.4% which is 34 times higher than that in general population [4].

Mode of Inheritance

The mode of inheritance in MMD is unclear but it is most likely multifactorial. MMD may be caused by several different mechanisms (disease heterogeneity). The mode of inheritance of familial moyamoya disease (FMMD) is autosomal dominant with incomplete penetrance [5]. As for the proportion of affected people among total offspring, 50% indicates an autosomal dominant mode and 25% indicates an autosomal recessive mode of inheritance.

The ratio of maternal transmission to parenteral transmission was 3.44 showing maternal predominance and mother to daughter transmission was commonly seen (60%). Adult onset and asymptomatic patients were more commonly seen with mother to daughter transmission. The proportion of monozygotic twinning is higher in MMD than general population. Most monozygotic twin pairs were female [5].

Diagnosis and Clinical Aspect

Diagnosis of MMD is highly dependent on imaging with MRI and cerebral angiography. Noninvasive MRI and MRA can detect the disease in almost 100% of affected patients including asymptomatic patients during screening studies [6].

Screening with MRA play important role for high-risk familial members of MMD. Clinical presentation of FMMD will be same as that of MMD in general population; transient ischemic attacks (TIA) or cerebral infarction in children and intracranial bleeding in adults, which will not be described in detail in this chapter.

Research and Genetics on FMMD

To clarify the genetic background of MMD several nonparametric linkage analysis using mainly affected sibling pairs were done, which showed linkage to 3p24.2-p26, 6q23, 12p12, and 17q25. A gene for FMMD is located in chromosome 17q25 [7].

The microsatellite polymorphism D353050 mapped to chromosome 3p24.2-p26 showed strong evidence of linkage by nonparametric analysis with NPL score of 3.46 [8].

The association analysis of tissue inhibitor of metalloproteinase-2 in17q25 showed that a polymorphism in promoter region was markedly associated with familial MMD. This result suggested that presence of G/C heterozygous genotype at position-418 in TIMP2 promotor region could be a genetic predisposing factor for FMMD [9].

References

1. Kuriyama S, Kusaka Y, Fujimura M et al (2008) Prevalence and clinicoepidemiological features of moyamoya disease in Japan. Stroke 39:42–47
2. Fukuyama S, Kanai M, Osawa M (1991) Clinical genetic analysis on the moyamoya disease. In: Fukui M (ed) Annual report 1990. The Research Committee on Spontaneous Occlusion of the Circle of Willis (Moyamoya Disease) of the Ministry of Health and Welfare, Fukuoka, Japan, pp 53–59, 141-146
3. Seol HJ, Wang KC, Kim SK et al (2006) Familial occurrence of moyamoya disease: a clinical study. Childs Nerv Syst 22:1143–1148
4. Kitahara T, Ariga N, Yamaura A et al (1979) Familial occurrence of moyamoya disease: report of three Japanese families. J Neurol Neurosurg Psychiatry 42:208–214
5. Mineharu Y, Tukenaka K, Yamakawa H et al (2006) Inheritance pattern of familial moyamoya disease: autosomal dominant mode and genomic imprinting. J Neurol Neurosurg Psychiatry 77:1025–1029
6. Houkin K, Tanaka N, Takahashi A et al (1994) Familial occurrence of moyamoya disease: magnetic resonance angiography as a screening test for high risk subjects. Childs Nerv Syst 10:421–425
7. Yamauchi T, Tada M, Houkin K et al (2000) Linkage of familial moyamoya disease (spontaneous occlusion of the circle of Willis) to chromosome 17q25. Stroke 31:930–935
8. Ikeda H, Sasaki T, Yoshimoto T et al (1999) Mapping of a familial moyamoya disease gene to chromosome 3p24.2-p26. Am J Hum Genet 64:533–537
9. Kang HS, Kim SK, Cho BK et al (2006) Single nucleotide polymorphisms of tissue inhibitor of metalloproteinase gene in familial moyamoya disease. Neurosurgery 58:1074–1080

Part III
Genetics

Overview

Shigeo Kure

Four Lines of Evidence for Involvement of Genetic Factors in the Etiology of Moyamoya Disease

The Presence of Familial Cases

Most patients with moyamoya disease are sporadic cases, but in Japan, 10–15% of patients with moyamoya disease have affected first-degree relatives [1–3]. In the United States, 6% of patients have a family history of the disease [4, 5]. The presence of familial cases in many countries suggests that genetic factors participate in the etiology of moyamoya disease. There may be some minor differences of clinical presentations between familial and sporadic cases. The ratio of women to men is 5.0 in familial cases and 1.6 in sporadic cases. Age of onset (mean ± SD) was 11.8 ± 11.7 in familial cases while in sporadic cases it was 30.0 ± 20.9 [6].

Concordance in Identical Twins

Hashikata et al. reported that concordance in the affection status of moyamoya disease has been proven in 80% of identical twins [7]. Tanghetti et al. described moyamoya disease in only one of two identical twins [8]. Concordance of moyamoya disease in identical twins appears higher than that in dizygotic twins, but not 100%, suggesting that moyamoya disease is a genetic disorder with incomplete penetrance, and/or that other factors may participate in its etiology.

S. Kure (✉)
Department of Pediatrics, Tohoku University School of Medicine,
Seiryomachi, Aobaku, Sendai 980-8574, Japan
e-mail: skure@mail.tains.tohoku.ac.jp

B.-K. Cho and T. Tominaga (eds.), *Moyamoya Disease Update*,
DOI 10.1007/978-4-431-99703-0_6, © Springer 2010

Ethnic Differences in Incidence

The prevalence of moyamoya disease shows an ethnic difference. It is high in East Asian countries, especially in Japan and Republic of Korea, while it is low in Western countries [9]. In Japan, the annual prevalence and incidence of moyamoya disease were estimated at 3.16 and 0.35/1,00,000, respectively [2]. Baba et al. have reported an update of an epidemiological study of Japanese patients, in which the prevalence and incidence are three times higher than in the previous report, at 10.5 and 0.94/1,00,000, respectively [10]. The incidence of moyamoya disease in the United States was examined during 1987–1998 by Uchino et al. [11]. They found 298 patients in California and Washington, and estimated the incidence at 0.086/1,00,000. Yonekawa et al. reported that the incidence in European countries is approximately one-tenth of that in Japan [12]. The incidence of moyamoya disease in Japan is, therefore, considered to be approximately ten times higher than in Western countries. In Asian Americans, the incidence of moyamoya disease is four times higher than in non-Asian Americans, providing compelling evidence that genetic factors play a dominant role compared with environmental factors [11].

Congenital Disorders with Moyamoya-Like Findings on Angiography

Many congenital disorders caused by genome mutations, chromosomal mutations, or gene mutations can sometimes be associated with cerebrovascular angiopathy, with angiographic features similar to moyamoya disease. A typical example of a congenital disease with genome mutations is Down syndrome. Children with Down syndrome have increased risk for stroke. Some of them have presented moyamoya-like angiographic findings with occlusive changes in the circle of Willis and collateral neovascularization. In patients with Down syndrome, the incidence of moyamoya-like disease is 30 times higher than in the general population [13]. Williams' syndrome is an example of a congenital disease with chromosomal mutations, which is sometimes associated with moyamoya-like disease. This syndrome is caused by a 2-Mb deletion in chromosome 7q11.23, in which about 20 genes exist, including elastin gene, *ELN*. Overexpression of *ELN* was reported in smooth muscle cells (SMCs) derived from patients with moyamoya disease, suggesting a role in its etiology [14]. Neurofibromatosis type I is an example of a disease with gene mutations similar to moyamoya. This disorder is also referred to as von Recklinghausen's disease, which is caused by mutations in fibrillin genes located on chromosome 17q11.

Approaches to Identify the Moyamoya Disease Genes

A multifactorial mode of inheritance may be involved in the occurrence and susceptibility of moyamoya disease. Because of the lack of highly aggregated families with moyamoya disease, its mode of inheritance remained undetermined. Recently, the mode of inheritance has been investigated in 15 highly aggregated Japanese families without consanguinity, all of which had more than three generations [15]. All types of transmission, including father-to-son, were observed in these families, and 59 of 135 (43.7%) offspring of the patients with moyamoya disease were affected or were obligate carriers. The authors concluded that the mode of inheritance of familial moyamoya disease is either autosomal dominant with incomplete penetrance or polygenic.

Two approaches have been used for the identification of predisposing genes to moyamoya disease: linkage analysis and candidate gene analysis. All the linkage studies have been performed in Japan, using affected sibling pairs and small nuclear families with moyamoya disease, but have been unable to identify replicable chromosomal loci [16–19]. Recently, Mineharu et al. reported on a genome-wide parametric linkage analysis in 15 three-generation pedigrees, and successfully mapped the moyamoya disease gene on chromosome 17q25.3 [20]. Candidate gene approaches consist of association and/or mutational analyzes of genes, which are supposed to be functionally related, with pathologic conditions of moyamoya disease. Abnormal regulation of migration and proliferation of vascular SMCs is supposed to underlie the etiology of moyamoya disease [21, 22]. SMCs produce both matrix metallo proteinase (MMP)-2 and MMP-9, and genetic deficiency in either may decrease SMC invasion in vitro and the formation of intimal hyperplasia in vivo [23], suggesting that MMP-related genes are good candidates for moyamoya disease genes. Kang et al. reported genetic polymorphism in TIMP4, a gene-encoding tissue inhibitor of MMP type 4 on chromosome 17q25, was significantly associated with familial moyamoya disease [24].

Identification of the First Gene Mutated in Moyamoya Disease

Recently, the first gene mutated in moyamoya disease has been found by a unique approach. The SMC-specific isoform of alpha-actin (*ACTA2*) is a major component of the contractile apparatus in SMCs located throughout the arterial system. Guo et al. have performed linkage analysis of seven families with thoracic aortic aneurysm and dissections (TAAT), and have mapped the TAAT gene to chromosome 10q23-24, in which *ACTA2* is located. Mutations in *ACTA2* were successfully identified in 14% of families with TAAT [25]. The authors hypothesized that the heterozygous carriers of *ACTA2* mutations predispose to vascular diseases other than TAAT. They scrutinized the medical records of the members of the TAAT families, and found that the mutation carriers had various types of vascular disease, coronary artery disease, and premature-onset strokes including moyamoya disease [26]. In the study, they presented three cases with moyamoya disease, in which there was severe stenosis of the terminal internal carotid arteries but absence of a vascular collateral network in the MRI angiography. It will be interesting if *ACTA2* mutation is found in other moyamoya patients with typical angiographic presentations.

Conclusions

There is strong evidence that genetic factors are involved in the etiology of moyamoya disease. The mode of inheritance of familial moyamoya disease has been identified to be autosomal dominant with incomplete penetrance by analysis of highly aggregated families with moyamoya disease. Recently, it has been reported that individuals with *ACTA2* mutations presented stenosis of the terminal internal carotid arteries. This finding is interesting, but requires replication in other patients with typical moyamoya disease, who have both the bilateral steno-occlusive lesions and the formation of a fine collateral network.

References

1. Ikezaki K, Han DH, Kawano T et al (1997) A clinical comparison of definite moyamoya disease between South Korea and Japan. Stroke 28:2513–2517
2. Wakai K, Tamakoshi A, Ikezaki K et al (1997) Epidemiological features of moyamoya disease in Japan: findings from a nationwide survey. Clin Neurol Neurosurg 99:S1–S5
3. Yamauchi T, Houkin K, Tada M et al (1997) Familial occurrence of moyamoya disease. Clin Neurol Neurosurg 99:S162–S167
4. Fukui M, Kono S, Sueishi K et al (2000) Moyamoya disease. Neuropathology 20:S61–S64
5. Scott RM, Smith JL, Robertson RL et al (2004) Long-term outcome in children with moyamoya syndrome after cranial revascularization by pial synangiosis. J Neurosurg 100 (2 Suppl Pediatrics): 142–149
6. Nanba R, Kuroda S, Tada M et al (2006) Clinical features of familial moyamoya disease. Childs Nerv Syst 22:258–262
7. Hashikata H, Liu W, Mineharu Y et al (2008) Current knowledge on the genetic factors involved in moyamoya disease. Brain Nerve 60:1261–1269
8. Tanghetti B, Capra R, Giunta F et al (1983) Moyamoya syndrome in only one of two identical twins. Case report. J Neurosurg 59:1092–1094
9. Ikezaki K (2001) Clinical manifestation: epidemiology, symptoms and signs, laboratory findings. In: Ikezaki K, Loftus C (eds) Moyamoya disease. Thieme, New York, p43–75
10. Baba T, Houkin K, Kuroda S (2008) Novel epidemiological features of moyamoya disease. J Neurol Neurosurg Psychiatry 79:900–904
11. Uchino K, Johnston SC, Becker KJ et al (2005) Moyamoya disease in Washington State and California. Neurology 65:956–958
12. Yonekawa Y, Ogata N, Kaku Y et al (1997) Moyamoya disease in Europe, past and present status. Clin Neurol Neurosurg 99:S58–S60
13. Ikezaki k, Loftus C (2001) Quasi-moyamoya disease: definition, classification, and therapy. In: Ikezaki k, Loftus C (eds) Moyamoya disease. Thieme, New York, p 2341
14. Yamamoto M, Aoyagi M, Tajima S et al (1997) Increase in elastin gene expression and protein synthesis in arterial smooth muscle cells derived from patients with moyamoya disease. Stroke 28:1733–1738
15. Mineharu Y, Takenaka K, Yamakawa H et al (2006) Inheritance pattern of familial moyamoya disease: autosomal dominant mode and genomic imprinting. J Neurol Neurosurg Psychiatry 77:1025–1029
16. Ikeda H, Sasaki T, Yoshimoto T et al (1999) Mapping of a familial moyamoya disease gene to chromosome 3p24.2-p26. Am J Hum Genet 64:533–537
17. Inoue TK, Ikezaki K, Sasazuki T et al (1997) DNA typing of HLA in the patients with moyamoya disease. Jpn J Hum Genet 42:507–515
18. Sakurai K, Horiuchi Y, Ikeda H et al (2004) A novel susceptibility locus for moyamoya disease on chromosome 8q23. J Hum Genet 49:278–281
19. Yamauchi T, Tada M, Houkin K et al (2000) Linkage of familial moyamoya disease (spontaneous occlusion of the circle of Willis) to chromosome 17q25. Stroke 31:930–935
20. Mineharu Y, Liu W, Inoue K et al (2008) Autosomal dominant moyamoya disease maps to chromosome 17q25.3. Neurology 70:2357–2363
21. Yamamoto M, Aoyagi M, Fukai N et al (1998) Differences in cellular responses to mitogens in arterial smooth muscle cells derived from patients with moyamoya disease. Stroke 29:1188–1193
22. Yamamoto M, Aoyagi M, Fukai N et al (1999) Increase in prostaglandin E(2) production by interleukin-1beta in arterial smooth muscle cells derived from patients with moyamoya disease. Circ Res 85:912–918
23. Johnson C, Galis ZS (2004) Matrix metalloproteinase-2 and -9 differentially regulate smooth muscle cell migration and cell-mediated collagen organization. Arterioscler Thromb Vasc Biol 24:54–60
24. Kang HS, Kim SK, Cho BK et al (2006) Single nucleotide polymorphisms of tissue inhibitor of metalloproteinase genes in familial moyamoya disease. Neurosurgery 58:1074–1080; discussion-80

25. Guo DC, Pannu H, Tran-Fadulu V et al (2007) Mutations in smooth muscle alpha-actin (ACTA2) lead to thoracic aortic aneurysms and dissections. Nat Genet 39:1488–1493
26. Guo DC, Papke CL, Tran-Fadulu V et al (2009) Mutations in smooth muscle alpha-actin (ACTA2) cause coronary artery disease, stroke, and moyamoya disease, along with thoracic aortic disease. Am J Hum Genet 84:617–627

Genetic Linkage Study

Shigeo Kure

Chromosome 3p24-26

Ikeda et al. performed a genome-wide linkage study using 16 Japanese families with moyamoya disease and 371 microsatellite markers [1]. In the study 13 of 16 families had sibling cases and the rest of them included parent–children transmission of the disease. Maximum nonparametric linkage (NPL) score of 3.4 was found at the marker D3S3050. NPL score of greater than 3.0 was observed at the three microsatellite markers, D3S2387, D3S3050, and D3S1560, which are located on chromosome 3p24.2-p26 (Fig. 1). In moyamoya disease, abnormal vascular formation is observed mainly in brain. Marfan syndrome is an extracellular matrix disorder with cardinal manifestations in the cardiovascular and skeleton systems. Moyamoya-like angiographic findings are sometimes associated with Marfan syndrome. Most patients with Marfan syndrome have mutations in fibrillin gene (*FRN*) on chromosome 15q21 [2]. The second locus for Marfan syndrome has been mapped at chromosome 3p25-24.2 [3]. Recently, *TGFBR2,* a putative tumor-suppressor gene implicated in several malignancies, has been identified for the second gene for Marfan syndrome [4]. Mutational analysis of *TGFBR2* in patients with moyamoya disease has not been reported. Yamamoto et al. hypothesized that paternally imprinted gene might be associated with this disorder because of a high incidence of maternal inheritance in familial moyamoya disease. Although they screened genes with monoallelic expressions on chromosome 3, no imprinting gene was identified in this region [5].

Chromosome 6

Various autoimmune diseases have been associated with human leukocyte antigen (HLA), which is located on chromosome 6p21. Aoyagi et al. found a significant association of HLA-B51 using 32 Japanese patients with nonfamilial moyamoya disease [6]. Inoue et al.

S. Kure (✉)
Department of Pediatrics, Tohoku University School of Medicine, Seiryomachi, Aobaku, Sendai 980-8574, Japan
e-mail: skure@mail.tains.tohoku.ac.jp

B.-K. Cho and T. Tominaga (eds.), *Moyamoya Disease Update*,
DOI 10.1007/978-4-431-99703-0_7, © Springer 2010

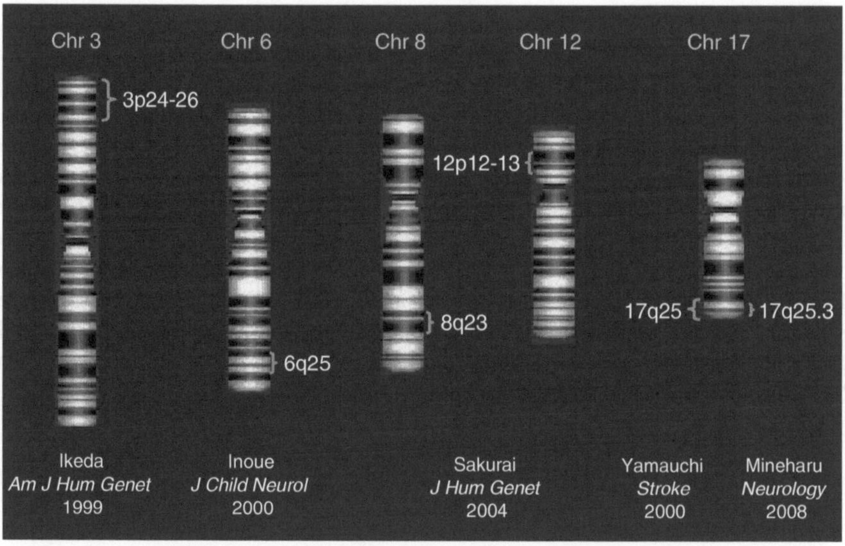

Fig. 1 Chromosomal loci for moyamoya disease gene revealed by linkage study of familial cases. First candidate region for moyamoya disease was reported in 1999 from Tohoku University. Dr Ikeda and colleagues mapped the responsible gene on chromosome 3p24-26 using 16 moyamoya families. The maximum nonparametric linkage (NPL) score was 3.5. After this study, four additional loci were reported on chromosomes 6, 8, 12, and 17

reported significant association between moyamoya disease and several HLA class II alleles by genotyping of HLA locus [7]. Frequency of patients with the single haplotype of DRB1*1510-DQA1*01021-DQB1*0602 was significantly lower than that in control subjects. The same group further studied chromosome 6 by genotyping 15 microsatellite makers in 20 affected sibling pairs, and found that one particular haplotype was shared by affected members in 19 of 20 families [8].

Han et al. reported the association of moyamoya disease and HLA alleles in Korean patients [9]. They performed the case control study using 28 patients with moyamoya disease and 198 control subjects, and found that the frequency of HLA-B35 allele was significantly increased in patient group compared to the control group (32.1 vs. 10.1%, $P<0.008$). The frequency of the HLA allele was most significantly increased among the female patients with late-onset moyamoya disease. They concluded that HLA-B35 is a useful genetic marker for moyamoya disease in Republic of Korea.

Chromosome 8q21-22

Sakurai et al. performed a genome-wide linkage analysis in 12 nuclear families with affected sibling pairs using 428 polymorphic microsatellite markers [10]. Maximum LOD score (MLS) of 2.8 was found at the marker D8S546 and MLS > 2.0 was observed at three markers, D8S1119, D8S559, and D8S546, which are located on chromosome 8q21.2-22. The authors suggested *TIEG* on chromosome 8q22.3 as a candidate gene for moyamoya disease, which encodes transforming growth factor-beta (TGF beta) inducible early gene-1. TGFβ1 is supposed to play a role in the etiology of moyamoya disease. Expression of TGFβ1 gene in cultured smooth muscle cells (SMC) derived from the superficial temporal arteries of the patients with moyamoya disease was significantly increased compared with those from controls [11]. TGFβ1 is a potent inducer of elastin gene in arterial SMC. The maximum levels of elastin synthesis and elastin mRNA in response to exogenous TGFβ1 was significantly greater in moyamoya SMCs than control SMCs [11]. Furthermore, levels of TGFβ1 in serum of patients with moyamoya disease are significantly higher than those of controls [12]. Other candidate genes in this locus suggested by the authors were *ANGPT1*, *EBAG9*, and *DD5*. *ANGPT1* encodes a secreted ligand for a receptor-like tyrosin kinase. *EBAG9* encodes estrogen receptor-binding site-associated antigen 9. *DD5* encodes a progestin-induced protein. Progestin regulates angiogenesis through vascular endothelial growth factor expression. In this study, a suggestive linkage level with MLS of 2.3 and NPL of 2.5 was also detected at the marker D12S1690, which is located on chromosome 12p13.2.

Chromosome 17q25

Yamauchi et al. performing the linkage analysis focusing on chromosome 17 because the characteristic lesions of moyamoya disease are occasionally seen in neurofibromatosis type 1 and its causative gene *NF1* is located on 17q11.2 [13]. A total of 24 families with moyamoya disease with multiple affected family members were analyzed with 22 microsatellite markers on chromosome 17. The result indicates that the MLS was 3.1 at the marker D17S939, and that the disease locus was encompassed within the 9-cM region between D17S785 and D17S836 on chromosome 17q25. The same group selected nine candidate genes, *DNA2, AANAT, PSP, HCNGP, HN1, SGSH, SYNGR2, EVPL*, and *TIMP2,* in the 9-cM region for mutational analysis by exon sequencing method [14]. No causative mutation was identified in the nine genes. Recently, Kang et al. performed the mutational and association analyzes of *TIM2* that encodes tissue inhibitor of metalloproteinase type 2 [15]. Although they found no causative mutations in the protein-coding regions, a significantly higher frequency of a heterozygous genotype was found in the *TIMP2* promoter region at position 418 in familial moyamoya disease, compared with nonfamilial moyamoya disease or control group. Vascular SMCs produce matrix metalloproteinase type 2, which plays a role in invasion and proliferation of SMCs [16]. Dysregulation of TIMP2 may, therefore, lead to abnormal proliferation and intimal thickening.

Chromosome 17q25.3

Mineharu et al. reported the genome-wide parametric linkage analysis for moyamoya disease in 15 extended Japanese families by using 382 polymorphic markers [17]. They collected three-generation pedigrees and applied an affected member-only analysis after MRI and MR angiography examinations. They use two diagnostic criteria, narrow and broad. Only patients with definite moyamoya disease was assigned under narrow criteria while patients with faint steno-occlusive lesions around the terminals of the internal carotid arteries were classified as affected under broad criteria. Significant evidence of linkage was observed only on chromosome 17q25.3 with maximum multipoint LOD score of 6.57 using narrow diagnostic criteria and 8.07 using broad criteria. The moyamoya disease locus has been finally mapped to a 3.5 Mb region between D17S1806 to the telomere, which is close to the previously-reported moyamoya locus with 9-cM, but not overlapping [13]. The authors discussed that steno-occlusive changes of the middle cerebral artery and unilateral moyamoya disease can be considered to be in the spectrum of moyamoya disease since high linkage scores was observed under both the narrow and broad diagnostic criteria. They selected four candidate genes in the responsible region based on their gene functions, *TIMP2, BAIAP2, RAC3*, and *RAB40B*. A promoter polymorphism of TIMP2 reported by the Korean group [15] was not polymorphic in the families. *BAIAP2* interacts with brain-specific angiogenesis inhibitor-1, which is an inhibitor of basic fibroblast growth factor (bFGF)-induced angiogenesis [18]. RAC3 and RAB40B are members of the ras oncogene family and important regulators of cell growth and cytoskeletal recognition. The authors performed the mutational analysis, but they found no causative mutation in the four candidate genes.

Conclusions

Recent linkage analysis has provided compelling evidence that the pathogenic gene of moyamoya disease would be identified on chromosome 17q25.3. A complete genetic characterization of the linked region, including comprehensive sequencing of each gene and copy number analysis, is imperative to identify the moyamoya disease gene [19]. Identification of the moyamoya disease gene would permit presymptomatic screening for high-risk individuals.

References

1. Ikeda H, Sasaki T, Yoshimoto T et al (1999) Mapping of a familial moyamoya disease gene to chromosome 3p24.2-p26. Am J Hum Genet 64:533–537
2. Dietz HC, Cutting GR, Pyeritz RE et al (1991) Marfan syndrome caused by a recurrent de novo missense mutation in the fibrillin gene. Nature 352:337–339
3. Collod G, Babron MC, Jondeau G et al (1994) A second locus for Marfan syndrome maps to chromosome 3p24.2-p25. Nat Genet 8:264–268
4. Mizuguchi T, Collod-Beroud G, Akiyama T et al (2004) Heterozygous TGFBR2 mutations in Marfan syndrome. Nat Genet 36:855–860
5. Yamamoto T, Akasaka Y, Ohtani K et al (2005) Molecular screening for moyamoya disease by use of expressed sequence tag on chromosome 3p. No To Hattatsu 37:20–25
6. Aoyagi M, Ogami K, Matsushima Y et al (1995) Human leukocyte antigen in patients with moyamoya disease. Stroke 26:415–417
7. Inoue TK, Ikezaki K, Sasazuki T et al (1997) DNA typing of HLA in the patients with moyamoya disease. Jpn J Hum Genet 42:507–515
8. Inoue TK, Ikezaki K, Sasazuki T et al (2000) Linkage analysis of moyamoya disease on chromosome 6. J Child Neurol 15:179–182
9. Han H, Pyo CW, Yoo DS et al (2003) Associations of moyamoya patients with HLA class I and class II alleles in the Korean population. J Korean Med Sci 18:876–880
10. Sakurai K, Horiuchi Y, Ikeda H et al (2004) A novel susceptibility locus for moyamoya disease on chromosome 8q23. J Hum Genet 49:278–281
11. Yamamoto M, Aoyagi M, Fukai N et al (1998) Differences in cellular responses to mitogens in arterial smooth muscle cells derived from patients with moyamoya disease. Stroke 29:1188–1193
12. Hojo M, Hoshimaru M, Miyamoto S et al (1998) Role of transforming growth factor-beta1 in the pathogenesis of moyamoya disease. J Neurosurg 89:623–629
13. Yamauchi T, Tada M, Houkin K et al (2000) Linkage of familial moyamoya disease (spontaneous occlusion of the circle of Willis) to chromosome 17q25. Stroke 31:930–935

14. Nanba R, Tada M, Kuroda S (2005) Sequence analysis and bioinformatics analysis of chromosome 17q25 in familial moyamoya disease. Childs Nerv Syst 21:62–68
15. Kang HS, Kim SK, Cho BK et al (2006) Single nucleotide polymorphisms of tissue inhibitor of metalloproteinase genes in familial moyamoya disease. Neurosurgery 58:1074–1080; discussion-80
16. Johnson C, Galis ZS (2004) Matrix metalloproteinase-2 and -9 differentially regulate smooth muscle cell migration and cell-mediated collagen organization. Arterioscler Thromb Vasc Biol 24:54–60
17. Mineharu Y, Liu W, Inoue K et al (2008) Autosomal dominant moyamoya disease maps to chromosome 17q25.3. Neurology 70:2357–2363
18. Shiratsuchi T, Oda K, Nishimori H et al (1998) Cloning and characterization of BAP3 (BAI-associated protein 3), a C2 domain-containing protein that interacts with BAI1. Biochem Biophys Res Commun 251:158–165
19. Meschia JF, Ross OA (2008) Heterogeneity of moyamoya disease:after a decade of linkage, is there new hope for a gene? Neurology 70:2353–2354

Single Nucleotide Polymorphism and Moyamoya Disease

Hyun-Seung Kang and Kyu-Chang Wang

Introduction

Single nucleotide polymorphisms (SNPs) are unique genetic differences between individuals that can contribute to disease susceptibility. Although more than 12 million SNPs have been identified, most of them are not associated with disease susceptibility [1]. Moyamoya disease (MMD) is more common in Asian populations; however, we do not know the reason for this. Genetic studies using SNPs may provide the answer. For example, an SNP in the promoter region of the tissue inhibitor of metalloproteinase 2 gene (*TIMP2*) is related to the occurrence of familial MMD [2]. High-throughput SNP genotyping may be fruitful in this field of research.

Single Nucleotide Polymorphisms: A Brief Review

SNPs are single base-pair positions in genomic DNA at which different sequence alternatives (alleles) exist in normal individuals in some populations, where the least frequent allele has an abundance of 1% or greater [3]. There are four basic SNP alternatives: C↔T (G↔A), C↔A (G↔T), C↔G (G↔C), and T↔A (A↔T). Among these, about two-thirds of all SNPs are of the C↔T (G↔A) variety. This is probably because of the frequent 5-methylcytosine formation at CpG dinucleotides, where CpG represents cytosine and guanine separated by a phosphate. 5-Methylcytosine undergoes spontaneous deamination to thymidine [4]. Genomic DNA sequence variations are continuously created at a rate of 100 new single base changes per individual [5, 6]. The rate is low (about 10^{-8} changes per nucleotide per generation), and the nature is random, which make single-base alleles very stable [6, 7]. Because there are so many SNPs to be gathered, it is difficult to know which ones will be useful, except for those

H.-S. Kang (✉)
Department of Neurosurgery, Seoul National University Hospital, Seoul National University College of Medicine, 101 Daehangno, Jongno-gu, Seoul 110-744, Republic of Korea
e-mail: hsk4428@yahoo.com

K.-C. Wang
Division of Pediatric Neurosurgery, Pediatric Clinical Neuroscience Center, Seoul National University Children's Hospital, Seoul National University College of Medicine, 101 Daehangno, Jongno-gu, Seoul 110-744, Republic of Korea

B.-K. Cho and T. Tominaga (eds.), *Moyamoya Disease Update*,
DOI 10.1007/978-4-431-99703-0_8, © Springer 2010

found in complementary DNA (cDNA), which are called cSNPs, and those in promoter regions of genes. *Nonsynonymous* SNPs, resulting in amino acid changes in proteins, and *regulatory* SNPs, causing deregulation of gene transcription, can play a role in disease processes [8]. The database dbSNP (http://www.ncbi.nlm.nih.gov/projects/SNP/) is an archive designed to provide full details of genomic and cDNA SNPs discovered from many species and is freely available to the public. From the clinical viewpoint, SNP alleles are considered to modify the risk for a disease rather than to cause a disease. For an effective association study using SNPs, careful preselection is important: which SNPs are tested for pathogenic effect [3]? First, we need to focus on biologically defined candidate genes or positional candidates from previous linkage investigations. Second, it is sensible to use SNPs that are likely to have functional consequences, such as nonsynonymous or regulatory SNPs. Having a homogenous and well-defined test population is also an important prerequisite.

Moyamoya Disease and Single Nucleotide Polymorphisms

Although the cause of MMD is unknown, genetic predisposition has been strongly suggested to play a role in the development of this disease. Loci for familial MMD have been found by linkage analyses and include chromosomes 3p24.2-p26, 6q25, 8q23, 12p12, and 17q25 [9–13]. In a study with the hypothesis that the deregulation of TIMPs would disrupt the balance between matrix metalloproteinases (MMPs) and TIMPs and result in erroneous smooth muscle cell (SMC) dynamics that induce MMD, sequences of *TIMP2* (in 17q25) and *TIMP4* (in 3p25) genes were compared between familial patients with MMD, nonfamilial patients with MMD, and normal controls [2]. This study identified an SNP at the Sp1 binding site in the *TIMP2* promoter region as a risk factor for familial MMD. Recently, increased expression of serum MMP-9 was demonstrated in patients with MMD, which might contribute to MMD pathogenesis in a similar way to *TIMP2* polymorphisms [14]. Moreover, the importance of chromosome 17q25 for MMD has been emphasized again in a subsequent study [13]. We believe other genes pertinent to SMC dynamics need to be included in future genetic studies, including studies involving SNPs. Examples are the smooth muscle alpha-actin gene (*ACTA2*) and a series of genes related to SMC differentiation [15].

Conclusion

SNP studies are valuable in the research into MMD, which has a strong genetic background. They can provide data supporting a hypothesis for the disease pathogenesis and produce valuable information in accordance with other studies demonstrating protein expression. As efficient analysis methods and extensive databases for SNPs become available, more important and interesting data are anticipated to be revealed.

References

1. Voisey J, Morris CP (2008) SNP technologies for drug discovery: a current review. Curr Drug Discov Technol 5:230–235
2. Kang HS, Kim SK, Cho BK et al (2006) Single nucleotide polymorphisms of tissue inhibitor of metalloproteinase genes in familial moyamoya disease. Neurosurgery 58:1074–1080

3. Brookes AJ (1999) The essence of SNPs. Gene 234:177–186
4. Holliday R, Grigg GW (1993) DNA methylation and mutation. Mutat Res 285:61–67
5. Kondrashov AS (1995) Contamination of the genome by very slightly deleterious mutations: why have we not died 100 times over? J Theor Biol 175:583–594
6. Crow JF (1995) Spontaneous mutation as a risk factor. Exp Clin Immunogenet 12:121–128
7. Li W, Sadler LA (1991) Low nucleotide diversity in man. Genetics 129:513–523
8. Chorley BN, Wang X, Campbell MR et al (2008) Discovery and verification of functional single nucleotide polymorphisms in regulatory genomic regions: current and developing technologies. Mutat Res 659:147–157
9. Ikeda H, Sasaki T, Yoshimoto T et al (1999) Mapping of a familial moyamoya disease gene to chromosome 3p24.2-p26. Am J Hum Genet 64:533–537
10. Inoue TK, Ikezaki K, Sasazuki T et al (2000) Linkage analysis of moyamoya disease on chromosome 6. J Child Neurol 15:179–182
11. Yamauchi T, Tada M, Houkin K et al (2000) Linkage of familial moyamoya disease (spontaneous occlusion of the circle of Willis) to chromosome 17q25. Stroke 31:930–935
12. Sakurai K, Horiuchi Y, Ikeda H et al (2004) A novel susceptibility locus for moyamoya disease on chromosome 8q23. J Hum Genet 49:278–281
13. Mineharu Y, Liu W, Inoue K et al (2008) Autosomal dominant moyamoya disease maps to chromosome 17q25.3. Neurology 70:2357–2363
14. Fujimura M, Watanabe M, Narisawa A et al (2009) Increased expression of serum matrix metalloproteinase-9 in patients with moyamoya disease. Surg Neurol (In press)
15. Guo DC, Papke CL, Tran-Fadulu V et al (2009) Mutations in smooth muscle alpha-actin (ACTA2) cause coronary artery disease, stroke, and moyamoya disease, along with thoracic aortic disease. Am J Hum Genet 84:617–627

HLA Studies in Moyamoya Disease

Myoung Hee Park, Seok Ho Hong, and Kyu-Chang Wang

Introduction

Although the pathogenesis of moyamoya disease (MMD) is still unclear [1], several pieces of evidence suggest the involvement of genetic factors in this disease [2]. Over 10% of MMD patients have affected blood relatives, and concordance in the affection status has been proven in 80% of identical twins. Moreover, there is an ethnic predisposition to MMD, the incidence of the disease being the highest in East Asian populations, such as Japanese and Koreans. Data from an epidemiological study of familial MMD have suggested that MMD is probably inherited in a polygenic or autosomal dominant mode with a low penetrance [3]. Microsatellite linkage analysis has identified genetic loci that are associated with MMD on chromosomes 3, 6, 8, and 17 [4–8]. However, the relevant genes have not so far been identified [1, 8].

In relation to genetic loci associated with MMD on chromosome 6, human leukocyte antigen (HLA) genes have been studied. There have been several studies investigating the associations of HLA genes with MMD. Associations of various HLA class I or class II alleles with the disease have been reported in several different studies of Japanese or Korean MMD patients with conflicting results [9–13]. It is noteworthy that most of the associations were relatively weak, and none of the HLA class I or class II alleles has been corroborated by more than one report.

This chapter describes the genomic organization of HLA genes, underlying mechanisms of HLA and disease associations, statistical methods evaluating HLA and disease associations, and HLA studies thus far reported in MMD patients and their implications.

M.H. Park (✉)
Department of Laboratory Medicine, Seoul National University College of Medicine, 101 Daehangno, Jongno-gu, Seoul 110–744, Republic of Korea
e-mail: parkmhee@snu.ac.kr

S.H. Hong
Department of Neurosurgery, Asan Medical Center, University of Ulsan College of Medicine, Seoul, Republic of Korea

K.-C. Wang
Division of Pediatric Neurosurgery, Pediatric Clinical Neuroscience Center, Seoul National University Children's Hospital, Seoul National University College of Medicine, Seoul, Republic of Korea

B.-K. Cho and T. Tominaga (eds.), *Moyamoya Disease Update*,
DOI 10.1007/978-4-431-99703-0_9, © Springer 2010

HLA and Disease Associations

Genomic Organizations of HLA Genes

HLA genes, which are located in the short arm of chromosome 6 (6p21), represent the major histocompatibility complex (MHC) of the human (Fig. 1). The human MHC spans approximately 4 Mb and contains over 200 identified loci. The MHC genes are clustered in three regions, namely class I, class II, and class III regions. The MHC class I and class II genes encode proteins that are expressed on cell surface, the class I and class II molecules, which are essential to immune recognition. In the human, the class I molecules include HLA-A, HLA-B, and HLA-C, and the class II molecules include HLA-DR, HLA-DQ, and HLA-DP [14]. These are the classical HLA molecules playing an important role in immune recognition and represent the classical transplantation antigens. Other molecules encoded within the MHC are the class III molecules (nonclassical HLA molecules), which are not expressed on cell surface but present as soluble plasma proteins. These include the MHC-linked complement components (C2, C4, and Bf), 21-hydroxylase (CYP21), heat shock protein (Hsp) 70, and tumor necrosis factor (TNF) [14].

Mechanisms of HLA and Disease Associations

The MHC (HLA) genes have been reported to be associated with various diseases, especially those diseases with underlying autoimmune pathogenesis. In addition to autoimmune diseases (e.g., Goodpasture's disease), immune-complex-mediated diseases (e.g., systemic lupus erythematosus) and nonimmune diseases (e.g., narcolepsy, for which autoimmune pathogenesis has

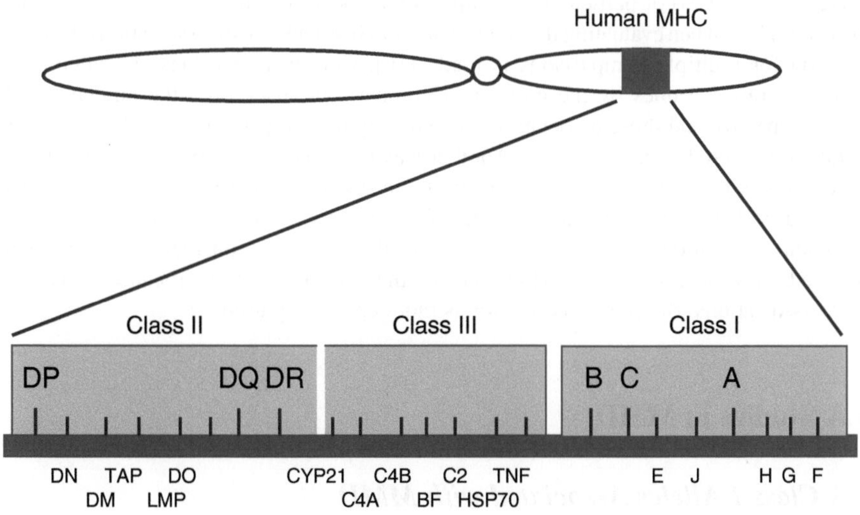

Fig. 1 Human major histocompatibility complex (MHC) genes. Human MHC is located in the short arm of chromosome 6 (6p21), and spans approximately 4 Mb containing over 200 identified loci. The MHC genes are clustered in three regions, class I, class II, and class III regions, containing HLA-A, B, C; HLA-DR, DQ, DP; and TNF, HSP70, C2, BF, C4, CYP21 genes, respectively

been recently suggested) also show HLA associations [15]. The possible mechanisms of HLA and disease associations are (1) molecular mimicry, (2) role of HLA molecules acting as receptors for microbes and drugs, and (3) role of HLA genes as disease-associated markers, closely linked with disease-related non-HLA genes [15]. When molecular mimicry is present between microbial antigens and autoantigens, cross-reactions can arise and immune response to microbial antigens can lead to an autoimmune disease. Another possible mechanism is that HLA molecules (cell-surface glycoproteins) may contribute to the uptake of certain pathogens by cells, or even act as cell-surface receptors for certain bacteria or virus (e.g., HLA-B27 and *Salmonella*, thus explaining reactive arthritis). Another important mechanism of HLA and disease associations is the involvement of non-HLA genes closely linked with HLA genes in the pathogenesis of the disease. Genes in the MHC region show strong linkage disequilibrium, and HLA and disease associations can be related with nonclassical HLA genes (e.g., complement components C2, C4, and Bf, TNF, and Hsp70) that encode proteins with obvious functions in the immune system (Fig. 1).

Statistical Analysis of HLA and Disease Associations

When HLA genes are associated with a particular disease, they may be associated with susceptibility to or protection against the development of the disease. When an HLA allele (or antigen) is associated with disease susceptibility, its frequency is increased, and when an HLA allele is associated with disease protection, its frequency is decreased in the patients compared to controls. HLA and disease associations are conventionally presented with relative risk (RR) values. The RR value indicates how many times more frequently the disease develops in the individuals possessing the HLA allele than in individuals not possessing the allele [16]. Thus, RR value of >1 is associated with disease susceptibility, and RR value of <1 is associated with disease protection.

HLA genes are the most polymorphic genes in the human genome, and weak statistical associations ($P<0.05$) of particular HLA alleles may occur by chance alone and may not be significant. Thus, when evaluating the significance of HLA and disease associations, Bonferroni correction for multiple comparisons is made [16]. Corrected P values are calculated by multiplying raw P values by the number of comparisons made (i.e., the number of HLA alleles compared), and those associations showing significant corrected P values (<0.05) are generally considered to be significant. Another way to correct for the bias due to the multiple comparisons is to do a second study on the same disease. If the HLA allele significantly associated with a particular disease in the first study with a P value of <0.05 shows a significant association in a second study, that HLA allele is considered as significantly associated with the disease [16]. However, for the evaluation of significance of HLA and disease associations, Bonferroni correction is more commonly used.

HLA Studies in MMD

HLA Class I Alleles Associated with MMD

Reported associations of HLA class I alleles with MMD are presented in Table 1. Kitahara et al. reported weak associations of HLA-A24, B46, and B54 ($P<0.05$ or <0.025) in Japanese MMD patients in the early 1980s [9]. When they reanalyzed a total of 49 cases including their

Table 1 Reported associations of HLA class I alleles with moyamoya disease

			MMD associations			
Ethnic	MMD patients	HLA alleles	Risks	*P*	*P* corr	References
Japanese	Unrelated ($n=18$)	A24	RR 3.83	<0.05		Kitahara et al. [9]
		B46	RR 6.50	<0.05		
		B54	RR 3.58	<0.025		
	Unrelated ($n=49$)[a]	B54	RR 3.80	<0.005		
		B61	RR 3.80	<0.005		
Japanese	Unrelated ($n=32$)	B51	RR 3.7	<0.002	<0.05	Aoyagi et al. [10]
		B67	RR 12.6	<0.01		
		Cw1	RR 0.3	<0.05		
Japanese	Total ($n=68$)	A*2602	RR 2.33	NS		Inoue et al. [11]
	Early-onset ($n=48$)	A*2602	RR 3.42	<0.05		
Korean	Total ($n=28$)	B35	RR 4.2	<0.008		Han et al. [13]
	Late-onset ($n=22$)	B35	RR 6.2	<0.002	<0.05[b]	
	Female ($n=17$)	B35	RR 7.9	<0.0007	<0.05[b]	

MMD moyamoya disease; *P corr* corrected *P* value; *RR* relative risk; *NS* not significant
[a]Including 18 cases of the authors' study and 31 reviewed cases
[b]*P* corr values were calculated from the data presented in the paper

own cases and 31 reviewed cases from two different reports, weak associations of B54 and B61 were observed ($P<0.005$, each). Another study of Japanese MMD patients by Aoyagi et al. showed associations of B51 (RR 3.7, corrected $P<0.05$) and B67 ($P<0.01$) [10]. They found Cw1 was weakly protective against the disease ($P<0.05$). Inoue et al. analyzed HLA class I alleles by molecular typing in Japanese MMD patients and reported a weak association of A*2602 allele with early-onset MMD (onset at ≤10 years of age, $P<0.05$) [11]. Han et al. reported an association of B35 in Korean MMD patients, and the association was somewhat stronger in late-onset (onset at >10 years of age, RR 6.2, corrected $P<0.05$) and in female patients (RR 7.9, corrected $P<0.05$) [13].

HLA Class II Alleles Associated with MMD

Reported associations of HLA class II alleles with MMD are presented in Table 2. Aoyagi et al. reported a weak association of HLA-DR1 with MMD ($P<0.05$) in Japanese patients by serological typing [10]. Inoue et al. reported weak associations of HLA-DR and DQ alleles in Japanese MMD patients by molecular typing [11, 12]. When they analyzed early-onset and late-onset patients separately, different HLA associations were observed. In early-onset patients, DRB1*0405 was a protective and DRB1*1501 and DQB1*0602 were susceptible alleles, whereas in late-onset patients, DQB1*0502 was a susceptible allele for the development of MMD [11].

Most of the studies on the HLA and MMD associations have been performed with relatively small numbers of patients, and familial and nonfamilial (sporadic) MMD patients have not been analyzed separately. Recently, we have found that HLA-DRB1*1302 [odds ratio (OR) 12.76, corrected *P* 0.008] and a closely linked DQB1*0609 allele (OR 14.67, corrected *P* 0.02) were very strongly associated with familial MMD, but not with nonfamilial cases in Koreans (unpublished data). These associations of HLA-DRB1*1302 and DQB1*0609 alleles with familial MMD are much stronger than any other association thus far reported for MMD.

Table 2 Reported associations of HLA class II alleles with moyamoya disease

Ethnic	MMD patients	HLA alleles	MMD associations Risks	*P*	*P* corr	References
Japanese	Unrelated ($n=32$)	DR1	RR 9.1	<0.05		Aoyagi et al.[10]
Japanese	Total ($n=71$)	DRB1*0405	RR 0.35	<0.01		Inoue et al.[11]
		DQB1*0401	RR 0.40	<0.025		
		DQB1*0502	RR 3.27	<0.025		
	Early-onset ($n=49$)	DRB1*0405	RR 0.38	<0.05		
		DRB1*1501	RR 2.3	<0.05		
		DQB1*0602	RR 2.42	<0.025		
	Late-onset ($n=22$)	DQB1*0502	RR 4.72	<0.05		
Korean	Total ($n=64$)	DRB1*1302	OR 1.67	0.14		Hong et al.[a]
	Familial ($n=10$)	DRB1*1302	OR 12.76	0.0003	0.008	
		DQB1*0609	OR 14.67	0.001	0.02	

OR odds ratio
[a] Unpublished data (submitted for publication)

We suggest that other MHC gene(s) closely linked with HLA-DRB1*1302 and DQB1*0609 alleles in Koreans might be associated with the susceptibility to familial MMD. As a candidate genetic factor, TNF-α, high producer allele closely linked with DRB1*1302-DQB1*0609 haplotype in this population, might be involved in the pathogenesis of the disease.

Implications of HLA Associations with MMD

Most of the HLA associations reported in MMD patients are rather weak in the strength of association and the results do not correlate with each other. Although Japanese and Koreans are very close in the distribution of HLA alleles [17], HLA studies in MMD patients failed to reveal common HLA alleles associated with the disease between Japanese and Koreans. Moreover, different studies in Japanese MMD patients also failed to reveal common HLA alleles associated with the disease. HLA class I or class II alleles may be simply disease-associated markers and are not directly associated with disease susceptibility or disease protection in MMD. It is more probable that other gene(s) closely linked with those HLA alleles showing associations with MMD are responsible for the pathogenesis of the disease.

Although we have no definite explanation for the pathogenesis of MMD, the final common pathway seems to involve proliferation of smooth muscle cells and their migration from the media to the intima in the carotid terminations of cerebral arteries in MMD patients [18]. This process is regulated by various growth factors, and the results from previous studies have shown that concentrations of certain growth factors or cytokines are increased in the cerebrospinal fluid and/or their expression is increased in the intracranial and extracranial arteries of patients with MMD: basic fibroblast growth factor, soluble adhesion molecules, cellular retinoic acid-binding protein I (CRABP-I), and hepatocyte growth factor [1]. In vascular injury and repair, a balance between the activities of connective tissue-degrading enzymes, matrix metalloproteinases (MMPs) and their endogenous inhibitors, and tissue inhibitors of metalloproteinases (TIMPs) is important [19], which might be deranged in MMD. It is of interest that a recent study of TIMP2 gene in Korean MMD patients suggested a difference in the genetic predisposition of familial and nonfamilial MMD [20], as we have found in the study of HLA-DR and -DQ genes in Korean patients.

Different subsets of MMD patients might differ in the genetic predisposition to develop the disease. Different subsets of MMD may be associated with different susceptibility genes and their products leading to the final common pathway involving proliferation of smooth muscle cells and their migration in the affected cerebral arteries in MMD patients. As one of the genetic factors, whether TNF-α high producer allele is associated with familial form of the disease has to be further studied.

References

1. Kuroda S, Houkin K (2008) Moyamoya disease:current concepts and future perspectives. Lancet Neurol 7:1056–1066
2. Hashitaka H, Liu W, Mineharu Y et al (2008) Current knowledge on the genetic factors involved in moyamoya disease. Brain Nerve 60:1261–1269 (in Japanese)
3. Mineharu Y, Takenaka K, Yamakawa H et al (2006) Inheritance pattern of familial moyamoya disease: autosomal dominant mode and genomic imprinting. J Neurol Neurosurg Psychiatry 77:1025–1029
4. Ikeda H, Sasaki T, Yoshimoto T et al (1999) Mapping of a familial moyamoya disease gene to chromosome 3p24.2-p26. Am J Hum Genet 64:533–537
5. Inoue TK, Ikezaki K, Sasazuki T et al (2000) Linkage analysis of moyamoya disease on chromosome 6. J Child Neurol 15:179–182
6. Sakurai K, Horiuchi Y, Ikeda H et al (2004) A novel susceptibility locus for moyamoya disease on chromosome 8q23. J Hum Genet 49:278–281
7. Yamauchi T, Tada M, Houkin K et al (2000) Linkage of familial moyamoya disease (spontaneous occlusion of the circle of Willis) to chromosome 17q25. Stroke 31:930–935
8. Mineharu Y, Liu W, Inoue K et al (2008) Autosomal dominant moyamoya disease maps to chromosome 17q25.3. Neurology 70:2357–2363
9. Kitahara T, Okumura K, Semba A et al (1982) Genetic and immunologic analysis on moya-moya. J Neurol Neurosurg Psychiatry 45:1048–1052
10. Aoyagi M, Ogami K, Matsushima Y et al (1995) Human leukocyte antigen in patients with moyamoya disease. Stroke 26:415–417
11. Inoue TK, Ikezaki K, Sasazuki T et al (1997) DNA typing of HLA in the patients with moyamoya disease. Jpn J Hum Genet 42:507–515
12. Inoue TK, Ikezaki K, Sasazuki T et al (1997) Analysis of class II genes of human leukocyte antigen in patients with moyamoya disease. Clin Neurol Neurosurg 99 (Suppl 2):S234–237
13. Han H, Pyo CW, Yoo DS et al (2003) Associations of moyamoya patients with HLA class I and class II alleles in the Korean population. J Korean Med Sci 18:876–880
14. Massey HD, McPherson RA (2007) Human leukocyte antigen: the major histocompatibility complex of man. In: McPherson RA, Pincus AR (eds) Henry's clinical diagnosis and management by laboratory methods, 21st edn. Saunders, Philadelphia
15. Warrens AN, Lechler RI (2000) Mechanisms of HLA and disease associations. In: Lechler R, Sarrens A (eds) HLA in health and disease, 2nd edn. Academic, San Diego
16. Tiwari JL, Terasaki PI (1985) HLA and disease associations. Springer, New York
17. Park MH, Hwang YS, Park KS et al (1998) HLA haplotypes in Koreans based on 107 families. Tissue Antigens 51:347–355
18. Aoyagi M, Fukai N, Yamamoto M et al (1996) Early development of intimal thickening in superficial temporal arteries in patients with moyamoya disease. Stroke 27:1750–1754
19. Shi Y, Patel S, Niculescu R et al (1999) Role of matrix metalloproteinases and their tissue inhibitors in the regulation of coronary cell migration. Arterioscler Thromb Vasc Biol 19:1150–1155
20. Kang HS, Kim SK, Cho BK et al (2006) Single nucleotide polymorphisms of tissue inhibitor of metalloproteinase genes in familial moyamoya disease. Neurosurgery 58:1074–1080

Part IV
Pathophysiology I: Protein, Cell, and Immunology

Proteins, Cells, and Immunity in the Moyamoya Disease: An Overview

Seung-Ki Kim, Kyu-Chang Wang, and Byung-Kyu Cho

Introduction

The pathogenesis of moyamoya disease (MMD) has not been fully clarified. A multifactorial mode of inheritance may be involved in disease occurrence or susceptibility.

The rare incidence and low mortality rate of the disease, the limited availability of surgical specimens from affected internal carotid arteries, and the lack of animal models of MMD represent obstacles to the basic research of MMD. Because of these limitations, the analysis of peripheral blood and cerebrospinal fluid (CSF) of patients has been an effective means of investigating the pathogenesis of this disease.

This chapter describes the role of proteins, cells, and immunity in the pathogenesis of MMD.

Proteins

The histopathological changes in the MMD stenotic/occluded major intracranial arteries are eccentric fibrocellular thickening of the intima that result from the proliferation of smooth muscle cells (SMCs) and fibrosis, which suggests the involvement of growth factors in this disease [1, 2]. In addition, the formation of extensive collateral vessels and neovascularization by indirect revascularization from a simply placed vascularized tissue indicate that angiogenic factors play an important role in the disease process. Based on these findings, many investigators have focused on the study of growth factors, cytokines, and their receptors (Table 1).

Previous studies have shown that certain growth factors or cytokines are elevated in the intracranial artery, extracranial artery (superficial temporal artery), serum, and CSF of patients

S.-K. Kim (✉)
Division of Pediatric Neurosurgery, Pediatric Clinical Neuroscience Center, Seoul National University Children's Hospital, Research Center for Rare Disease, Seoul National University College of Medicine, 101 Daehangno, Jongno-gu, Seoul 110-744, Republic of Korea
e-mail: nsthomas@snu.ac.kr

K.-C. Wang and B.-K. Cho
Division of Pediatric Neurosurgery, Pediatric Clinical Neuroscience Center,
Seoul National University Children's Hospital, Seoul National
University College of Medicine, 101 Daehangno, Jongno-gu, Seoul 110-744, Republic of Korea

B.-K. Cho and T. Tominaga (eds.), *Moyamoya Disease Update*,
DOI 10.1007/978-4-431-99703-0_10, © Springer 2010

Table 1 Cytokines, cells, and immunological factors in MMD

Items	Findings	Specimens
Cytokines		
bFGF	Elevated	Major intracranial cerebral arteries, STA, CSF
TGF-β	Elevated	Cultured SMCs from STA, serum
	No significant increase	CSF
PDGF	Fewer receptors and altered response to PDGF	Cultured SMCs from STA
	No significant increase	CSF
HGF	Expressed	Major intracranial cerebral arteries
	Elevated	CSF
CRABP-I	Elevated	CSF
HIF-1α, endoglin	Overexpressed	Middle cerebral artery
VEGF, IL-8	No significant increase	CSF
Cells		
Arterial SMCs	Increased TGF-β	STA
	Fewer receptors and altered response to PDGF	
	Increased elastin	
	Increased IL-1β-induced PGE_2	
Circulating EPCs	Decreased (colony-forming unit)	Peripheral blood
	Increased (FACS)	Peripheral blood
Immunological factors		
ICAM-1, VCAM-1, E-selectin	Increased	CSF
IL-1	TGF-β induction→elastin accumulation	SMC
	PGE_2 production	
	NO induction	
Autoantibodies	Detected	Serum, CSF

bFGF Basic fibroblast growth factor; *TGF-β* transforming growth factor-β; *PDGF* platelet-derived growth factor; *HGF* hepatocyte growth factor; *CRABP-I* cellular retinoic acid-binding protein-I; *HIF-1α* hypoxia-inducing factor-1α; *VEGF* vascular endothelial growth factor; *IL-8* interleukin-8; *SMC* smooth muscle cell; *EPC* endothelial progenitor cell; *ICAM-1* intercellular adhesion molecule type 1; *VCAM-1* vascular cell adhesion molecule type 1; *IL-1* interleukin-1; PGE_2 prostaglandin E_2; *FACS* (VCAM-1); *FACS* fluorescence activated cell sorting; *NO* nitric oxide; *STA* superficial temporal artery; *CSF* cerebrospinal fluid

with MMD. Notable examples include the basic fibroblast growth factor (bFGF) [3–7], the transforming growth factor-β (TGF-β1) [8], and the platelet-derived growth factor (PDGF) [9].

The increased expression of bFGF in the major intracranial cerebral arteries, superficial temporal arteries, and CSF in MMD has been previously reported [3–7]. The elevation of bFGF in patients with MMD may be a major causative factor for the development of stenosis of the major intracranial arteries and angiogenesis of collateral circulation [7]. Conversely, bFGF was suggested to have therapeutic value, as its topical administration to the cortex at the time of the development of synangiosis promotes the formation of new vessels [10]. Independently of its neuroprotective role, bFGF has also been shown to have a direct vasodilator action on pial arterioles and to improve regional cerebral blood flow, both of which would be helpful in counteracting the hypoperfusion state seen in MMD [4]. Furthermore, the levels of bFGF expression may be a prognostic marker to predict the extent of angiogenesis, as this factor is apparently elevated in patients with well-developed neovascularization after indirect revascularization surgery [4, 7]. Elevation of bFGF in the CSF is not a feature that is exclusive to MMD. It is noteworthy that bFGF is significantly elevated in the CSF of patients with Chiari malformation, tethered cord, arteriovenous malformation, and brain tumors [4]. These findings suggest that CSF bFGF may play wide-ranging roles in a number of central nervous system (CNS) conditions associated with ischemia and hypervascularity. Therefore, the influence of cerebral ischemia, not specific for MMD, on the increased levels of expression of bFGF cannot be completely ruled out.

The levels of expression of TGF-β are increased in cultured SMCs derived from superficial temporal arteries and in the serum of MMD patients [8]. It is suggested that TGF-β plays a role in elastin accumulation, which is responsible for the intimal thickening observed in MMD [11]. However, the CSF of MMD patients does not exhibit increased levels of TGF-β compared with the control group [6, 7].

SMCs derived from the superficial temporal arteries of patients with MMD express fewer PDGF receptors and show an altered response to PDGF [9]. However, the levels of PDGF in the CSF of MMD patients are normal [7].

The hepatocyte growth factor (HGF) is strongly expressed in the carotid fork, and its levels are markedly elevated in the CSF [12]. HGF is somewhat elevated in the CSF of patients with good development of collateral circulation through indirect synangiosis compared with that of patients with poor results [7]. Therefore, it is suggested that the level of HGF in the CSF is a reliable indicator for predicting the efficacy of revascularization after indirect bypass surgery, similar to what was described for bFGF.

Recently, the cellular retinoic acid-binding protein-I (CRABP-I) was identified in the CSF of patients with MMD [13]. As CRABP-I attenuates the inhibitory effect of retinoic acid on the growth factor-stimulated SMC proliferation, the high expression of CRABP-I in CSF may be associated with intimal thickening in MMD [13]. It remains to be determined how the retinoid pathway is involved in intimal thickening in MMD and whether retinoids are an efficacious treatment for MMD. Similar to bFGF, elevated CRABP-I levels were also noted in the CSF of patients with cavernous malformations. Therefore, CRABP-I may be related to cerebrovascular disease in general.

The hypoxia-inducing factor-1α (HIF-1α) and endoglin are overexpressed in the intima of middle cerebral artery specimens from patients with MMD [14]. These molecules are associated with TFG-β. Furthermore, bFGF and HGF may play a role in the induction of HIF-1α and in proliferative responses in MMD.

Notably, the CSF of MMD patients exhibits no significant increase in the levels of angiogenic factors, including PDGF, TGF-β, interleukin-8, and vascular endothelial growth factor (VEGF), compared with the control group [7].

Cells

Histopathological findings from the scalp arteries of MMD patients revealed the presence of a pronounced neointima similar to that found in the intracranial arteries [1]. Therefore, SMCs cultured from superficial temporal arteries were studied to evaluate the pathogenesis of vascular occlusion and abnormal vasculogenesis. Pathological findings suggest the presence of systemic factors that promote the migration and proliferation of SMCs from the media to the intima in MMD [1]. In addition, SMCs overexpress TGF-β, express fewer PDGF receptors, and exhibit a diminished response to serum mitogens, especially to PDGF [9]. Intimal thickening may be associated with morphological and biochemical alterations of extracellular matrix components, which include elastin, collagen, and other proteoglycans [1]. Elastin mRNA and protein levels are elevated in SMCs derived from the superficial temporal arteries of MMD patients compared with control SMCs, which suggests the occurrence of abnormal elastogenesis in vivo [11].

Circulating endothelial progenitor cells (EPCs) play an important role in physiological and pathological neovascularization and may be involved in the attenuation of ischemic disease. In MMD patients, EPCs may play a direct role in neovascularization and/or perform regulatory roles as a source of growth/angiogenic factors [15]. Angiogenesis, which is the paradigm of postnatal neovascularization, is a process whereby new vessels and endothelial cells are derived by sprouting from preexisting differentiated endothelial cells [16]. However, in MMD, some of these new vessels and endothelial cells may be derived from EPCs of bone marrow origin, which is a process referred to as postnatal vasculogenesis [17].

Flow cytometry and colony-forming assays are the main methods used to count and assess the function of EPCs. Although the characteristics of EPCs have been studied in MMD patients, there is a lack of consensus regarding the role of these cells in this disease [15, 18, 19]. One study that used colony-forming assays reported lower levels of EPCs in MMD patients versus controls [18], and another study that used flow cytometry found increased levels of EPCs in MMD patients versus controls [19]. Although these findings suggest that EPCs induce vaso-occlusive changes and/or recruit the compensatory vascular network, it is unclear whether this effect is causative or simply associated with pathologic arterial changes. The mechanisms underlying the occurrence of intimal thickening in a limited portion of the arterial occlusion, such as the circle of Willis, are not clear. Further studies are required to elucidate the exact functional roles of EPCs in the pathogenesis of MMD.

Immunity

Immunological factors, inflammation, or thrombosis may be associated with the development of obstruction/stenosis of the intracranial internal carotid arteries.

The presence of macrophages and T lymphocytes in the surface layer of the thickened intima suggest the possibility of chronic inflammation in SMC proliferation [20].

Endothelial adhesion molecules, which include the intercellular adhesion molecule type 1 (ICAM-1), the vascular cell adhesion molecule type 1 (VCAM-1), and E-selectin, were previously reported to be increased in the CSF of MMD patients, which suggests the presence of ongoing immunological activation in the CNS [21]. Endothelial adhesion molecules are not only associated with inflammation but also activated by tissue ischemia and neovascularization [21]. Endothelial cells are the primary source of soluble ICAM-1 and VCAM-1 in various brain disorders. The elevated levels of these soluble adhesion molecules in the CSF may be the result of their increased expression in vascular endothelial cells [21]. However, the possibility of passive leakage from the systemic circulation or ongoing cerebral ischemia as a source of these adhesion molecules among this group of patients cannot be excluded [21]. The levels of the soluble isoforms of VCAM-1 and ICAM-1 are increased in the CSF of patients with stroke, subarachnoid hemorrhage, or traumatic head injuries [12]. There is no difference in the serum levels of these adhesion molecules between the MMD and control groups [21].

A possible interaction between the immune system and the vessel wall has been suggested in MMD. Inflammatory stimuli can induce cytokines, which include interleukin-1 (IL-1) and TGF-β [11]. IL-1 induces release of TGF-β1 from SMCs and from inflammatory cells in MMD patients. TGF-β1 may modulate the expression of the elastin gene and elastin accumulation in arterial SMCs in MMD patients [11]. The stimulation of cells with interleukin-1β (IL-1β) led to a significantly greater release of prostaglandin E_2 (PGE_2) into the medium (compared with control SMCs) via the activation of cyclooxygenase-2 (COX-2) from MMD SMCs [22]. Excessive amounts of PGE_2 may increase vascular permeability and decrease vascular tone, thus facilitating exposure of the vessels to blood constituents, including growth factors and cytokines that might induce and promote the development of intimal thickening in MMD [22]. Excessive amounts of PGE_2 also inhibit the migration and proliferation of SMCs that might be necessary for the rapid repair of vascular wall injury, which results in the continued increase in vascular permeability and facilitates the prolonged exposure of vessels to blood constituents [22]. The stimulation of SMCs with IL-1 led to the expression of inducible nitric oxide (NO) synthetase and the release of NO [22]. NO is an endothelium-derived relaxing factor that regulates vascular tone and inhibits SMC migration [23].

Autoimmunity may also be relevant to MMD, as autoantibodies are more frequently detected in the serum and CSF of these patients than in those of control subjects [1, 24]. The histological findings in the vessels are also considered similar to the chronic inflammatory changes observed in polyarteritis or in Kawasaki's disease [1]. However, the paucity of other inflammatory features, both histological and biochemical, opposes this view [1]. Even though an autoimmune process has been implicated in MMD, further studies are required to elucidate the direct participation of autoimmunity in the pathological changes of this disease.

Thrombogenesis has been implicated in MMD as a causative factor [1]. Systematic analyses seeking evidence of a thrombotic tendency in MMD have revealed that one-third of the patients examined had either congenital or acquired tendencies that favored thrombosis [25]. Prothrombotic states or thrombophilia sometimes accompany angiographic findings similar to MMD and result in cerebral infarction. These findings suggest that thrombi may play either an essential role or a contributory role in MMD and in the consequent cerebral ischemia.

In spite of enthusiastic research efforts, the pathogenesis of MMD remains enigmatic. It is not clear whether these factors are causative or are simply associated with disease pathogenesis; for example, they may contribute to the angiogenesis associated with this disease or may be an epiphenomenon that results from recurrent strokes. Further studies are required to determine whether these factors represent potential diagnostic or therapeutic targets for the management of MMD.

References

1. Ikezaki K, Kono S, Fukui M (2001) Etiology of moyamoya disease: pathology, pathophysiology, and genetics. In: Ikezaki K, Loftus CM (eds) Moyamoya disease. Rolling Meadows: American Association of Neurological Surgeons
2. Kono S, Oka K, Sueishi K (1990) Histopathologic and morphometric studies of leptomeningeal vessels in moyamoya disease. Stroke 21:1044–1050
3. Hoshimaru M, Takahashi JA, Kikuchi H et al (1991) Possible roles of basic fibroblast growth factor in the pathogenesis of moyamoya disease: an immunohistochemical study. J Neurosurg 75:267–270
4. Malek AM, Connors S, Robertson RL et al (1997) Elevation of cerebrospinal fluid levels of basic fibroblast growth factor in moyamoya and central nervous system disorders. Pediatr Neurosurg 27:182–189
5. Suzui H, Hoshimaru M, Takahashi JA et al (1994) Immunohistochemical reactions for fibroblast growth factor receptor in arteries of patients with moyamoya disease. Neurosurgery 35:20–25

6. Takahashi A, Sawamura Y, Houkin K et al (1993) The cerebrospinal fluid in patients with moyamoya disease (spontaneous occlusion of the circle of Willis) contains high level of basic fibroblast growth factor. Neurosci Lett 160:214–216
7. Yoshimoto T, Houkin K, Takahashi A et al (1996) Angiogenic factors in moyamoya disease. Stroke 27:2160–2165
8. Hojo M, Hoshimaru M, Miyamoto S et al (1998) Role of transforming growth factor-beta1 in the pathogenesis of moyamoya disease. J Neurosurg 89:623–629
9. Aoyagi M, Fukai N, Sakamoto H et al (1991) Altered cellular responses to serum mitogens, including platelet-derived growth factor, in cultured smooth muscle cells derived from arteries of patients with moyamoya disease. J Cell Physiol 147:191–198
10. Kubo H (1993) Angiogenesis on encephalo-myo-synangiosis. The effect of basic fibroblast growth factor. Nippon Geka Hokan 62:82–91 (in Japanese)
11. Yamamoto M, Aoyagi M, Tajima S et al (1997) Increase in elastin gene expression and protein synthesis in arterial smooth muscle cells derived from patients with Moyamoya disease. Stroke 28: 1733–1738
12. Nanba R, Kuroda S, Ishikawa T et al (2004) Increased expression of hepatocyte growth factor in cerebrospinal fluid and intracranial artery in moyamoya disease. Stroke 35:2837–2842
13. Kim SK, Yoo JI, Cho BK et al (2003) Elevation of CRABP-I in the cerebrospinal fluid of patients with Moyamoya disease. Stroke 34:2835–2841
14. Takagi Y, Kikuta K, Nozaki K et al (2007) Expression of hypoxia-inducing factor-1 alpha and endoglin in intimal hyperplasia of the middle cerebral artery of patients with Moyamoya disease. Neurosurgery 60:338–345
15. Yoshihara T, Taguchi A, Matsuyama T et al (2008) Increase in circulating CD34-positive cells in patients with angiographic evidence of moyamoya-like vessels. J Cereb Blood Flow Metab 28:1086–1089
16. Folkman J, Shing Y (1992) Angiogenesis. J Biol Chem 267:10931–10934
17. Isner JM, Asahara T (1999) Angiogenesis and vasculogenesis as therapeutic strategies for postnatal neovascularization. J Clin Invest 103:1231–1236
18. Jung KH, Chu K, Lee ST et al (2008) Circulating endothelial progenitor cells as a pathogenetic marker of moyamoya disease. J Cereb Blood Flow Metab 28:1795–1803
19. Rafat N, Beck GCh, Peña-Tapia PG et al (2009) Increased levels of circulating endothelial progenitor cells in patients with Moyamoya disease. Stroke 40:432–438
20. Masuda J, Ogata J, Yutani C (1993) Smooth muscle cell proliferation and localization of macrophages and T cells in the occlusive intracranial major arteries in moyamoya disease. Stroke 24:1960–1967
21. Soriano SG, Cowan DB, Proctor MR et al (2002) Levels of soluble adhesion molecules are elevated in the cerebrospinal fluid of children with moyamoya syndrome. Neurosurgery 50:544–549
22. Yamamoto M, Aoyagi M, Fukai N et al (1999) Increase in prostaglandin E(2) production by interleukin-1beta in arterial smooth muscle cells derived from patients with moyamoya disease. Circ Res 85:912–918
23. Noda A, Suzuki Y, Takayasu M et al (2000) Elevation of nitric oxide metabolites in the cerebrospinal fluid of patients with moyamoya disease. Acta Neurochir (Wien) 142:1275–1280
24. Kim J, Kim SK, Wang KC et al (2004) SEREX identification of the autoantibodies that are prevalent in the cerebrospinal fluid of patients with moyamoya disease. Biotechnol Lett 26:585–588
25. Tsuda H, Hattori S, Tanabe S et al (1997) Thrombophilia found in patients with moyamoya disease. Clin Neurol Neurosurg 99 (Suppl 2):S229–233

Vascular Smooth Muscle Cell-Related Molecules and Cells

Yasushi Takagi

The characteristic findings of intimal thickening and resulting steno-occlusion at the terminal portion of the internal carotid artery (ICA) along with pathological changes in neighboring arteries have been enumerated in the guidelines for the diagnosis of moyamoya disease [1, 2]. Fibrocellular thickening of the intima, an irregular disruption of the internal elastic lamina, and the attenuation of the media are the main findings [1, 3]. These findings have been observed not only in the carotid fork but also in cortical branches of the middle cerebral artery (MCA) [1, 3, 4]. In perforating arteries, microaneurysm formation and fragmented elastic lamina have been detected, and these are considered to be one of the reasons for intracerebral hemorrhage [1]. Sometimes, extracranial arteries such as superior temporal arteries (STA) and renal arteries have also been shown to be affected by the same stenotic changes, so that moyamoya disease can be considered to be a kind of systemic diseases [5].

Increased level of several growth factors and their receptors including basic fibroblast growth factor (bFGF), transforming growth factor-beta (TGF-beta), and hepatocyte growth factor (HGF) have been detected in the STA and ICA [5–8]. Using immunohistochemical methods, these factors were elevated in vascular walls [5–8]. In previous studies, expressions of growth factors and cytokines in cerebrospinal fluid (CSF) have been analyzed. According to these reports, bFGF, TGF-beta, and HGF were also elevated in CSF [5–8]. These observations indicate that elevated growth factors may affect the surrounding tissue and cells. Growth factors may affect the growth and characteristic change of vascular smooth muscle cells and induce thickening of intima. In addition, it is possible that they influence the formation of transdural anastomosis which is a special characteristic of moyamoya disease.

Besides the growth factors, several cytokines were supposed to be involved in moyamoya disease. Overproduction of prostaglandin E(2) and nitric oxide metabolite was reported by different analyzes in previous studies [9, 10]. Concentrations of soluble vascular-cell adhesion molecule type 1, intracellular adhesion molecule type 1, and E-selection in the CSF are also increased in moyamoya disease [6]. These factors are related to the inflammatory process and known to be induced in activated endothelial cells. During atherogenesis, they are induced in endothelial cells. Thus, they may be closely related with intimal hyperplasia in moyamoya

Y. Takagi (✉)
Department of Neurosurgery, Kyoto University Graduate School of Medicine,
54 Kawahara-cho, Sakyo, Kyoto, 606-8507, Japan
e-mail: ytakagi@kuhp.kyoto-u.ac.jp

B.-K. Cho and T. Tominaga (eds.), *Moyamoya Disease Update*,
DOI 10.1007/978-4-431-99703-0_11, © Springer 2010

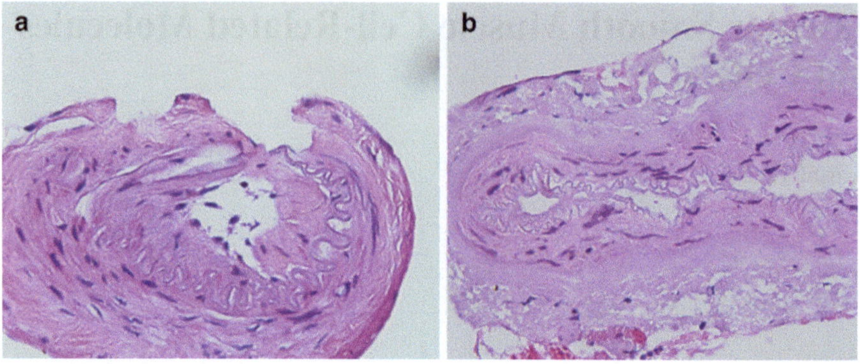

Fig. 1 Photographs of specimens of the middle cerebral artery taken from patients with or without moyamoya disease (hematoxylin and eosin stain). The sample from a patient with moyamoya disease shows intimal hyperplasia (**a**) and that from the control patient does not (**b**). Original magnification ×100

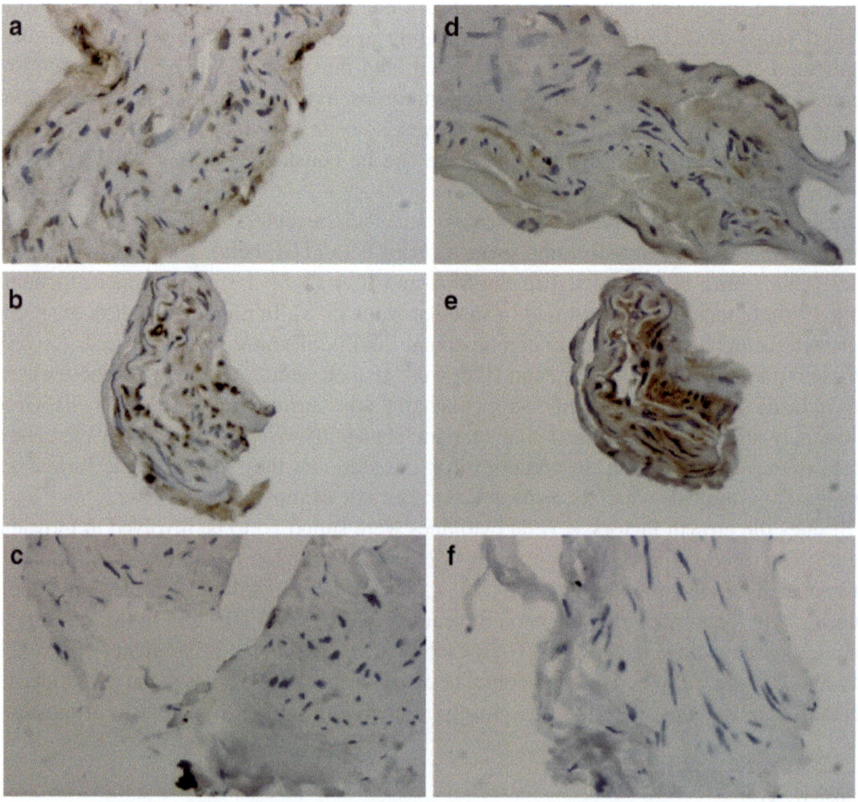

Fig. 2 Immunohistochemical analysis for single-stranded DNA (ssDNA). Immunopositive cells from ssDNA were detected in the specimens from a patient with moyamoya disease (**a**, **b**) but not in those from the control patient (**c**). Immunohistochemical analysis for cleaved caspase-3. Immunopositive cells for cleaved caspase-3 were detected in the specimens from moyamoya disease (**d**, **e**) but not in those from the control patient (**f**). Original magnification, ×100

disease. Concerning the molecules related to the extracellular matrix which plays a role in cerebral hemorrhage and angiogenesis, matrix metalloproteinase-9 (MMP-9) has been analyzed. Serum level of MMP-9 was elevated in moyamoya disease [7].

Several studies using cultured smooth muscle cells from the patients with moyamoya disease have been reported [2, 10–12]. Among them, the involvement of platelet-derived growth factor (PDGF), prostaglandin E(2), and elastin in moyamoya disease were clarified [8, 9, 13]. Prostaglandin E(2) production stimulated by interleukin-1 beta was elevated in smooth muscle cells from patients with moyamoya disease [8]. Responses to PDGF and IL-1 beta in migration and DNA synthesis were different between smooth muscle cells from those with moyamoya disease and from control patients [8, 14]. In addition, smooth muscle cells derived from patients with moyamoya disease show increased elastin synthesis stimulated by TGF-beta [9]. These observations indicates that intracellular signal transduction in the cells of moyamoya disease differs from that in normal cells. The different expressions growth factors, other molecules and intracellular signal transduction have the possibility to affect the extent of angiogenesis and intimal hyperplasia of intracranial and extracranial arteries.

Recently, surgical specimens obtained at bypass surgery were used in histopathological studies [15–17]. In these studies, the specimens from the distal part of the MCA were analyzed. Intimal hyperplasia, disruption of internal elastic lamina, and thinning of media were obvious in the distal part of the MCA as well as in the ICA (Fig. 1) [4]. Furthermore, apoptosis related to caspase-3 was detected in intima and media of distal MCA from patients with moyamoya disease (Fig. 2) [18]. Concerning intimal hyperplasia, hypoxia-inducing factor 1-α was reported to be induced in hyperplastic intima of moyamoya disease [15].

In summary, intimal hyperplasia and medial thinness in patients with moyamoya disease are affected by expressions of growth factors, cytokines, and adhesion molecules. In addition, cellular response against stimuli is also changed from the normal condition. This phenomenon is not limited to the terminal portion of internal cerebral artery but also occurs in the peripheral portion of the MCA.

References

1. Kuroda S, Houkin K (2008) Moyamoya disease: current concepts and future perspectives. Lancet Neurol 7:1056–1066
2. Scott RM, Smith ER (2009) Moyamoya disease and moyamoya syndrome. N Engl J Med 360:1226–1237
3. Achrol AS, Guzman R, Lee M et al (2009) Pathophysiology and genetic factors in moyamoya disease. Neurosurg Focus 26:E4
4. Takagi Y, Kikuta K, Nozaki K et al (2007) Histological features of middle cerebral arteries from patients treated for moyamoya disease. Neurol Med Chir (Tokyo) 47:1–4
5. Aoyagi M, Fukai N, Yamamoto M et al (1996) Early development of intimal thickening in superficial temporal arteries in patients with moyamoya disease. Stroke 27:1750–1754
6. Soriano SG, Cowan DB, Proctor MR et al (2002) Levels of soluble adhesion molecules are elevated in the cerebrospinal fluid of children with moyamoya syndrome. Neurosurgery 50:544–549
7. Fujimura M, Watanabe M, Narisawa A et al (2009) Increased expression of serum matrix metalloproteinase-9 in patients with moyamoya disease. Surg Neurol [Epub ahead of print]
8. Yamamoto M, Aoyagi M, Fukai N et al (1999) Increase in prostaglandin E(2) production by interleukin-1beta in arterial smooth muscle cells derived from patients with moyamoya disease. Circ Res 85:912–918
9. Yamamoto M, Aoyagi M, Tajima S et al (1997) Increase in elastin gene expression and protein synthesis in arterial smooth muscle cells derived from patients with Moyamoya disease. Stroke 28:1733–1738

10. Nanba R, Kuroda S, Ishikawa T et al (2004) Increased expression of hepatocyte growth factor in cerebrospinal fluid and intracranial artery in moyamoya disease. Stroke 35:2837–2842
11. Houkin K, Yoshimoto T, Abe H et al (1998) Role of basic fibroblast growth factor in the pathogenesis of moyamoya disease. Neurosurg Focus 5:e2
12. Noda A, Suzuki Y, Takayasu M et al (2000) Elevation of nitric oxide metabolites in the cerebrospinal fluid of patients with moyamoya disease. Acta Neurochir (Wien) 142:1275–1279
13. Aoyagi M, Fukai N, Matsushima Y et al (1993) Kinetics of 125I-PDGF binding and down-regulation of PDGF receptor in arterial smooth muscle cells derived from patients with moyamoya disease. J Cell Physiol 154:281–288
14. Yamamoto M, Aoyagi M, Fukai N et al (1998) Differences in cellular responses to mitogens in arterial smooth muscle cells derived from patients with moyamoya disease. Stroke 29:1188–1193
15. Takagi Y, Kikuta K, Nozaki K et al (2007) Expression of hypoxia-inducing factor-1 alpha and endoglin in intimal hyperplasia of the middle cerebral artery of patients with moyamoya disease. Neurosurgery 60:338–345
16. Hojo M, Hoshimaru M, Miyamoto S et al (1998) Role of transforming growth factor-beta1 in the pathogenesis of moyamoya disease. J Neurosurg 89:623–629
17. Hoshimaru M, Takahashi JA, Kikuchi H et al (1991) Possible roles of basic fibroblast growth factor in the pathogenesis of moyamoya disease: an immunohistochemical study. J Neurosurg 75:267–270
18. Takagi Y, Kikuta K, Sadamasa N et al (2006) Caspase-3-dependent apoptosis in middle cerebral arteries in patients with moyamoya disease. Neurosurgery 59:894–900

Ischemia/Angiogenesis-Related Molecules and Cells

Jin Hyun Kim, Seung-Ki Kim, and Kyu-Chang Wang

Ischemia/Angiogenesis-Related Molecules

Fibroblast Growth Factor

Twenty-three fibroblast growth factors (FGFs) and four tyrosine kinase receptors (FGFRs) have been identified. FGF-1 and FGF-2 are potent stimulators of endothelial cell proliferation, migration, sprouting, and tube formation and bind to all four FGFRs [1] (Table 1). Ten isoforms have been identified in the brain. In particular, FGF-2 increases the expression of the vascular endothelial growth factor (VEGF) and proteases, and upregulates the expression of $\alpha_v\beta_3$ integrin complexes and other adhesion molecules in endothelial cells. Sections of the superficial temporal artery (STA) from patients with moyamoya disease (MMD) exhibit dense and strong FGFR signal and basic FGF immunoreactivity in endothelial cells, in cells scattered in the thickened intima, and in smooth muscle cells (SMCs) in the media [2]. It is reported that FGF-2 is also elevated (by ~tenfold) in the cerebrospinal fluid (CSF) of patients with MMD and is also increased in patients with good outcomes after surgical revascularization [3, 4]. The upregulation of FGF-2 can be interpreted as either promoting collateral vascularization or as the causative agent in progressive stenosis. FGF-4 has been demonstrated to increase the production of matrix metalloproteases 1 (MMP-1) and to decrease the levels of the tissue inhibitor of MMP-1 (TIMP-1) via the upregulation of VEGF by FGF-4.

J.H. Kim (✉)
Clinical Research Institute, Gyeongsang National University Hospital, 90 Chilam-dong, Jinju, Gyeongnam 660-702, Republic of Korea
e-mail: ajini7044@paran.com

S.-K. Kim and K.-C. Wang
Division of Pediatric Neurosurgery, Seoul National University Children's Hospital, Seoul, Republic of Korea

B.-K. Cho and T. Tominaga (eds.), *Moyamoya Disease Update*,
DOI 10.1007/978-4-431-99703-0_12, © Springer 2010

Table 1 Molecules and cells involved in angiogenesis

Molecules		
Factor	Related roles	Reports in MMD
FGF	Proliferation, migration, and tube formation in ECs, PCs, and SMCs	Takahashi et al. (1993), Suzui et al. (1994), Yoshimoto et al. (1996)
VEGF	Proliferation, migration, and tube formation in ECs, PCs, and SMCs	Yano et al. (2005)
Angiopoietins	Proliferation and migration in ECs, PCs, and SMCs	None
PDGF	Proliferation, migration, and tube formation in ECs, PCs, SMCs	None
EGF	Proliferation in uncertain cells	None
TGF-β	Proliferation, migration, and tube formation in ECs	Hojo et al. (1998)
TNF-α	Proliferation, migration, and tube formation in ECs and SMCs	None
Integrins	Tube formation in ECs	None
VE-cadherin	Maintenance of the stable monolayer of ECs	None
PECAM-1	Organization of ECs	None
MMPs	Proliferation, migration, and tube formation in ECs and PCs	Cunningham et al. (2005), Kang et al. (2006), Fujimura et al. (2009)
MicroRNAs	Proliferation, migration, and angiogenesis in ECs	None
Cells		
Cells	Related roles	Reports in MMD
EPCs	Endothelial regeneration and vascular repair	Rafat et al. (2009)Yoshihara et al. (2008)
ECs	Vascular homeostasis	None
Mural cells	Stabilization of the vascular tube and vessel maturation	Yamamoto et al. (1998)

ECs Endothelial cells; *PCs* pericytes; *SMCs* smooth muscle cells

Vascular Endothelial Growth Factor

VEGF is the best characterized and the most important of the inducers of angiogenesis. The molecule is involved in the regulation of multiple steps of angiogenesis. In the central nervous system (CNS), astrocytes secrete VEGF when exposed to hypoxic conditions [5]. VEGF contributes to initial vasodilatation by inducting the activity of nitric oxide synthase in endothelial cells and increases the permeability of these cells. Therefore, VEGF was originally classified as a permeability factor. There are six families of VEGF proteins that differ in their properties and functions: VEGF-A, VEGF-B, VEGF-C, VEGF-D, VEGF-E, and placental growth factor. VEGF-A is the most common VEGF family and has four splice variants: $VEGF_{121}$, $VEGF_{189}$, $VEGF_{206}$, and $VEGF_{165}$. $VEGF_{165}$ is the splice variant most common in the CNS [6]. The two VEGF receptors (VEGFRs) with tyrosine kinase activity, i.e., VEGFR1 (also known as Flt-1) and VEGFR2 (also referred to as Flk-1 or KDR), are found on endothelial cells of the CNS. The binding of VEGF to VEGFRs activates a receptor tyrosine kinase pathway that affects the replication, migration, differentiation, and survival of endothelial cells. Until recently, VEGF was known as a specific mitogen that promotes behaviors of endothelial cells together with angiopoietins (Angs). Interestingly, VEGF levels are also elevated in the CSF of patients with MMD; however, they do not correlate with surgical outcomes [3]. Recently, Rafat et al. [7] reported that serum VEGF concentrations in MMD patients are significantly higher than those detected in healthy controls. These increased levels of VEGF correlated with the increased number of circulating endothelial progenitor cells (EPCs) in MMD patients. However, the inverse correlation was also found in the MMD group. It has been suggested that the increased circulating EPC mobilization in MMD may not be entirely mediated by VEGF, although the increase in the number of circulating EPCs in MMD may play a role in the increased angiogenesis in MMD [7]. The role of circulating EPCs in MMD angiogenesis will be further discussed in the next paragraph.

Angiopoietins

Like VEGF, Angs act specifically on endothelial cells and play a crucial role in vessel maturation [8]. Four forms of Ang have been described, i.e., Ang-1, -2, -3 and -4. All of them function as paracrine growth factors on endothelial cells. These are ligands of the tunica interna endothelial cell kinase (Tie2/Tek) receptor. However, it is not clear whether they activate the Tie 1 receptor. There are no reports on the correlation between MMD and Angs; however, this subject may be worthy of future study.

Angiopoietin 1

Ang-1 is secreted by vascular SMCs and promotes sprouting of endothelial cells. However, it does not induce the proliferation of, or tube formation in, endothelial cells in vitro. It has been suggested that the interaction of Ang-1 with Tie2 in endothelial cells is essential for the maturation and stabilization of the developing vasculature and for normal remodeling.

Angiopoietin 2

Originally, Ang-2 was described as an antagonist of Ang-1, as it blocks Ang-1-induced autophosphorylation of Tie-2 in endothelial cells. The role of Ang-2 in endothelial cells is complicated, as this molecule acts as a pro- or anti-angiogenic factor depending on the nature of co-stimulatory molecules. In the presence of VEGF, Ang-2 mediates the increase in capillary diameter, induces migration and proliferation of endothelial cells, and stimulates sprouting of new blood vessels. However, Ang-2 causes apoptosis in endothelial cells and regression of blood vessels in the absence of VEGF. In addition, Ang-2 participates in vessel destabilization and matrix degradation, together with a number of proteases, which include MMPs and the plasminogen activator. This process is required for angiogenesis, and for endothelial cell basement degradation and vessel remodeling by pericytes and SMCs.

Angiopoietins 3 and 4

Few studies are reported for Ang-3 and -4. Ang-3 is expressed in a variety of tissues. Ang-4 is highly expressed in the lungs and activates the Tie2 receptor, whereas Ang-3 does not.

Platelet-Derived Growth Factor

Although the PDGF was originally isolated from platelets, various cell types express this molecule. There are four different PDGF families (PDGF-A, -B, -C and -D) and two different PDGF receptors (PDGFR-α and PDGFR-β), which activate a receptor tyrosine kinase pathway. Similar to VEGF and the Angs, PDGF initially induces cells proliferation via the activation of a receptor tyrosine kinase pathway and can also affect endothelial cells and induce angiogenesis. Endothelial cells express PDGFR-β exclusively, which interacts with PDGF-B. Stimulation of endothelial cells with PDGF-B induces tube formation, sprouting, and proliferation in vitro. In particular, PDGF-B acts with VEGF to promote stability between endothelial cells and SMCs in newly formed vessels [9]. Studies of MMD and PDGF revealed that PDGF-AA and PDGF-BB stimulate cell migration, but not DNA synthesis, in MMD SMCs. In contrast, in control SMCs, PDGF-AA stimulates DNA synthesis exclusively and PDGF-BB clearly stimulates both cell migration and DNA synthesis. These results suggest that PDGF is involved in intimal thickening in MMD SMCs [10].

Epidermal Growth Factor

Epidermal growth factor (EGF) signaling is required for physiological angiogenesis and is triggered by binding of EGF to the EGF-receptor (EGFR). EGF acts as a mitogen for endothelial cells and has been demonstrated to promote angiogenesis in vivo. Treatment with EGF-blocking antibodies results in decreased vascular density and increased apoptosis of endothelial cells [11]. One study reported EGF-related angiogenesis in MMD, showed that the EGF level in CSF of the MMD patients was below the limits for measurement [3].

Transforming Growth Factor-β

Endothelial cells produce transforming growth factor-β (TGF-β) and express TGF-β receptors. Like Ang-2, TGF-β acts as an angiostatic or angiogenic molecule. TGF-β stimulates or inhibits the proliferation of endothelial cells and tube formation in vitro, in a dose-dependent manner. Of note, TGF-β-induced angiogenesis in endothelial cells in vivo is indirectly achieved and occurs preferentially via the recruitment of inflammatory cells, which in turn release pro-angiogenic cytokines. TGF-β is also involved in the differentiation of endothelial cells and vascular SMCs, which includes the formation of adequate tubes and stable vessel walls, whereas it is not involved in the migration and proliferation of precursor cells. TGF-β1, in particular, is associated with the pathogenesis of MMD, which includes abundant neovascularization. The serum level of TGF-β1 is significantly higher in patients with MMD than in controls. The expression of TGF-β1 is significantly higher in cultured SMCs derived from the STAs of patients with MMD than in those derived from the STAs of patients with arteriosclerotic cerebrovascular disease [12].

Tumor Necrosis Factor-α

The effect of the tumor necrosis factor-α (TNF-α) on angiogenesis is similar to that of TGF-β. TNF-α promotes or inhibits endothelial cell proliferation and tube formation at low (0.1–0.5 ng/ml) and high (1–10 ng/ml) doses, respectively. In addition, TNF-α, similarly to TGF-β, induces the formation of new vessels in vivo via its pro-inflammatory properties. TNF-α-mediated angiogenesis has not been studied in MMD.

Integrins

Integrins, a family of heterodimeric proteins that consist of different α and β chain isoforms, are the major cell surface receptors that mediate the adhesion of endothelial cells to the extracellular matrix (ECM) and to adjacent cells. The α subunit has an extracellular domain that binds matrix molecules, and the β subunit has a cytoplasmic domain that interacts with several signaling mediators. VEGF and FGF-2 increase the expression of several members of the integrin family in endothelial cells [13]. One integrin family member, $\alpha_v\beta_3$, is upregulated in endothelial cells of newly sprouting blood vessels within tumors, such as glioblastomas, and is highly expressed at the tips of sprouting vessels during wound healing. Integrins $\alpha_1\beta_1$ and $\alpha_2\beta_1$ also affects VEGF-induced angiogenesis [14]. These effects were identified using antibodies and peptides for each integrin. Integrin-related angiogenesis has not been studied in MMD.

Vascular Endothelial Cadherin

Vascular endothelial cadherin (VE-cadherin) is an endothelial cell-specific cadherin localized at the intercellular adhesion junctions between endothelial cells. The functions of cadherins are modulated by catenins (directly by β-catenin, γ-catenin, and p120-catenin, and indirectly by α-catenin,). β-, γ-, and p120-catenin become highly phosphorylated after stimulation with VEGF. This modification leads to a destabilization of the cell–cell junction, which allows cells to proliferate and modulates VEGFR functions [15]. Therefore, VE-cadherin contributes to the maintenance of the stable monolayer of endothelial cells in the vessel wall. Until recently, the role of VE-cadherin on MMD angiogenesis was unknown.

Platelet Endothelial Cell Adhesion Molecule 1

The platelet endothelial cell adhesion molecules (PECAMs) are members of the immunoglobulin super family, which mediates cell-to-cell adhesion. PECAM-1 (also known as CD31) is expressed on endothelial cells, platelets, and leukocytes. Similar to VE-cadherin, PECAM-1 is necessary for the organization of endothelial cells into tubular networks in vitro [16]. Blocking antibodies directed against PECAM-1, were used to demonstrate that this molecule is an important factor for in vivo angiogenesis [16]. There are no studies on the relationship between PECAM-1 and MMD.

Matrix Metalloproteinases

MMPs are matrix-degrading enzymes that play an important role in ECM degradation and endothelial cell invasion. Several MMPs are expressed in the CNS. They are associated with ECM remodeling in pathophysiological conditions [1]. A major function of MMP activity is the opening of the blood–brain barrier after cerebral ischemia [17]. VEGF increases the expression of MMPs. MMP-1, -2, and -9 are produced during endothelial cell migration and tube formation. Recent studies demonstrated a combined effect for MMPs and TIMPs during the repair process of cerebral ischemia, especially angiogenesis. One finding suggests that the G/C heterozygous genotype at position -418 in the TIMP2 promoter may be a genetic predisposing factor for familial MMD [18]. Recently, the serum level of MMP-9 was reported to be significantly higher in MMD patients than in healthy controls. This is not true for serum MMP-2 levels. Immunohistochemical analysis of surgical specimens showed a significant increase in MMP-9 expression within the arachnoid membrane of MMD samples [19]. This result suggests that the increased levels of MMP-9 may contribute to pathologic angiogenesis and/or to the instability of the vascular structure in MMD.

Other Angiogenic Factors

In addition to the angiogenic factors mentioned above, several other factors are involved in angiogenesis. These include the granulocyte and granulocyte/macrophage colony-stimulating factor, angiogenin, insulin-like growth factor, tissue factor, factor V, and erythropoietin. However, it is not well understood whether these factors are involved in MMD angiogenesis. One study reported that the hepatocyte growth factor (HGF) is densely found in the carotid fork, and that its CSF level is markedly elevated in MMD, which suggests that HGF may be a key protein in the pathogenesis of MMD [20].

Angiostatic Factors

Among the angiostatic factors, angiostatin and endostatin are inhibitors of the proliferation, migration, and tube formation of endothelial cells and MMPs and inducers of apoptosis in endothelial cells in vivo [21]. Ang-2, as described previously, induces vessel destabilization by antagonizing Ang-1 signaling and apoptosis in endothelial cells. In addition, TNF-α, TGF-β, thrombospondin-1, thrombospondin-2, and pigment epithelium-derived factor are involved in decreased proliferation and migration and increased apoptosis in endothelial cells. The roles played by these factors in MMD angiogenesis remain unknown.

MicroRNAs

MicroRNAs were originally described as short noncoding RNAs that function as negative regulators of gene expression. Over 500 human microRNAs have been identified to date, and increasing evidence indicates that microRNAs have distinct expression profiles and play crucial roles in various physiological and pathological processes, which include cardiogenesis, hematopoietic lineage differentiation, and oncogenesis. Very recently, it has been reported that the response of the vascular endothelium to angiogenic stimuli is modulated by microRNAs. A few specific microRNAs have been described that regulate endothelial cell functions and angiogenesis. Let7-f, miR-27b, and mir-130a were identified as pro-angiogenic microRNAs. In contrast, miR-221 and miR-222 inhibit endothelial cell migration, proliferation, and angiogenesis in vitro. The endothelial cell-specific miR-126 microRNA also promotes angiogenesis in response to angiogenic growth factors, which include VEGF and bFGF, by repressing negative regulators of signal transduction pathways. Additional microRNAs have been implicated in the regulation of various aspects of angiogenesis [22]. Thus, targeting the expression of microRNAs may be a novel therapeutic approach for diseases that involve excess or insufficient vasculature. Studies of the effect of microRNAs on angiogenesis have just started. Therefore, the application of microRNAs on MMD angiogenesis will be valuable and novel.

Ischemia/Angiogenesis-Related Cells

Endothelial Progenitor Cells

EPCs are involved in physiological and pathological angiogenesis, as they are actively recruited at sites of new vessel growth. Moreover, circulating EPCs contribute to endothelial regeneration and vascular repair. Several lines of evidence indicate that EPCs also play a role in adult neovascularization, as well as in the maintenance of endothelial integrity and function. EPCs normally circulate in peripheral blood and replace injured endothelial cells for vessel repair. Cerebrovascular disease and cardiovascular and peripheral atherosclerosis, have been associated with lower numbers of circulating EPCs. In addition, low EPC levels have been shown to represent an independent risk factor for future cardiovascular events. Although the characteristics of EPCs have been studied in various vascular diseases, there are only a few studies on the role of these cells in patients with MMD [7, 23].

Endothelial Cells

The endothelium regulates vascular homeostasis and is responsible for angiogenesis, which is a process mediated by the sprouting of endothelial cells from pre-existing vessels. The proliferation and migration of endothelial cells in response to molecular signals are major components of newly formed vessels in adults [1]. Endothelial cells are heterogeneous in morphology, function, and gene expression profiles. Physically, endothelial cells have been shown to differ in size and thickness. The most important characteristic that differentiates these cells is the integrity of the tight junctions. The blood–brain barrier, composed of continuous endothelial cell tight junctions, is an important protective factor for the CNS. The tight junctions are modulated by factors that include VEGF. Mitotically, the endothelial cells in the brain are tightly downregulated. Hence, they are upregulated during angiogenesis [24]. Some studies suggest that endothelial cells play an important role in the initiation of angiogenesis, whereas other studies suggest that these cells are induced to replicate and migrate to complete the angiogenic process [24]. A practical relationship between endothelial cells and MMD angiogenesis has not been described.

Mural Cells: Pericytes and Smooth Muscle Cells

The vascular tube must be stabilized by mural cells. The recruitment of mural cells (i.e., pericytes and SMCs) of blood vessels is an important step of vessel maturation [25]. The initial step of maturation is the fusion of the newly formed capillaries with other vessels. The process of vessel maturation includes a step-by-step transition from the growing vessel bed to the quiescent, fully formed, and functional network. Therefore, the recruitment of pericytes and accumulation of ECM proteins in the adjacent basement membrane contributes to vessel maturation and to its transition to the quiescent state. To achieve this, mesenchymal cells in the surrounding tissue proliferate and migrate to the abluminal surface of the premature vessels. These mesenchymal cells subsequently differentiate either into pericytes, located within the basement membrane, or into vascular SMCs, found abluminally of the basement membrane. Pericytes are in direct intercellular contact with endothelial cells and form the walls of capillaries and immature blood vessels, whereas the walls of mature blood vessels and those of large-diameter vessels (i.e., arteries and veins) are formed by several layers of SMCs separated from the endothelium by a layer of basement membrane [26]. SMCs derived from the STAs of MMD patients, together with PDGF, are actually involved in intimal thickening [10]. In MMD SMCs, PDGF-AA and -BB stimulate cell migration but not DNA synthesis.

References

1. Fan Y, Yang GY (2007) Therapeutic angiogenesis for brain ischemia: a brief review. J Neuroimmune Pharmacol 2:284–289
2. Suzui H, Hoshimaru M, Takahashi JA et al (1994) Immunohistochemical reactions for fibroblast growth factor receptor in arteries of patients with moyamoya disease. Neurosurgery 35:20–24
3. Yoshimoto T, Houkin K, Takahashi A et al (1996) Angiogenic factors in moyamoya disease. Stroke 27:2160–2165
4. Takahashi A, Sawamura Y, Houkin K et al (1993) The cerebrospinal fluid in patients with moyamoya disease (spontaneous occlusion of the circle of Willis) contains high level of basic fibroblast growth factor. Neurosci Lett 160:214–216
5. Yano A, Shingo T, Takeuchi A et al (2005) Encapsulated vascular endothelial growth factor-secreting cell grafts have neuroprotective and angiogenic effects on focal cerebral ischemia. J Neurosurg 103:104–114
6. Takahashi T, Kalka C, Masuda H et al (1999) Ischemia- and cytokine-induced mobilization of bone marrow-derived endothelial progenitor cells for neovascularization. Nat Med 5:434–438
7. Rafat N, Beck GCh, Peña-Tapia PG et al (2009) Increased levels of circulating endothelial progenitor cells in patients with Moyamoya disease. Stroke 40:432–438
8. Yancopoulos GD, Davis S, Gale NW et al (2000) Vascular-specific growth factors and blood vessel formation. Nature 407 (6801): 242–248
9. Hellstrom M, Gerhardt H, Kalen M et al (2001) Lack of pericytes leads to endothelial hyperplasia and abnormal vascular morphogenesis. J Cell Biol 153:543–553
10. Yamamoto M, Aoyagi M, Fukai N et al (1998) Differences in cellular responses to mitogens in arterial smooth muscle cells derived from patients with moyamoya disease. Stroke 29:1188–1193
11. Kedar D, Baker CH, Killion JJ et al (2002) Blockade of the epidermal growth factor receptor signaling inhibits angiogenesis leading to regression of human renal cell carcinoma growing orthotopically in nude mice. Clin Cancer Res 8:3592–3600
12. Hojo M, Hoshimaru M, Miyamoto S et al (1998) Role of transforming growth factor-beta1 in the pathogenesis of moyamoya disease. J Neurosurg 89:623–629
13. Smyth SS, Patterson C (2002) Tiny dancers: the integrin-growth factor nexus in angiogenic signaling. J Cell Biol 158:17–21

14. Senger DR, Claffey KP, Benes JE et al (1997) Angiogenesis promoted by vascular endothelial growth factor: regulation through alpha1beta1 and alpha2beta1 integrins. Proc Natl Acad Sci USA 94:13612–13617
15. Vestweber D (2008) VE-cadherin: the major endothelial adhesion molecule controlling cellular junctions and blood vessel formation. Arterioscler Thromb Vasc Biol 28(2):223–232
16. Cao G, O'Brien CD, Zhou Z et al (2002) Involvement of human PECAM-1 in angiogenesis and in vitro endothelial cell migration. Am J Physiol Cell Physiol 282:C1181–1190
17. Cunningham LA, Wetzel M, Rosenberg GA (2005) Multiple roles for MMPs and TIMPs in cerebral ischemia. Glia 50:329–339
18. Kang HS, Kim SK, Cho BK et al (2006) Single nucleotide polymorphisms of tissue inhibitor of metalloproteinase genes in familial moyamoya disease. Neurosurgery 58:1074–80
19. Fujimura M, Watanabe M, Narisawa A et al (2009) Increased expression of serum matrix metalloproteinase-9 in patients with moyamoya disease. Surg Neurol Jan 13 [Epub ahead of print]
20. Nanba R, Kuroda S, Ishikawa T et al (2004) Increased expression of hepatocyte growth factor in cerebrospinal fluid and intracranial artery in moyamoya disease. Stroke 35:2837–2842
21. Distler JH, Hirth A, Kurowska-Stolarska M et al (2003) Angiogenic and angiostatic factors in the molecular control of angiogenesis. Q J Nucl Med 47:149–161
22. Suárez Y, Sessa WC (2009) MicroRNAs as novel regulators of angiogenesis. Circ Res 104:442–454
23. Yoshihara T, Taguchi A, Matsuyama T et al (2008) Increase in circulating CD34-positive cells in patients with angiographic evidence of moyamoya-like vessels. J Cereb Blood Flow Metab 28:1086–1089
24. Harrigan MR (2003) Angiogenic factors in the central nervous system. Neurosurgery 53:639–660
25. Gerhardt H, Betsholtz C (2003) Endothelial-pericyte interactions in angiogenesis. Cell Tissue Res 314:15–23
26. Jain RK (2003) Molecular regulation of vessel maturation. Nat Med 9:685–693

Immunological Aspects of Moyamoya Disease

Ji Hoon Phi, Seung-Ki Kim, Kyu-Chang Wang, and Byung-Kyu Cho

Introduction

Immunological phenomena have pervasive effects on the human body. Many physiological and pathological processes involve the immune system. Because of this pervasiveness, it is often difficult to know whether an observed immunological reaction truly underlies a process or whether it is simply an epiphenomenon. The role of the immune system in moyamoya disease is a controversial issue. The etiology of moyamoya disease is currently unknown. Various etiologies, genetic and environmental, have been proposed; however, none have been definitively proven. There is a lot of evidence for immunological abnormalities in patients with moyamoya disease. However, much of the evidence is indirect and lacks a solid causal relationship. Nonetheless, it is strongly believed that immunological processes play an important role at least in the progression of moyamoya disease. In this chapter, the pathological and epidemiological evidence that supports the immunological origin of moyamoya disease is discussed.

Pathological Evidence

Atherosclerosis, which is primarily a degenerative and metabolic lesion, can be viewed as an inflammatory process in the blood vessel walls. Local and systemic inflammation is associated with the development of atherosclerosis. Macrophages, dendritic cells, T lymphocytes, and other inflammatory cells, especially lipid-laden foam cells, have been found in atherosclerotic vessel walls [1]. Chronic systemic inflammation, manifested as elevated C-reactive protein, is

J.H. Phi (✉), K.-C. Wang, and B.-K. Cho
Division of Pediatric Neurosurgery, Pediatric Clinical Neuroscience Center, Seoul National University Children's Hospital, Seoul National University College of Medicine,
101 Daehangno, Jongno-gu, Seoul, Republic of Korea
e-mail: eages@paran.com

S.-K. Kim
Division of Pediatric Neurosurgery, Pediatric Clinical Neuroscience Center, Seoul National University Children's Hospital, Research Center for Rare Disease, Seoul National University College of Medicine,
101 Daehangno, Jongno-gu, Seoul 110-744, Republic of Korea

B.-K. Cho and T. Tominaga (eds.), *Moyamoya Disease Update*,
DOI 10.1007/978-4-431-99703-0_13, © Springer 2010

a strong risk factor of cardiovascular disease and stroke [2, 3]. In laboratory studies and clinics, treatments that target inflammatory cells or proinflammatory cytokines are under investigation [4, 5].

Although it is difficult to obtain pathological specimens of the affected arteries from patients with moyamoya disease, several autopsy studies have provided a consistent description of the vascular pathology of moyamoya disease. Intimal thickening, undulation and thickening of the internal elastic lamina, thinning of the media, and proliferation of smooth muscle cells are characteristic features of the vascular pathology of moyamoya disease [6, 7]. A lack of lipid-laden foamy macrophages is a notable finding that distinguishes the vascular changes in moyamoya disease from those of atherosclerosis [6]. Evidence for inflammation in the vascular wall is sparse in patients with moyamoya disease. Smooth muscle cells are the predominant cellular component of the thickened vascular wall. The presence of intramural macrophages and T lymphocytes has also been reported; however, they were small in number and scattered in the superficial layer of the intimal thickening [8]. Despite the paucity of evidence for immune cell infiltration in the vascular lesions of patients with moyamoya disease, the roles of cytokines in smooth muscle cell proliferation and migration have been intensively investigated.

The expression of basic fibroblast growth factor (b-FGF) is elevated in the vascular walls and cerebrospinal fluid (CSF) of patients with moyamoya disease [9]. Elevated levels of soluble endothelial adhesion molecules, such as vascular cell adhesion molecule type 1, intercellular adhesion molecule, and E-selectin, have been reported in the CSF of patients with moyamoya disease and linked to ongoing inflammation of the central nervous system [10]. Hepatocyte growth factor, a potent angiogenic factor and inducer of smooth muscle cell migration, is also elevated in the CSF of patients with moyamoya disease [11]. Proteomic analysis of the CSF of patients with moyamoya disease revealed that cellular retinoic-acid-binding protein 1 (CRABP-1) was significantly elevated [12]. CRABP-1 attenuates the activity of retinoids that negatively regulate proangiogenic and mitogenic cytokines, thereby allowing smooth muscle cell proliferation and intimal thickening. The observed elevation of various cytokines provides theoretical models explaining the peculiar vascular changes associated with moyamoya disease [11, 12]. However, they tell little about what initiates the pathological process. It is also unclear whether the elevated cytokines are active perpetuators of moyamoya pathogenesis or simple bystanders.

Association with Autoimmune Diseases

An autoimmune disease involves immune attack of the organ of interest, the presence of circulating autoantibodies, and epidemiological marks indicative of immune activation such as a previous infectious episode. At present, there is insufficient evidence for these mechanisms in moyamoya disease. However, some patients with moyamoya-like vascular changes have an overt association with autoimmune diseases or autoimmune phenomena in other organs (these patients are duly classified as having moyamoya syndrome), supporting the role of an autoimmune mechanism in the moyamoya pathogenesis in at least some patients.

Graves' disease is an autoimmune thyrotoxicosis predominantly affecting women. More than 20 patients with Graves' disease have been reported to have associated moyamoya-like vascular changes [13]. In these patients, acute thyrotoxic states can exert hemodynamic stress on the brain, exacerbating ischemic injury [14]. Common immune dysregulation that results in autoimmune cerebral vasculitis has been proposed for the concurrence of Graves' disease and moyamoya-like vascular changes [15]. There is an interesting report of a patient with

Graves' disease and moyamoya-like vascular changes that resolved after treatment with steroids and plasmapheresis [16]. However, there is no direct evidence that the vascular changes in these patients are immune-mediated. The hemodynamic stress caused by the thyrotoxicosis rather than immune attacks may contribute to the vascular changes in these patients [13].

Antiphospholipid syndrome (APS) includes the presence of a heterogeneous group of antiphospholipid (APL) autoantibodies, such as lupus anticoagulant and anticardiolipin antibody, and repeated thrombotic episodes. There are several reports of patients with moyamoya-like vascular changes and documented APS [17, 18]. In a study of ten patients with moyamoya syndrome, three had APL antibodies [19]. However, the incidence and significance of detectable APL antibodies are unknown for patients with primary moyamoya disease. It is noteworthy that one of the three patients with APL antibodies in the previous study had Down syndrome as the underlying disease. The association of Down syndrome and moyamoya syndrome is well established [20]. Patients with Down syndrome have an increased frequency of malignancy and autoimmune diseases, such as autoimmune thyroiditis and type 1 diabetes mellitus, indicating the presence of immune dysregulation [21, 22]. Leno et al. [23] reported a patient with Down syndrome, Graves' disease, APL antibodies, and moyamoya-like vascular changes with ischemic stroke. Therefore, autoimmunity may underlie all these three autoimmune phenomena. However, this scheme could be applied to only a small proportion of patients with moyamoya disease, because at present evidence for autoimmunity is lacking for the majority of them.

Association with Infectious Diseases

Infectious agents can directly invade intracranial arteries and cause inflammation and vasculitis. Moreover, infectious agents can elicit autoimmune responses by molecular mimicry, chronic inflammation, and immune dysregulation. Several infectious agents have been suspected to underlie the etiology of moyamoya disease. In one study, patients with moyamoya disease had a higher titer of antibody to *Propionibacterium acnes* compared to normal control subjects [24]. Because *P. acnes* is a major species of microflora of the head and neck, the possible association of *P. acnes* infection and moyamoya disease was raised. A similar study on cytomegalovirus and Epstein–Barr virus (EBV) revealed that patients with moyamoya disease had a higher titer of anti-EBV antibodies and a higher frequency of EBV DNA in serum than did normal controls [25]. However, the statistical power of these studies was rather weak and the causal relationships revealed were obscure. Several case reports exist for childhood stroke associated with *Mycoplasma pneumonia* infection [26–29]. All reported patients had unilateral occlusion of an intracranial vessel except for one patient with a typical radiological feature of moyamoya disease [30]. Therefore, although an infectious etiology of moyamoya disease is a tempting possibility, there is currently little evidence supporting this hypothesis.

Kawasaki, Takayasu, and Moyamoya Disease

Primary systemic vasculitis (PSV) is a group of diseases characterized by blood vessel inflammation that may lead to stenosis, occlusion, aneurismal formation, and rupture of the involved vessels [31]. Kawasaki disease is a self-limiting PSV of childhood that predominantly attacks medium-sized vessels, notably coronary arteries [32]. Takayasu arteritis is a PSV of adolescents and young adults that predominantly involves large-sized vessels, such as the aorta and its branches [33]. These diseases are thought to be primarily immune-mediated and presumably caused by infectious and autoimmune mechanisms.

There are several common characteristics between moyamoya disease and these PSVs. First, the incidence of these diseases is highest in Asia, especially in Japan and Republic of Korea. Second, there is a strong predilection for arteries of specific regions in these diseases: cerebral arteries for moyamoya disease, coronary arteries for Kawasaki disease, and the aorta and its large branches for Takayasu arteritis. Third, despite the predilection for cerebral arteries, there is evidence for systemic involvement in moyamoya disease like PSVs; for example, renal artery stenosis and hypertension are frequently observed in patients with moyamoya disease [34].

Nonetheless, a substantial difference exists between moyamoya disease and PSVs. First, Kawasaki disease and Takayasu arteritis have overt acute phases with fever and other systemic symptoms. In this acute phase, laboratory studies have revealed an elevated erythrocyte sedimentation rate, C-reactive protein, and immune cytokines, indicating an active inflammation in these diseases. However, there is virtually no active phase or serological evidence for active inflammation in moyamoya disease. Second, inflammatory cell infiltration and progression of the lesion in the affected vessel walls are well documented for Kawasaki disease and Takayasu arteritis compared to moyamoya disease. Third, there is a large body of evidence supporting infectious etiologies for Kawasaki disease and Takayasu arteritis, although the etiologic agents have not yet been specified. For moyamoya disease, an infectious etiology has been proposed; however, there is scant evidence to support it. Finally, immunosuppression by intravenous immunoglobulin, corticosteroids, and other agents is largely effective for Kawasaki disease and Takayasu arteritis, whereas it has no proven role for moyamoya disease. Therefore, more evidence is needed to consider moyamoya disease as a variant of PSVs in which immunological processes play a major role.

Conclusions

Elevated immune cytokines and signaling molecules have been reported in the vascular wall and CSF of patients with moyamoya disease. These molecules may contribute to the smooth muscle cell proliferation that constitutes the major cellular component of the pathological lesions in moyamoya disease. Some patients with moyamoya-like vascular changes have concurrent autoimmune diseases such as Graves' thyrotoxicosis and APS. Association of moyamoya disease with *P. acnes* and EBV infection has been proposed by serological evidence. All these findings support the role of immunological processes in the development and progression of moyamoya disease. However, at least at present, moyamoya disease cannot be considered as a bona fide vasculitis, and further research is required to elucidate the role of the immune system in this enigmatic disease.

References

1. Galkina E, Ley K (2009) Immune and inflammatory mechanisms of atherosclerosis. Annu Rev Immunol 27:165–197
2. Ridker PM, Hennekens CH, Buring JE et al (2000) C-reactive protein and other markers of inflammation in the prediction of cardiovascular disease in women. N Engl J Med 342(12):836–843
3. Andersson J, Johansson L, Ladenvall P et al (2009) C-reactive protein is a determinant of first-ever stroke: prospective nested case-referent study. Cerebrovasc Dis 27(6):544–551
4. Mach F, Schonbeck U, Sukhova GK et al (1998) Reduction of atherosclerosis in mice by inhibition of CD40 signalling. Nature 394(6689):200–203
5. Saha P, Modarai B, Humphries J et al (2009) The monocyte/macrophage as a therapeutic target in atherosclerosis. Curr Opin Pharmacol 9(2):109–118

6. Takebayashi S, Matsuo K, Kaneko M (1984) Ultrastructural studies of cerebral arteries and collateral vessels in moyamoya disease. Stroke 15(4):728–732
7. Takekawa Y, Umezawa T, Ueno Y et al (2004) Pathological and immunohistochemical findings of an autopsy case of adult moyamoya disease. Neuropathology 24(3):236–242
8. Masuda J, Ogata J, Yutani C (1993) Smooth muscle cell proliferation and localization of macrophages and T cells in the occlusive intracranial major arteries in moyamoya disease. Stroke 24(12):1960–1967
9. Houkin K, Yoshimoto T, Abe H et al (1998) Role of basic fibroblast growth factor in the pathogenesis of moyamoya disease. Neurosurg Focus 5(5):e2
10. Soriano SG, Cowan DB, Proctor MR et al (2002) Levels of soluble adhesion molecules are elevated in the cerebrospinal fluid of children with moyamoya syndrome. Neurosurgery 50(3):544–549
11. Nanba R, Kuroda S, Ishikawa T et al (2004) Increased expression of hepatocyte growth factor in cerebrospinal fluid and intracranial artery in moyamoya disease. Stroke 35(12):2837–2842
12. Kim SK, Yoo JI, Cho BK et al (2003) Elevation of CRABP-I in the cerebrospinal fluid of patients with Moyamoya disease. Stroke 34(12):2835–2841
13. Sasaki T, Nogawa S, Amano T (2006) Co-morbidity of moyamoya disease with Graves' disease. report of three cases and a review of the literature. Intern Med 45(9):649–653
14. Im SH, Oh CW, Kwon OK et al (2005) Moyamoya disease associated with Graves disease: special considerations regarding clinical significance and management. J Neurosurg 102(6):1013–1017
15. Tendler BE, Shoukri K, Malchoff C et al (1997) Concurrence of Graves' disease and dysplastic cerebral blood vessels of the moyamoya variety. Thyroid 7(4):625–629
16. Utku U, Asil T, Celik Y et al (2004) Reversible MR angiographic findings in a patient with autoimmune Graves disease. Am J Neuroradiol 25(9):1541–1543
17. Booth F, Yanofsky R, Ross IB et al (1999) Primary antiphospholipid syndrome with moyamoya-like vascular changes. Pediatr Neurosurg 31(1):45–48
18. Bakdash T, Cohen AR, Hempel JM, Hoagland J, Newman AJ (2002) Moyamoya, dystonia during hyperventilation, and antiphospholipid antibodies. Pediatr Neurol 26(2):157–160
19. Bonduel M, Hepner M, Sciuccati G et al (2001) Prothrombotic disorders in children with moyamoya syndrome. Stroke 32(8):1786–1792
20. Jea A, Smith ER, Robertson R et al (2005) Moyamoya syndrome associated with Down syndrome: outcome after surgical revascularization. Pediatrics 116(5):e694–701
21. Kusters MA, Verstegen RH, Gemen EF et al (2009) Intrinsic defect of the immune system in children with Down syndrome: a review. Clin Exp Immunol 156(2):189–193
22. Goldacre MJ, Wotton CJ, Seagroatt V et al (2004) Cancers and immune related diseases associated with Down's syndrome: a record linkage study. Arch Dis Child 89(11):1014–1017
23. Leno C, Mateo I, Cid C et al (1998) Autoimmunity in Down's syndrome: another possible mechanism of moyamoya disease. Stroke 29(4):868–869
24. Yamada H, Deguchi K, Tanigawara T et al (1997) The relationship between moyamoya disease and bacterial infection. Clin Neurol Neurosurg 99(Suppl 2):S221–224
25. Tanigawara T, Yamada H, Sakai N et al (1997) Studies on cytomegalovirus and Epstein-Barr virus infection in moyamoya disease. Clin Neurol Neurosurg 99(Suppl 2):S225–228
26. Visudhiphan P, Chiemchanya S, Sirinavin S (1992) Internal carotid artery occlusion associated with *Mycoplasma pneumoniae* infection. Pediatr Neurol 8(3):237–239
27. Leonardi S, Pavone P, Rotolo N et al (2005) Stroke in two children with *Mycoplasma pneumoniae* infection. A causal or casual relationship? Pediatr Infect Dis J 24(9):843–845
28. Fu M, Wong KS, Lam WW et al (1998) Middle cerebral artery occlusion after recent *Mycoplasma pneumoniae* infection. J Neurol Sci 157(1):113–115
29. Tanir G, Aydemir C, Yilmaz D et al (2006) Internal carotid artery occlusion associated with *Mycoplasma pneumoniae* infection in a child. Turk J Pediatr 48(2):166–171
30. Greco F, Castellano Chiodo D, Sorge A et al (2006) Multiple arterial ischemic strokes in a child with moyamoya disease and *Mycoplasma pneumoniae* infection. Minerva Pediatr 58(1):63–68
31. Eleftheriou D, Dillon MJ, Brogan PA (2009) Advances in childhood vasculitis. Curr Opin Rheumatol 21(4):411–418
32. Pinna GS, Kafetzis DA, Tselkas OI et al (2008) Kawasaki disease: an overview. Curr Opin Infect Dis 21(3):263–270
33. Tann OR, Tulloh RM, Hamilton MC (2008) Takayasu's disease: a review. Cardiol Young 18(3):250–259
34. Togao O, Mihara F, Yoshiura T et al (2004) Prevalence of stenoocclusive lesions in the renal and abdominal arteries in moyamoya disease. Am J Roentgenol 183(1):119–122

Part V
Pathophysiology II: Hemodynamics, Biomechanical Aspect

Hemodynamics

Jeong Chul Kim and Eun Bo Shim

Introduction

Blood is composed of blood cells suspended in plasma. The viscosity of blood varies with clinical conditions that influence blood cell aggregation and the hematocrit, and involves hemodynamic changes in vessels directly [1–3]. Generally, in arteries with diameters larger than 3 mm, the viscosity of blood is essentially constant when the shear rate exceeds 100 s^{-1} [4]. By contrast, in capillaries with diameters smaller than 400 μm, the decrease in the vessel diameter reduces the viscosity of blood by redistributing blood cells at the center of the vessel [5]. Therefore, we should consider non-Newtonian blood flow behavior according to the flow conditions in blood vessels. This section briefly describes the basics of fluid mechanics that might be useful for understanding cerebral hemodynamics.

Definition of a Fluid

A fluid is defined as a substance that deforms continuously under the application of a shear (tangential) stress no matter how small the shear stress may be [6]. In most cases, fluids comprise the liquid and gas phases of the physical forms in which matter exists. The distinction between fluid and solid phases is clear when we compare their deformation over time when a shear stress is applied (Fig. 1). When the shear force F is applied to a plate, the deformation of the block continues to increase with time, whereas that of a solid is proportional to the shear stress applied.

J.C. Kim
Institute of Medical and Biological Engineering, Medical Research Center, Seoul National University College of Medicine, 199-1 Dongsoong-dong, Jongno-gu, Seoul 110-744, Republic of Korea

E.B. Shim (✉)
Department of Mechanical and Biomedical Engineering, Kangwon National University, Chuncheon, Kangwon 200-701, Republic of Korea
e-mail: ebshim@kangwon.ac.kr

B.-K. Cho and T. Tominaga (eds.), *Moyamoya Disease Update*,
DOI 10.1007/978-4-431-99703-0_14,

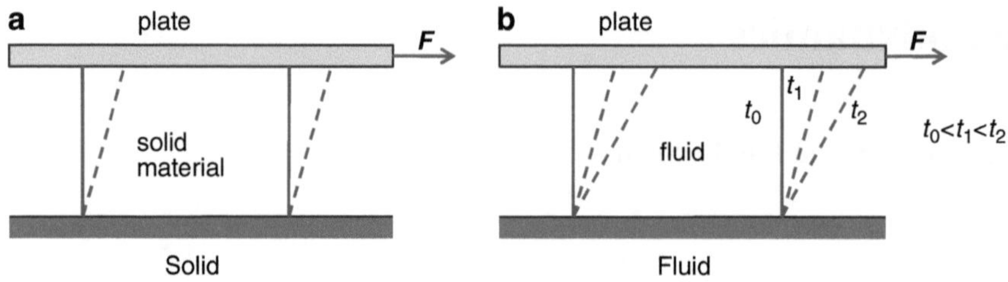

Fig. 1 Behavior of a solid (**a**) and fluid (**b**) under the action of a constant shear force

Fig. 2 Shear stress as a function of the shear rate for one-dimensional flow

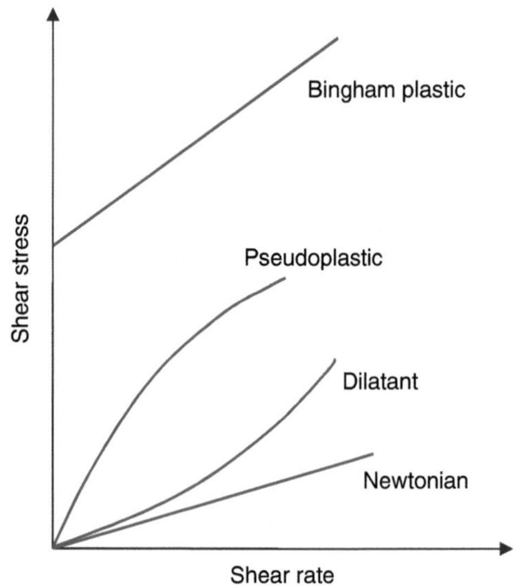

Viscosity

Fluids may be classified as Newtonian and non-Newtonian fluids according to the relationship between the applied shear stress and the shear rate (Fig. 2). Fluids in which the shear stress is directly proportional to the shear rate are Newtonian fluids. All fluids in which the shear stress is not directly proportional to the rate of deformation (the shear rate) are non-Newtonian fluids. The most common Newtonian fluids are water and air under normal conditions. The relationship between shear stress (τ) and the shear rate (du/dy, x-velocity gradient in the y-direction) in a Newtonian fluid can be described as Newton's law of viscosity.

$$\tau_{yx} = k\frac{du}{dy}, \tag{1}$$

where the subscript yx denotes the vector normal to the plane in which the shear stress is applied (xz-plane) and the direction of deformation (the x-direction). The constant of proportionality, μ, is the dynamic viscosity. In the absolute metric system, the basic unit of viscosity is the poise [1 poise = 1 g/(cm·s)] and in the System International of Units (SI) it is kg/(m · s) or Pa · s [1 Pa · s = 1 N · s/m²]. The dynamic viscosity of water is 1.0 centipoise (cP) at 20°C, and that of blood with a normal hematocrit is 3.5–4.0 cP at body temperature.

Many common fluids exhibit non-Newtonian behavior. Two familiar examples are toothpaste and Lucite paint. The latter is very thick when in the can, but becomes thin when sheared by brushing. This shear-thinning characteristic can be seen in the blood flow; in the low-wall-shear-stress region around bifurcations, the viscosity of blood increases through red blood cells aggregation, whereas in capillaries with diameters less than 400 μm, the viscosity decreases via the redistribution of red blood cells at the centerline of the vessel (Fahraeus–Lindqvist effect). Numerous empirical equations have been proposed to describe non-Newtonian fluid flow [7]. The power law model, one of the simplest, can adequately represent the relationship between shear stress and the shear rate:

$$\tau_{yx} = k\left(\frac{du}{dy}\right)^n, \tag{2}$$

where the exponent n is the flow behavior index and the coefficient k is the consistency index; both are determined empirically.

Governing Equations (Poiseuille's Law)

General fluid flow can be described mathematically by the Navier–Stoke equation, which can be reduced to the following for steady pipe flow (Fig. 3) [8]

$$u = \frac{(P_1 - P_2)}{4\mu L}(R^2 - r^2), \tag{3}$$

where P_1 and P_2 are the pressures at the ends of the length (L), R is the internal radius, and r is the radius of the pipe. This is the equation for a parabola, where $u=0$ when $r=R$ and is a maximum when $r=0$ at the centerline of the pipe. The total volume rate of flow Q can be defined as

$$Q = \int_0^R u\mathrm{d}A = \int_o^R 2\pi ur\mathrm{d}r = \frac{2\pi(P_1 - P_2)}{4\mu L}\int_0^R r(R^2 - r^2)\mathrm{d}r = \frac{\pi R^4(P_1 - P_2)}{8\mu L}, \tag{4}$$

where dA is an element of area. This is commonly referred to as the Poiseuille equation. It is important to note that the volume flow is directly related to the fourth power of the radius, and

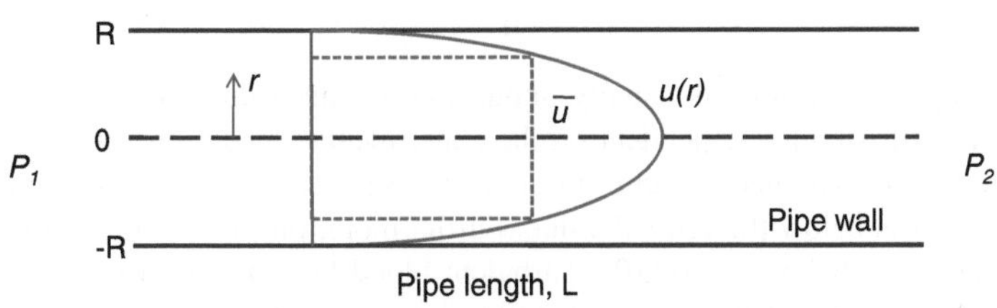

Fig. 3 Parabolic velocity profile of pipe flow driven by a pressure difference

that the flow increases exponentially with the radius of the pipe. The mean velocity is obtained by dividing the volume flow Q by the cross-sectional area πR^2, so that from (4) we get

$$\bar{u} = \frac{Q}{A} = \frac{R^2(P_1 - P_2)}{8\mu L} = \frac{1}{2}u_{\max}. \tag{5}$$

Finally, the wall shear stress is given by

$$\tau_w = \mu\frac{\mathrm{d}u}{\mathrm{d}r} = \frac{1}{2}R\left(\frac{P_1 - P_2}{L}\right) = \frac{4\mu\bar{u}}{R}. \tag{6}$$

Although the wall shear stress is proportional to the mean velocity in laminar flow, it is constant in turbulent flow. Recently, numerous studies have reported on the role of hemodynamic wall shear stress in atherosclerosis formed around the outer edge of vessel bifurcations by disturbed flow [9]. Arterial level shear stress (>15 dynes/cm^2) induces endothelial quiescence and an atheroprotective gene expression profile, whereas low shear stress (<4 dynes/cm^2), which is prevalent at atherosclerosis-prone sites, stimulates an atherogenic phenotype.

Laminar and Turbulent Flows

Viscous flow regimes are classified as laminar or turbulent based on the flow structure. In the lamina regime, the flow structure is characterized by smooth motion in laminae, or layers. The flow structure in the turbulent regime is characterized by random, three-dimensional motions of fluid particles in addition to the mean motion (Fig. 4). In laminar flow, no macroscopic mixing of adjacent fluid layers occurs. A thin filament of dye injected into a laminar flow appears as a single line, except for the slow diffusion due to molecular motion. By contrast, a dye filament injected into turbulent flow disperses quickly throughout the flow field; the line of dye breaks up into myriad entangled threads of dye. This behavior of turbulent flow is caused by velocity fluctuations. For steady laminar flow, the velocity at a point remains constant with time. In turbulent flow, the velocity trace indicates random fluctuations of the instantaneous velocity about the temporal mean velocity. We can consider the instantaneous velocity to be the sum of the temporal mean velocity and the fluctuating component.

Poiseuille's law relating steady flow and the pressure gradient in a pipe is no longer valid when the flow velocity exceeds a certain limit. The critical point is dependent on the diameter of the pipe, the mean velocity of the flow, and the density and viscosity of the liquid. This is expressed as a dimensionless quantity known as the Reynolds number (Re):

$$\mathrm{Re} = \frac{\rho\bar{u}D}{\mu}. \tag{7}$$

The critical Reynolds number is usually about 2,000. This value, however, is determined experimentally and is highly dependent on the experimental conditions. In the human body, the maximum Reynolds number in large arteries exceeds the critical value, although the average Reynolds number is below the critical value. Furthermore, pulsatile flow becomes unstable at Reynolds numbers below 2,000 [10]. Turbulent blood flow has been suggested to have a direct effect on the arterial wall. Post-stenotic dilation has been attributed to progressive weakening of the wall by turbulence, which has a potential role in atherogenesis.

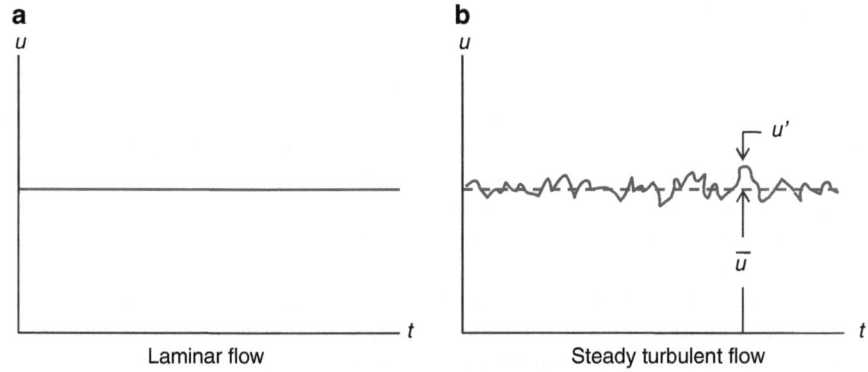

Fig. 4 Temporal variation in the velocity profile in laminar (**a**) and turbulent (**b**) flows

Blood Flow in Arteries

The most obvious feature of blood flow in arteries is that it is pulsatile. However, for a more realistic description of blood flow in arteries, the elasticity of the vessel and the flow resistance due to the complex network of peripheral vessels and internal organs should be considered. This section deals with the physics of pulsatile flow and its effects on hemodynamics in the arterial system according to the properties of the arterial wall.

Pulsatile Flow

One of conditions for the application of Poiseuille's equation (4) is that the flow is steady. Velocity profiles in pulsatile flow may differ greatly from the parabolic profile of steady Poiseuille flow. The flow profile depends on the frequency of oscillation, ω ($\omega = 2\pi f$, where f is the frequency) and on the vessel radius R, blood viscosity μ, and blood density ρ. These variables can be combined into a single dimensionless parameter called Womersley's alpha parameter:

$$\alpha^2 = \frac{R^2 \omega \rho}{\mu}. \quad (8)$$

When α is small, the effect of pulsatility on the flow profile is slight, and the flow is quasi-steady; at each instant, the flow is approximately the same as the steady flow. This means that, in the periphery of small vessels and with little oscillation, we can describe the pressure–flow relationship using Poiseuille's law. Conversely, the velocity profiles are strongly influenced by pulsatility when α is large. For the very large conduit arteries, where $\alpha > 10$, friction does not play a significant role, the pressure–flow relationship can be described using inertance alone. When $\alpha >> 1$, the velocity profiles in a pipe follow sinusoidal function with time only:

$$u = \frac{K}{\omega \rho}(\sin \omega t). \quad (9)$$

Properties of the Arterial Wall

In reality, an artery is a viscoelastic tube whose diameter varies with the pulsating pressure that is generated by a pulsating flow; in addition, it propagates pressure and flow waves at a certain velocity, which is largely determined by the elastic properties of the arterial wall. To study the hemodynamics of the arterial system, knowledge of the elastic properties of the arterial wall is of fundamental importance. This section deals with the basic concept of elasticity and the effects of its changes during circulation on the hemodynamic properties of the arterial wall.

When a force F is applied to a specimen with cross-sectional area A and length L, the length increases by ΔL. To obtain a unique characterization of the material, independent of sample size, we normalize the force by the area, and the stress is obtained as $\sigma = F/A$. Similarly, we normalize the length change to the starting length L_0 and obtain the strain as $\varepsilon = \Delta L/L_{0.}$ The relationship between stress and strain is given in Fig. 5a. The slope of the stress–strain curve in the region where a linear relationship holds is defined as the elastic modulus (Young's modulus of elasticity, $E = \sigma/\varepsilon$). The units of the elastic modulus are the same as units of pressure, i.e., $N/m^2 = Pa$ or mm Hg.

By contrast, a curved relationship between stress and strain can be observed in main vessels (Fig. 5b). Vascular tissue is composed of elastin, vascular smooth muscle, and collagen. Elastin fibers are highly extensible, and even at large deformations, they can be characterized by an almost constant Young's modulus. Conversely, collagen fibers are very stiff [11]. At low strains, collagen fibers are wavy and bear no load, and the elastin and smooth muscle mainly determine the wall elasticity. At larger strains, collagen starts bearing a load, leading to an increasingly stiff wall.

Elasticity plays an important role in circulation. All blood vessels are elastic, and their elastic moduli do not differ greatly. A typical value of the incremental elastic modulus of arteries in the normal human at a pressure of 100 mm Hg is about 5×10^6 dynes/cm^2 or 500 kPa (3,750 mm Hg). For diastolic heart tissue, the incremental elastic modulus at a filling pressure of 5 mm Hg is about 4×10^5 dynes/cm^2 or 40 kPa, and in systole, these values are 20 or more times larger. With the passage of time, certain histological changes that alter structure and function occur in the walls of the large central arteries. The principal changes occur in the intima and media [12, 13]; endothelial cells of the intima become more irregular in size and

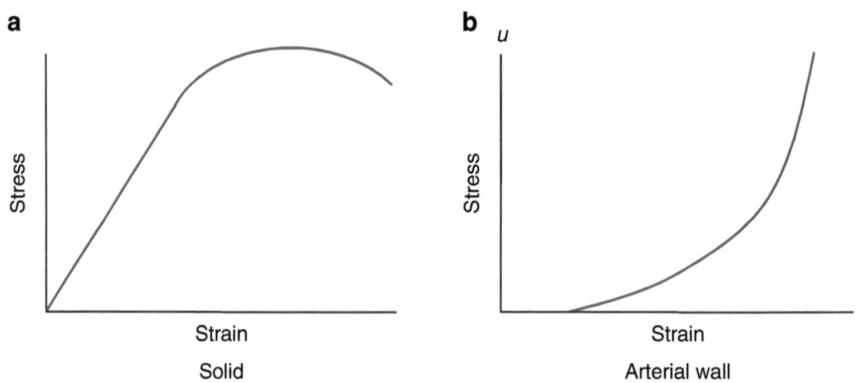

Fig. 5 Stress–strain relationship for general solid materials (**a**) and the arterial wall (**b**)

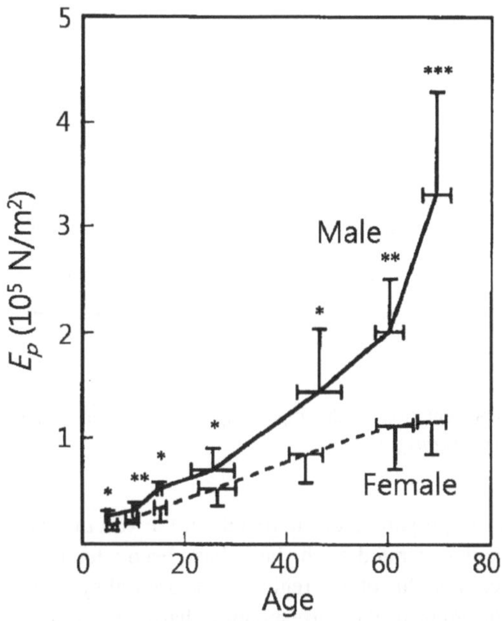

Fig. 6 Age-related increase in the abdominal aortic pressure–strain modulus (E_p) of females compared with males. Note that the increase in stiffness (E_p) is almost linear with age in females, whereas in males it is exponential in nature and of greater magnitude. *$P<0.05$, **$P<0.01$, ***$P<0.001$. Copied from [17]

shape, and their function is depressed progressively. These changes in arterial wall structure lead to an increased elastic modulus (Fig. 6) with age and a decrease in arterial distensibility and compliance [14, 15]. This increase in arterial rigidity increases the pulse wave velocity and reflected wave amplitude and causes an increase in systolic blood pressure; this, in turn, increases the incidence of stroke, cardiac failure, and all-cause mortality [16, 17]. Other macroscopic findings with aging are a progressive increase in artery diameter, wall thickness, intima–medial thickness, and pulse wave velocity [18]. The increase in the mean distal abdominal aortic stiffness and internal diameter with age was found to be gender dependent, with a greater increase occurring in males.

Vascular Impedance

As its name implies, the term "impedance" is a measure of the opposition to flow presented by a system. Etymologically, the term "resistance" conveys the same meaning as does impedance, but it is confined to non-oscillatory or steady motions. In another sense, clinicians frequently use the term "impedance" to refer to the impediment or hindrance to blood flow [19, 20]. When the general term is applied to the vascular system, it is usually in reference to the input impedance, this being the ratio between pulsatile pressure and pulsatile flow recorded in an artery feeding a particular vascular bed. The input impedance has to do with the input to the entire vascular tree beyond this site; it depends not only on the local arterial

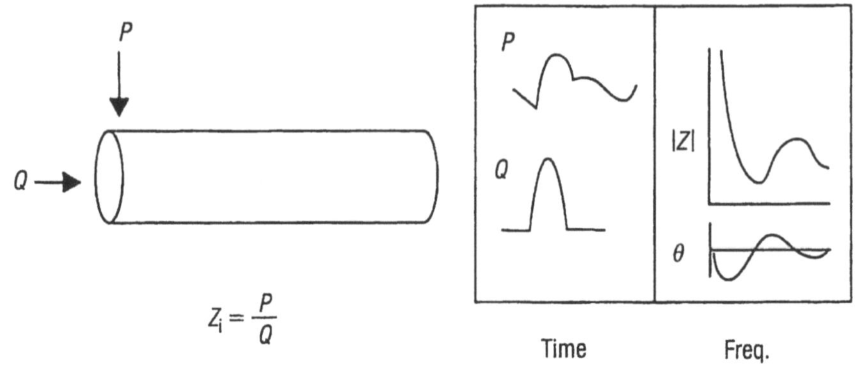

Fig. 7 Diagrammatic representation of the input impedance concept (*left*) and a representation of modulus (|Z|) and phase (θ) (*right*)

properties but also on the properties of all vessels in the vascular bed beyond, down to the point where all pulsations generated by the heart have been attenuated [10].

The input impedance modulus of any region of the arterial system is the ratio of harmonic terms of pressure at the input to the corresponding harmonic terms of flow. Therefore, the ratio of pulsatile pressure to pulsatile flow in the common carotid artery determines the input impedance of the cerebral arterial system. The simplest model of the arterial system is the Windkessel, with lumped capacitance and resistance elements [21, 22]. The term "Windkessel" means "air-chamber" in German. The input impedance can be expressed as the modulus and phase (Fig. 7). At the input of a Windkessel, the impedance modulus falls from its high value at zero frequency, which is determined by its resistive value, to low values at high frequency, which are determined by the magnitude of capacitance in relation to resistance, whereas the phase is zero at zero frequency and becomes progressively more negative (flow leading pressure) at higher frequencies.

Let us consider the effects of the elasticity of the arterial wall on the hemodynamics using an equivalent electrical circuit for the aortic system represented in Fig. 7. If we assume that the arterial wall is rigid, the value of the capacitance is zero, and we can analyze blood flow using the Poiseuille equation. The input flow to the arterial system equals the sum of the outflow of blood from the arterial system into the venous system and the rate of storage:

$$Q_{\text{in}} = Q_{\text{out}} + Q_{\text{stored}} = \frac{p(t)}{R} = 0. \tag{10}$$

If the arterial wall loses its elastic properties ($C=0$), the rate of storage is zero, and the blood from the heart flows into the capillaries directly. In this situation, no phase difference exists between the curves for flow and for pressure. Conversely, when the arterial wall has compliance, a portion of the ejected cardiac output flows into the arterial system, and the rest is stored in the arterial wall (i.e., the rate of storage is not zero). The remaining volume is supplied to the peripheral vessels during diastole. This process can be described mathematically as

$$Q_{\text{in}} = Q_{\text{out}} + Q_{\text{stored}} = \frac{p(t)}{R} + \frac{\text{dVolume}}{\text{d}t} = \frac{p(t)}{R} + C\frac{\text{d}p(t)}{\text{d}t}. \tag{11}$$

When the elasticity of an artery (capacitance, C) varies from 1.9 to 0.1 with constant resistance R, the peak blood pressure decreases markedly from 350 to near 100 mm Hg. Conversely, when the resistance varies from 10 to 100 with constant elasticity (C), only a minor increase in blood pressure is observed. These facts demonstrate the important role of the elasticity of the arterial wall in regulating blood pressure and the risk of hypertension due to atherosclerosis.

Conclusion

To understand hemodynamics in the cerebral arteries, the basic concepts of fluid mechanics are essential. Moyamoya disease is a cerebrovascular disease that involves, at least in part, hemodynamic factors. Recent advances in computer technology and medical imaging equipment have provided quantitative insight into the hemodynamics of complex arterial systems by combining these numerical and experimental techniques [23]. Phase-contrast magnetic resonance angiography and transcranial Doppler are noninvasive techniques for measuring regional cerebral blood flow in real time [24, 25]. The determination of the hemodynamics in cerebral arteries using these ultra-sophisticated technologies will contribute to the diagnosis and treatment of moyamoya disease.

References

1. Isogai Y, Yokose T, Maeda T et al (1984) The OP-Rheometer system, a new device for analysis of viscosity and viscoelasticity of blood: description and clinical application. Biorheology 1:s35–s41
2. De Backer TL, De Buyzere M, Segers P et al (2002) The role of whole blood viscosity in premature coronary artery disease in women. Atherosclerosis 165:367–373
3. von Tempelhoff G, Nieman F, Heilmann L et al (2000) Association between blood rheology, thrombosis and cancer survival in patients with gynecologic malignancy. Clin Hemorheol Microcirc 22:107–130
4. Brooks DE, Goodwin JW, Seaman GVF (1970) Interactions among erythrocytes under shear. J Appl Physiol 28:172–177
5. Gupta BB, Seshadri V (1977) Flow of red blood-cell suspensions through narrow tubes. Biorheology 14:133–143
6. Fox RW, McDonald AT (1998) Introduction to fluid mechanics, 5th edn. Wiley, New York
7. Cho YI, Kensey KR (1991) Effects of the non-Newtonian viscosity of blood on flows in a diseased arterial vessel. 1. Steady flows. Biorheology 28:241–262
8. White FM (1991) Viscous fluid flow. McGraw-Hill, Singapore
9. Malek AM, Alper SL, Izumo S (2009) Hemodynamic shear stress and its role in atherosclerosis. JAMA 282:2035–2042
10. Nichols WW, O'Rourke MF (2005) McDonald's blood flow in arteries, 5th edn. Oxford University Press, New York
11. Lanne T, Stale H, Bengtsson H et al (1992) Noninvasive measurement of diameter changes in the distal abdominal aorta in man. Ultrasound Med Biol 18:451–457
12. Celermajer DS, Sorensen KE, Bull C (1994) Endothelium-dependent dilation in the systemic arteries of asymptomatic subjects relates to coronary risk factors and their interaction. J Am Coll Cardiol 24:1468–1474
13. Smith AR, Hagen TM (2003) Vascular endothelial dysfunction in aging: loss of Akt-dependent endothelial nitric oxide synthase phosphorylation and partial restoration by (R)-alpha-lipoic acid. Biochem Soc Trans 31:1447–1449
14. Gozna ER, Marble AE, Shaw A (1974) Age-related changes in the mechanics of the aorta and pulmonary artery of man. J Appl Physiol 36:407–411
15. McGrath BP, Liang YL, Teede H (1998) Age-related deterioration in arterial structure and function in postmenopausal women: impact of hormone replacement therapy. Arterioscler Thromb Vasc Biol 18:1149–1156

16. Schram MT, Henry RM, van Dijk RA et al (2004) Increased central artery stiffness in impaired glucose metabolism and type 2 diabetes: the Hoorn Study. Hypertension 43:176–181
17. Sonesson B, Hansen F, Stale H et al (1993) Compliance and diameter in the human abdominal-aorta - the influence of age and sex. Eur J Vasc Surg 7:690–697
18. Agmon Y, Khandheria BK, Meissner I et al (2003) Is aortic dilatation an atherosclerosis-related process? J Am Coll Cardiol 42:1076–1083
19. Wilcken DEL, Guz A, Charlier AA et al (1964) Effects of alterations in aortic impedance on performance of ventricles. Circ Res 14:283–293
20. Finkelstein SM, Cohn JN, Collins VR et al (1985) Vascular hemodynamic impedance in congestive heart failure. Am J Cardiol 55:423–427
21. Stergiopulos N, Meister JJ, Westerhof N (1995) Evaluation of methods for estimation of total arterial compliance. Am J Physiol 268:H1540–1548
22. Van Huis GA, Sipkema P, Westerhof N (1987) Coronary input impedance during cardiac cycle as determined by impulse response method. Am J Physiol 253:H317–324
23. Lee SW, Antiga L, Spence JD et al (2008) Geometry of the carotid bifurcation predicts its exposure to disturbed flow. Stroke 39:2341–2347
24. Zhao M, Amin-Hanjani S, Ruland S et al (2007) Regional cerebral blood flow using quantitative MR angiography. Am J Neuroradiol 28:1470–1473
25. Tsivgoulis G, Alexandrov AV, Sloan MA (2009) Advances in transcranial Doppler ultrasonography. Curr Neurol Neurosci Rep 9:46–54

Regional Predilection of Lesions and Stages of Moyamoya Disease

Ho Jun Seol

Introduction

Moyamoya disease (MMD) is an idiopathic entity characterized by progressive occlusion of the distal internal carotid arteries (ICAs), as well as the proximal anterior artery (ACA) and middle cerebral artery (MCA). Although the vast majority of cases are sporadic, familial factors have been implicated in a small subset of cases. The frequency of familial occurrence of MMD is estimated to be approximately 7–10% of all reported cases [1] and the incidence among Asians is high. In addition, studies looking at the pathogenesis of MMD have uncovered both genetic predisposing factors as well as acquired factors. Single nucleotide polymorphism, sickle cell anemia, and neurofibromatosis are among some of the purported genetic factors. Acquired conditions such as tuberculosis meningitis infection and atherosclerosis have also been identified [2].

From an anatomical standpoint, the primary structural abnormalities in vessels afflicted with MMD entail smooth muscle cell proliferation and migration, which ultimately manifest as intimal thickening [3].

A similar phenomenon is observed in vessels of the heart, kidney, and other organs [4]. These observations might suggest that systemic factors could play a role in the pathogenesis of MMD. Such factors include nitric oxide (NO), vascular endothelial growth factor, platelet derived growth factor, and alpha-1 antitrypsin. Nevertheless, the etiology of MMD as well as its initial predilection for the distal ICA, proximal MCA, and proximal ACA remains unclear. Hemodynamic changes as well as factors within the intracranial vasculature have been hypothesized to play a role. Recent investigations have therefore focused on regional changes with respect to intracranial blood flow. This chapter will introduce computational modeling to study cerebral regional hemodynamic parameters with the goal of ascertaining why specific vascular regions are affected by MMD.

H.J. Seol (✉)
Department of Neurosurgery, Kangwon National University Hospital, 17-1, Hyoja 3-dong, Chuncheon, Kangwon-do, 200-722, Republic of Korea
e-mail: junoseol@kangwon.ac.kr

B.-K. Cho and T. Tominaga (eds.), *Moyamoya Disease Update*,
DOI 10.1007/978-4-431-99703-0_15, © Springer 2010

Methods and Hemodynamic Factors That are Crucial to the Study of Regional Predilection of MMD

Over the years, many different techniques have been employed to predict regional blood flow and hemodynamic changes in patients with MMD. These studies have included SPECT, perfusion MRI, EEG, and TCD, amongst others. However, while the above techniques provided useful data with respect to regional hemodynamics, they were not adept at elucidating why MMD had a preference for certain points of cerebral vessels. Furthermore, performing measurements on small vessels such as the cerebral arteries is usually fraught with significant technical challenges. The above dilemma therefore required construction of a simplified disease model for investigation of local hemodynamic factors in normal condition of brain. Computerized mathematical models have been very useful in this regards. Recently, it became possible to delineate most properties in all of the regions of interest, using a numerical analysis. Burleson et al. [5] reported that blood flow simulation results in intracranial saccular and lateral aneurysms. Moore et al. [6] analyzed the hemodynamics of cerebral arteries using three-dimensional models. In cardiovascular disease, shear stress is concerned with the automatic regulation of constriction and dilation of the arteries. In other words, from a mechanical point of view, autoregulation is defined as a mechanism to preserve shear stress to normal levels [7]. Biochemically, vasoconstrictors and vasodilators like endothelin and NOS_3 [8], respectively, play a critical in the autoregulation of vessels. The diameter of the vessel is regulated by the contraction or relaxation of smooth muscle. When the shear stress of the vessel decreases, endothelin is secreted which results in vascular smooth muscle contraction. This in turn results in narrowing of the vessel diameter, as well as increased velocity of flow. With increased velocity, the shear stress is eventually restored to normal levels. Therefore, the interplay between shear stress and biochemical mediators is very critical to the autoregulatory mechanism of cardiovascular contraction and dilation [9].

How Is the Hemodynamics in Distal ICA and/or BA?

Recently, the author and colleagues tried computational analysis of hemodynamic changes within predilection sites of MMD. We hypothesized that a state of continuous low shear stress may result to stimulation, proliferation as well as smooth muscle migration into the intima of the vessel. We used a commercial finite element package, Automatic Dynamics Incremental Nonlinear Analysis (ADINA, version 7.0; Watertown, MA) to simulate the fluid dynamics in the cerebral arteries. Using this method, we performed computational analysis for the major intracranial vessels related to MMD to investigate the possible relation between the hemodynamic factors and the arterial regions of stenosis in MMD.

Using normal reference data for diameter of cerebral arteries in the literature [10] and several normal CT angiographic data, we presented a two-dimensional model using Autocad (2005 version; AutoDesk, San Rafael, CA). Model geometry was performed using mesh system of Hypermesh (version 3.0; Altair, Troy, MI) and analyzed by a commercial finite element package, ADINA. We modeled the blood flow in cerebral arteries as transient, incompressible, and viscous fluid. Blood viscosity and density were assumed to be 0.403 kg $m^{-1} s^{-1}$ and 1,040 kg m^{-3}, respectively. Models of ICA and basilar artery (BA) are shown in Fig. 1, where the markings, indicated by each number in the figure, denote the points of interest for numerical comparison.

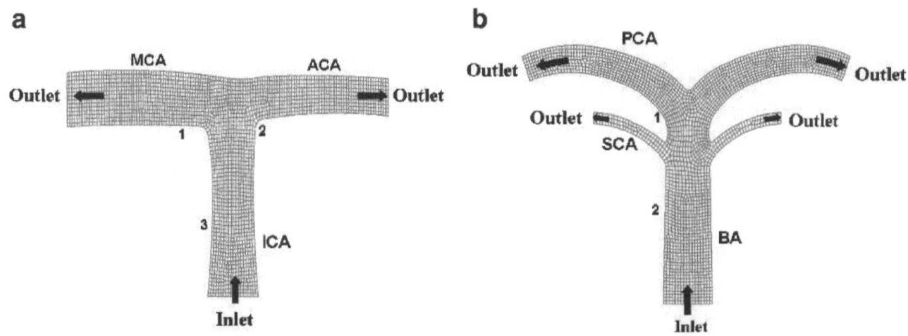

Fig. 1 Two-dimensional models. (**a**) ICA bifurcation model at an angle of 90° showing the calculating lattice, which was made up by Hypermesh. (**b**) BA bifurcation model, which was made by the same manner with the ICA model. *ACA* anterior cerebral artery, *MCA* middle cerebral artery, ICA internal carotid artery, *PCA* posterior cerebral artery, *SCA* superior cerebellar artery, *BA* basilar artery

Pulsatory waveform of 280 mm s^{-1} of maximum velocity was obtained by the analysis of the blood flow velocity. This maximum velocity was established as an inlet boundary condition for the ICA and BA. A fully developed velocity profile was assumed in the inlet. The formula for the velocity distribution in the inlet can be expressed as follows.

$$u(r) = V_C\left[1-\left(\frac{2r}{D}\right)^2\right] \tag{1}$$

Here, u and V_C are the velocity in the axial direction and the maximum axial velocity at the centerline of the vessel, respectively, r is a radial coordinate, whereas D is the diameter of the vessel. This axial velocity represents the parabolic distribution along radial direction at the inlet surface. We applied a traction-free boundary condition for the outlet.

In the ICA model of MMD, the predisposing areas of proximal MCA and proximal ACA (points 1 and 2, respectively) and the nonpredisposing area of ICA (point 3) were evaluated in view of shear stress (Fig. 2a).

In our simulation, points 1 and 2 in the ICA model showed lower values of shear stress. These points are located at the proximal MCA and ACA, which are the predisposing vascular areas in real MMD patients. This coincidence of low shear stress points and predisposing areas of MMD may suggest that the low shear stress or turbulent flow in a certain point can act as a stimulus for smooth muscle proliferation or migration. Furthermore, if there is a superimposed systemic factor such as a genetic or acquired vascular disorder associated with a local hemodynamic stimulus, that could synergistically contribute to smooth muscle proliferation and migration in a patient with MMD.

In the demonstration of velocity vector (Fig. 2b), a difference of velocity between proximal ACA and MCA was observed. This discrepancy might have been caused by the slightly larger diameter of MCA compared to that of ACA in this model. The velocity in the lower stream of MCA is lower than the velocity in the upper stream of MCA. Turbulent flow developed in the ACA by the MCA flow effect.

In the BA model of MMD (Fig. 3a, b), the predisposing area of proximal posterior cerebral artery (PCA; point 1) and the nonpredisposing area of mid-BA (point 2) were compared to each other. However, the difference of shear stress between points 1 and 2 in the BA model was not noticeably large, as it was comparable to that of the ICA model. Such a difference

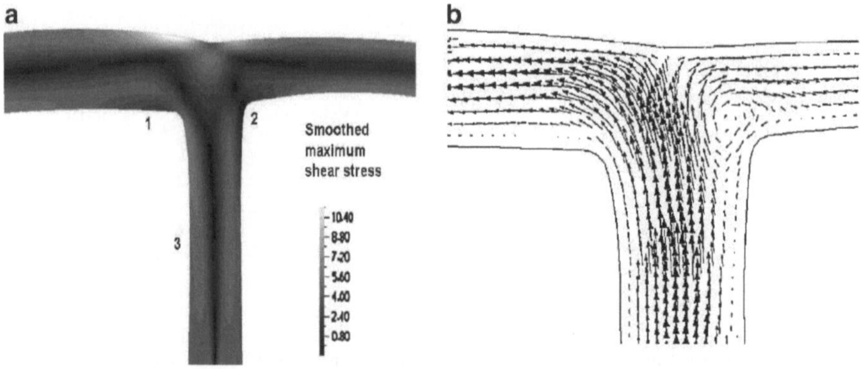

Fig. 2 Numerical data of the ICA bifurcation model. (**a**) Shear stress contour and the variable data according to the point were shown. (**b**) Velocity vector showing the lower velocity in the lower stream of MCA (near to the point 1) and turbulent flow on the point 2

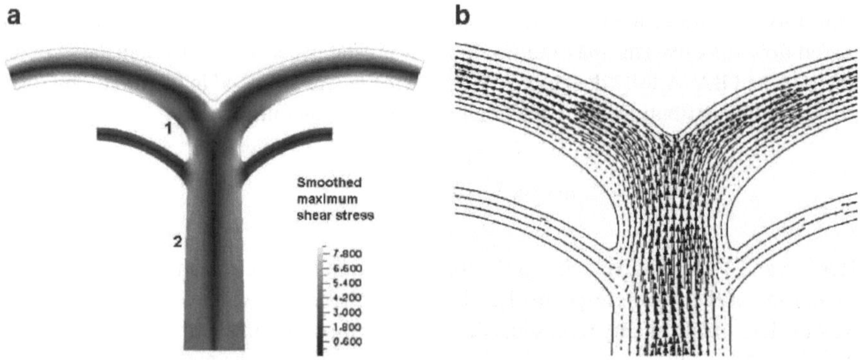

Fig. 3 Numerical data of the BA bifurcation model. (**a**) Shear stress contour and the variable data according to the point were demonstrated. (**b**) Velocity vector showing the symmetrical distribution

may be related to the real clinical condition, in which anterior circulation of ICA is involved first and posterior circulation of PCA is affected later in advanced stages.

Could This Hemodynamic Factor of Shear Stress Be an Etiology of This Predilection?

Intimal thickening is the histologic pathological hallmark of MMD. It is the aftermath of proliferation and migration of smooth muscle cells from the media to the intima by uncertain systemic factors [3].

The role of hemodynamics in intimal changes has been extensively studied in acquired cardiovascular artherosclerotic disease. In particular, changes related to shear stress have been implicated in this process. It has been demonstrated, for instance, that if shear stress levels are lowered below the physiological minimum threshold, morphologically changes can be appreciated within endothelial cells [11]. In the normal state, smooth muscle contraction serves as a means to preserve shear stress. Repeated contraction and relaxation from stimulation, can result in the proliferation of smooth muscle cells [11].

The mechanism of how this discrepancy between the ICA and the BA models developed can be explained by a three-dimensional study, which uses models more similar to real vessels. However, in the future, studies that incorporate more complex flow patterns could further enhance our understanding of MMD. For example, there is reverse flow into posterior circulation through the posterior communicating artery, as the stenosis of distal ICA progresses. Besides, there can be additional concurrent vascular diseases such as aortic arch syndrome or renal artery stenosis. These vessels may share a similar pathophysiology with the cerebrovascular predisposing points in MMD. The fluid–solid interface remodeling, which reflects thickness and property of the vessel wall, can be beneficial in the simulation of dynamic status in MMD.

How Is the Hemodynamic Change Higher According to the Stage of MMD?

Within the literature, there is only a single report assessing cerebral blood flow after surgical therapy [12]. The authors examined various conditions including direct and indirect bypass surgery. They calculated the possible additional blood flow associated with each condition and also ascertained the best treatment option.

Nonetheless, there are technical challenges associated with simulating the complex and dynamic situation. For instance, the flow of anterior system circulation would decrease as the obstruction of ICA progresses. In addition, posterior circulation would be more important in compensating the depletion of cerebral blood volume. Therefore, we have to simulate each Suzuki grade. Of course, three-dimensional models should be simulated before and after bypass surgery. To our knowledge, there is not yet any published paper concerning these points of view.

Even if further studies are necessary, analysis of hemodynamics by computational models of two-dimensional geometries of normal distal ICA suggests that a continuous low shear stress in predisposing areas may promote the stenosis via proliferation and migration of smooth muscle cells in MMD, especially in patients who have genetic predispositions or systemic factors.

References

1. Kaneko Y, Imamoto N, Mannoji H et al (1998) Familial occurrence of moyamoya disease in the mother and four daughters including identical twins. Neurol Med Chir (Tokyo) 38:349–354
2. Suzuki J, Kodama N (1983) Moyamoya disease – a review. Stroke 14:104–109
3. Aoyagi M, Fukai N, Yamamoto M et al (1997) Development of intimal thickening in superficial temporal arteries in patients with moyamoya disease. Clin Neurol Neurosurg 2(99 Suppl):213–217
4. Ikeda E, Hosoda Y (1992) Spontaneous occlusion of the circle of Willis (cerebrovascular moyamoya disease): with special reference to its clinicopathological identity. Brain Dev 14:251–253
5. Burleson AC, Strother CM, Turitto VT (1995) Computer modeling of intracranial saccular and lateral aneurysms for the study of their hemodynamics. Neurosurgery 37:774–782
6. Moore S, David T, Chase JG et al (2006) 3D models of blood flow in the cerebral vasculature. J Biomech 39:1454–1463

7. Wootton DM, Ku DN (1999) Fluid mechanics of vascular systems, diseases, and thrombosis. Annu Rev Biomed Eng 1:299–329
8. Rubanyi GM, Romero JC, Vanhoutte PM (1986) Flow-induced release of endothelium-derived relaxing factor. Am J Physiol 250:1145–1149
9. Chiu JJ, Chen LJ, Lee PL et al (2003) Shear stress inhibits adhesion molecule expression in vascular endothelial cells induced by coculture with smooth muscle cells. Blood 101:2667–2674
10. Krabbe-Hartkamp MJ, van der Grond J, de Leeuw FE et al (1998) Circle of Willis: morphologic variation on three-dimensional time-of-flight MR angiograms. Radiology 207:103–111
11. Davies PF, Spaan JA, Krams R (2005) Shear stress biology of the endothelium. Ann Biomed Eng 33:1714–1718
12. Charbel FT, Misra M, Clarke ME et al (1997) Computer simulation of cerebral blood flow in moyamoya and the results of surgical therapies. Clin Neurol Neurosurg 2(99 Suppl):68–73

Part VI
Clinical Features

Clinical Features of Moyamoya Disease: An Overview

Yong-Seung Hwang

Introduction

The two cardinal clinical features of moyamoya disease are ischemic attacks or intracranial hemorrhages. However, the main clinical presentations of moyamoya disease differ substantially between children and adults. Most children with moyamoya disease develop transient ischemic attacks (TIA) or cerebral infarction, whereas about half of the adult patients develop intracranial hemorrhage, and half develop TIA or cerebral infarction, or both [1]. Regarding the ethnic difference, clinical features and the course of moyamoya disease in whites clearly differ from moyamoya disease in Asians in the timing of the onset of vasculopathy and lower rate of hemorrhage [2].

Ischemic Attacks

The most frequently noticed clinical pattern of moyamoya disease, especially in pediatric patients, is recurrent TIAs without remaining neurologic sequelae. The focal neurologic findings, including hemiparesis that may alternate sides, dysarthria, aphasia, or sensory disturbance, resolve within a few hours. The TIAs are characteristically induced by hyperventilation or breath-holding, for example when crying or playing a wind instrument or harmonica [3]. Some patients may experience an attack after blowing on and eating hot and spicy noodles. These neurologic events appear to have a vasoreactive mechanism responsive to an acid–base imbalance, not simply thromboembolic mechanisms [4].

The EEG change produced by hyperventilation in moyamoya disease will be presented in the chapter by J. Chae, this volume. Young children often cannot specify the ischemic symptoms and complain just of vague weakness or fatigue.

The hemiparesis should be differentiated from the postictal Todd's palsy. Besides TIAs, recurrent infarcts and rapid disease progression are frequently seen in moyamoya disease

Y.-S. Hwang (✉)
Department of Pediatrics, Pediatric Clinical Neuroscience Center,
Seoul National University Children's Hospital, Seoul National University College of Medicine,
101 Daehangno, Jongno-gu, Seoul 110-744, Republic of Korea
e-mail: childnr@snu.ac.kr

B.-K. Cho and T. Tominaga (eds.), *Moyamoya Disease Update*,
DOI 10.1007/978-4-431-99703-0_16, © Springer 2010

presenting prior to age 6 years [5]. Over time, moyamoya disease can remain stable, but more typically follows a progressive course with severe motor impairment and intellectual deterioration [6].

Intracranial Hemorrhage

Although ischemic attacks may occur in adult patients, intracerebral, intraventricular, or subarachnoid hemorrhage occurs more frequently than in children. About half of adult patients with moyamoya disease develop intracranial bleeding. After cerebral hemorrhage, severely disabled and lethal outcomes may follow.

Two main causes of intracranial bleeding in moyamoya disease are rupture of dilated, fragile moyamoya vessels or rupture of saccular aneurysms in the circle of Willis. The hemorrhage due to persistent hemodynamic stress of the moyamoya vessels occurs in the basal ganglia, thalamus, or periventricular region. Intraventricular hemorrhage is frequently complicated [7]. Peripheral aneurysms in the collateral vessels or moyamoya vessels might be identified on cerebral angiography in some patients [8]. The second cause, rupture of saccular aneurysms located around the circle of Willis occurs most commonly at the basilar artery bifurcation or at the junction of the basilar artery and the superior cerebellar artery. The vertebrobasilar system has an important role in providing collateral circulation in patients with moyamoya disease. Thus, hemodynamic stress probably induces the formation of a saccular aneurysm in the vertebrobasilar system; rupture of a saccular aneurysm causes subarachnoid hemorrhage [8]. There is increasing evidence that moyamoya disease in adults might induce subarachnoid hemorrhage over the cerebral cortex despite the absence of an intracranial aneurysm [9]. A third cause of intracranial bleeding in adult patients with moyamoya disease is rupture of the dilated collateral arteries on the brain surface, although this is rare [10]. Pregnancy and childbirth might increase the risk of ischemic or hemorrhagic stroke in women who are treated either medically or surgically for moyamoya disease. This issue will be discussed in the chapter by J. Takahashi, this volume.

Seizure, Headache, Involuntary Movement and Other Neurologic Symptoms

Convulsion is the third most common manifestation of moyamoya disease in children [6]. About 20–30% of cases present with seizures [11]. Recurrent seizure attacks in moyamoya disease should be regarded as symptomatic localization-related epilepsy and may be manifested as secondarily generalized tonic–clonic convulsions [12]. The clinical features and course of moyamoya disease with epilepsy are the same as moyamoya disease with TIA or infarction [13]. Unusual absence epilepsy, intractable to medical therapy, associated with moyamoya disease has been reported [14].

Progressive cognitive decline and mental retardation is present in more than half of the cases, and patients with onset of cerebral ischemia before 5 years of age usually develop progressive mental retardation [15].

Headache and involuntary movement associated with moyamoya disease are discussed in the chapters by R. Shirane and S. Nogawa S, respectively, in this volume.

An atypical case of adult moyamoya disease with initial onset of brainstem ischemia has been reported. The patient initially presented with left hemisensory disturbance caused by a pontine lesion, followed by a myelopathy of the upper cervical spinal cord [16]. Visual disturbance and nonspecific psychic disturbance are listed in the signs and symptoms of moyamoya disease [6].

References

1. Kuroda S, Houkin K (2008) Moyamoya disease: current concepts and future perspectives. Lancet Neurol 7:1056–1066
2. Kraemer M, Heienbrok W, Berlit P (2008) Moyamoya disease in Europeans. Stroke 39:3193–3200
3. Fukui M, Kono S, Sueishi K et al (2000) Moyamoya disease. Neuropathology 20:S61–S64
4. Mikulis DJ, Krolczyk G, Desal H et al (2005) Preoperative and postoperative mapping of cerebrovascular reactivity in moyamoya disease by using blood oxygen level-dependent magnetic resonance imaging. J Neurosurg 103:347–355
5. Kim S, Seol HJ, Cho B et al (2004) Moyamoya disease among young patients: its aggressive clinical course and the role of active surgical treatment. Neurosurgery 54:840–846
6. Suzuki J, Kodama N (1983) Moyamoya disease – a review. Stroke 14:104–109
7. Irikura K, Miyasaka Y, Kurata I et al (1996) A source of haemorrhage in adult patients with moyamoya disease: the significance of tributaries from the choroidal artery. Acta Neurochir (Wien) 138:1282–1286
8. Kawaguchi S, Sakaki T, Morimoto T et al (1996) Characteristics of intracranial aneurysms associated with moyamoya disease. A review of 111 cases. Acta Neurochir (Wien) 138:1287–1294
9. Marushima A, Yanaka K, Matsuki T et al (2006) Subarachnoid hemorrhage not due to ruptured aneurysm in moyamoya disease. J Clin Neurosci 13:146–149
10. Osanai T, Kuroda S, Nakayama N et al (2008) Moyamoya disease presenting with subarachnoid hemorrhage localized over the frontal cortex: case report. Surg Neurol 69:197–200
11. Yonekawa Y, Kahn N (2003) Moyamoya disease. Adv Neurol 92:113–118
12. Manceau E, Giroud M, Dumas R (1997) Moyamoya disease in children. A review of the clinical and radiological features and current treatment. Childs Nerv Syst 13:595–600
13. Nakase H, Ohnishi H, Touho H et al (1993) Long-term follow-up study of "epileptic type" moyamoya disease in children. Neurol Med Chir (Tokyo) 33:621–624
14. Kikuta K, Takagi Y, Arakawa Y et al (2006) Absence epilepsy associated with moyamoya disease. Case report. J Neurosurg (4 Suppl Pediatrics) 104:265–268
15. Moritake K, Handa H, Yonekawa Y et al (1986) Follow-up study on the relationship between age at onset of illness and outcome in patients with moyamoya disease. No Shinkei Geka 14:957–963
16. Hirano T, Uyama E, Tashima K et al (1998) An atypical case of adult moyamoya disease with initial onset of brain stem ischemia. J Neurol Sci 157:100–104

Headache in Moyamoya Disease

Reizo Shirane and Miki Fujimura

Introduction

Moyamoya disease is a chronic, occlusive cerebrovascular disease with unknown etiology characterized by bilateral steno-occlusive changes at the terminal portion of the internal carotid artery and an abnormal vascular network at the base of the brain [1]. Clinical presentation of moyamoya disease includes transient ischemic attack (TIA), cerebral infarction, intracerebral hemorrhage, and seizure [2]. TIA is one of the most common clinical presentations of moyamoya disease both in pediatric and adult cases [2], while intracerebral hemorrhage is mostly seen among adult cases [3]. Recently, headache is also considered to be one of the common clinical presentations of moyamoya disease. Patients with moyamoya disease may complain of headache before and after revascularization surgery. In this chapter, the authors focus on headache as the clinical presentation of moyamoya disease, and discuss the incidence and mechanism of this symptom. We further discuss the efficacy of revascularization surgery for the improvement of headache.

Headache as the Common Clinical Presentation of Moyamoya Disease

The Research Committee on Spontaneous Occlusion of the Circle of Willis, of the Ministry of Health, Labor, and Welfare, Japan, has classified the onset-type of moyamoya disease to "hemorrhage," "epilepsy," "cerebral infarction," "TIA," and "crescendo TIA (more than two

R. Shirane
Department of Neurosurgery, Miyagi Children's Hospital, 4-3-17 Ochiai, Aoba-ku, Sendai 989-3126, Japan

M. Fujimura (✉)
Department of Neurosurgery, Kohnan Hospital, 4-20-1 Nagamachi-minami, Taihaku-ku, Sendai 982-8523, Japan
e-mail: fujimur@kohnan-sendai.or.jp

B.-K. Cho and T. Tominaga (eds.), *Moyamoya Disease Update*,
DOI 10.1007/978-4-431-99703-0_17, © Springer 2010

Table 1 Onset-type of 962 patients with moyamoya disease

Onset-type	Number of patients
Transient ischemic attack (TIA)	353 (37%)
Cresiendo TIA	63 (7%)
Cerebral infarction	165 (17%)
Intracranial hemorrhage	186 (19%)
Headache	57 (6%)
Seizure	29 (3%)
Asymptomatic	32 (3%)
Others	13 (1%)
Unclear	64 (7%)

attacks per month)." More recently, "headache" was included as one of the onset-type in 2003 by this committee. Based on the most recent survey by this committee, 57 patients (6%) suffered from headache as the initial symptom among 962 patients with moyamoya disease (Table 1) [2]. Besides these presentations, the recent advance in noninvasive diagnostic modalities such as magnetic resonance (MR) imaging and MR angiography has led to the realization that the incidence of asymptomatic moyamoya disease could be higher than previously thought [4], accounting for 3% (32 patients as the initial symptom) among 962 moyamoya patients [2]. Based on the author's experience, a substantial number of "asymptomatic" adult patients have headache as their potential complaint, though they are classified to "asymptomatic" patients. They are suspected to have suffered from TIA in their childhood, which spontaneously resolved during their adolescence by the decreasing demand of cerebral blood flow in their adolescence and adulthood. Such patients sometimes complain of headache without ischemic symptoms even after the disappearance of TIA. According to the survey by the association of patients with moyamoya disease and their families, more than 50% of the patients with moyamoya disease, including both preoperative and postoperative status, complain of headache.

Headache and Revascularization Surgery

Patients with moyamoya disease often complain of headache before surgery, after surgery, or in both periods, and the symptom is one of the major complaints in moyamoya disease. Preoperative headache was considered to be related to hypoperfusion because it has been reported that headaches could disappear after revascularization surgery [5]. Such phenomenon is especially documented after indirect pial synangiosis for pediatric moyamoya disease. It was considered to be a sort of migraine or to be derived from hemodynamic changes, while the exact cause was undetermined [6]. Seol and colleagues reviewed 204 consecutive surgical cases with pediatric moyamoya disease, and found that preoperative headache was present in 21.6% (44 of 204) of the patients and was one of their major symptoms [7]. Postoperative headache was seen in 63% (28 of 44) of the patients with preoperative headache, and in 6.3% (10 of 160) of those without preoperative headache. Notably, the aggravation on postoperative MR imaging or single-photon emission computed tomography scan did not correlate with this symptom, suggesting that progressive recruitment and redistribution

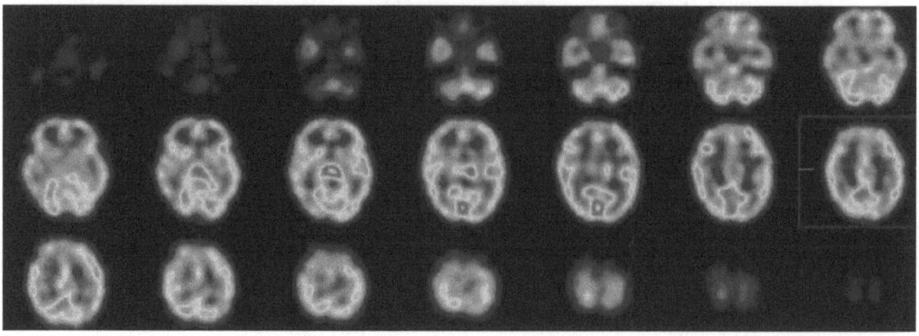

Fig. 1 *N*-isopropyl-*p*-[^{123}I] iodoamphetamine single-photon emission computed tomography in a 14-year-old female presenting with significant headache and weakness on her left lower extremity, indicating her cerebral blood flow at the vascular territory of right anterior cerebral artery was markedly compromised

of blood flow, as well as the hemodynamic compromise, could be the cause of headaches in patients with moyamoya disease [7]. The author performed direct revascularization surgery (superficial temporal artery–middle cerebral artery anastomosis) for 13 patients with significant headache with apparent hemodynamic compromise. As a result, 11 of 13 (84.6%) patients showed marked improvement of their symptom after surgery. A 14-year-old female was admitted to our clinic suffering from significant headache and weakness on her left lower extremity 6 years after successful direct/indirect revascularization during her childhood. Medication was not effective for her headache, and single-photon emission computed tomography scan demonstrated decreased cerebral blood flow at the vascular territory of right anterior cerebral artery (Fig. 1), while direct/indirect revascularization was well visualized by MR angiography (Fig. 2). Then she underwent right occipital artery–posterior cerebral artery anastomosis as the salvage surgery [8]. Her weakness and headache completely disappeared after surgery, indicating that direct revascularization surgery improved her cerebral hemodynamics and could thereby relieve headache. In light of the hypothesis that progressive recruitment of indirect pial synangiosis stimulates trigeminal nerve and thus causes headache, direct revascularization surgery may have more potential benefit for improving headache by rapid improvement of cerebral blood flow and ameliorating the demand for the development of pial synangiosis.

Conclusion

Headache is one of the common clinical presentations of moyamoya disease. Patients with moyamoya disease may complain of headache before and after revascularization surgery. Although the underlying mechanism and optimal treatment of such headache are undetermined, the decreased cerebral blood flow, and the progressive recruitment and redistribution of blood flow are thought to be a cause of headache in patients with moyamoya disease. The revascularization surgery, direct revascularization surgery in particular, may have potential benefit for improving headache by relieving the hemodynamic compromise.

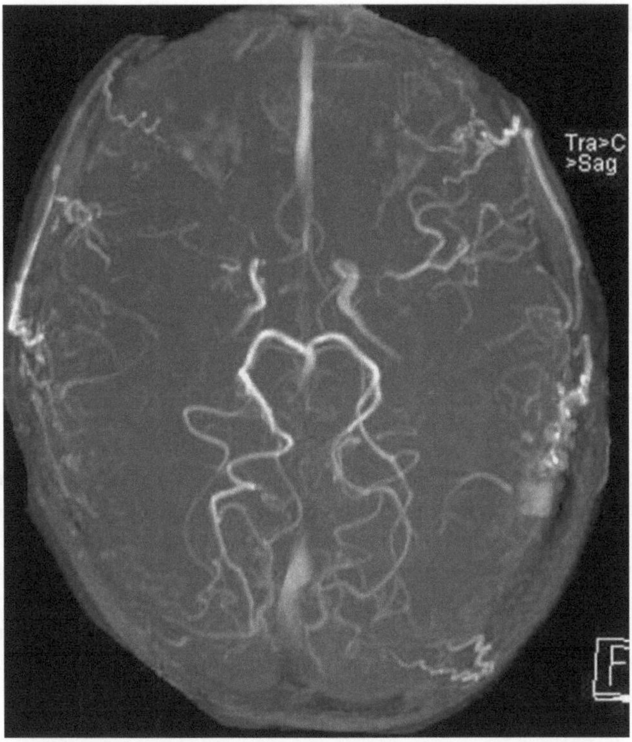

Fig. 2 A 14-year-old female presenting with significant headache and weakness on her left lower extremity. Magnetic resonance (MR) angiography, 6 years after direct/indirect revascularization surgery for ischemic-onset moyamoya disease, indicates that both direct and indirect anastomosis were well demonstrated

References

1. Suzuki J, Takaku A (1969) Cerebrovascular 'moyamoya' disease. Disease showing abnormal net-like vessels in base of brain. Arch Neurol 20:288–299
2. Oki K, Suzuki N (2007) In: Hashimoto N (ed) Report by the Research Committee on Spontaneous Occlusion of the Circle of Willis (Moyamoya Disease) pp. 4–5
3. Yoshida Y, Yoshimoto T, Shirane R et al. (1999) Clinical course, surgical management, and long-term outcome of moyamoya patients with rebleeding after an episode of intracerebral hemorrhage: an extensive follow-up study. Stroke 30:2272–2276
4. Kuroda S, Hashimoto N, Yoshimoto T et al. (2007) Radiological findings, clinical course, and outcome in asymptomatic moyamoya disease. Results of multi-center survey in Japan. Stroke 38:1430–1435
5. Matsushima Y, Aoyagi M, Niimi Y et al. (1990) Symptoms and their pattern of progression in childhood moyamoya disease. Brain Dev 12:784–789
6. Scott RM, Smith JL, Robertson RL et al. (2004) Long-term outcome in children with moyamoya syndrome after cranial revascularization by pial synangiosis. J Neurosurg 100(2 Suppl Pediatrics):142–149
7. Seol HJ, Wang KC, Kim SK et al. (2005) Headache in pediatric moyamoya disease: review of 204 consecutive cases. J Neurosurg 103(5 Suppl Pediatrics):439–442
8. Hayashi T, Shirane R, Tominaga T (2009) Additional surgery for postoperative ischemic symptoms in patients with moyamoya disease. The effectiveness of occipital artery-posterior cerebral artery bypass with an indirect procedure: technical case report. Neurosurgery 64:E95–96

Involuntary Movement

Shigeru Nogawa and Norihiro Suzuki

Introduction

Moyamoya disease is an idiopathic cerebrovascular disease characterized by progressive steno-occlusion of the arteries of the circle of Willis, accompanied by collateral vessel formation in the basal ganglia [1, 2]. Involuntary movements are relatively rare symptoms of this condition, and their frequency is estimated to range from 3 to 6% [3–5]. However, the incidence could be higher, if limb shaking, a specific type of transient ischemic attack (TIA), is also included. In this chapter, we focus on moyamoya disease-induced involuntary movements, and the patient characteristics, symptoms, underlying mechanisms, and treatment of this condition are discussed.

Characteristics of the Patients

In regard to the sex predilection of moyamoya disease associated with involuntary movements, females are more frequently affected than males, just as for the other subtypes of moyamoya disease (ratio 1:1.8) [6]. The female predominance appears to be particularly marked for the disease associated with chorea (ratio 1:4) [7]. Pregnancy might be a risk factor for movement disorders associated with this disease, as discussed below. The age at onset varies from infancy to young adulthood and is identical to that for the ischemic subtypes of the disease. Usually, severe occlusive changes in the terminal portion of the internal carotid artery are found on the side opposite to that of the affected limbs, or on both sides.

S. Nogawa (✉)
Department of Neurology, Tokyo Dental College Ichikawa General Hospital,
5-11-13 Sugano, Ichikawa, Chiba 272-8513, Japan
e-mail: snogawa@tdc.ac.jp

N. Suzuki
Department of Neurology, Keio University School of Medicine, 35 Shinanomachi, Shinjuku-ku,
Tokyo 160-8582, Japan

B.-K. Cho and T. Tominaga (eds.), *Moyamoya Disease Update*,
DOI 10.1007/978-4-431-99703-0_18, © Springer 2010

Symptoms

Association of a wide variety of movement disorders with moyamoya disease has been reported in the literature. The spectrum of these involuntary movements includes chorea [4, 5, 7, 8], choreo-athetosis [9], dyskinesia [7, 10], dystonia [9, 11–13], limb shaking [14], and epilepsia partialis continua [7]. Some of these occur in a paroxysmal manner, while others can be triggered by the initiation of some movement ("kinesigenic") [7], by some particular form of exercise [13], or by various types of hyperventilation maneuvers. The movements are usually transient, ranging in duration from several seconds to a few months, and rarely constant.

Mechanisms

The main mechanism of onset of these involuntary movements is thought to be cerebral ischemia induced by steno-occlusion of the arteries of the circle of Willis. Any exercises inducing hyperventilation, such as singing [8] and crying [5, 11], and any emotional excitement [5], may precipitate the symptom, because they produce cerebral vasoconstriction. This hypothesis is supported by the fact that revascularization surgery is associated with resolution of the involuntary movements [15] or at least a significant decrease in their frequency. Although the classical lesion sites in patients with choreo-athetosis are the basal ganglia [16, 17], especially the striatum [13, 18], recent evidence has revealed that any disconnection between the basal ganglia and the cerebral cortex, even subcortical white matter lesions, can cause involuntary movements [12, 19–22] by interrupting the "Alexander–Crutcher" circuits [23]. For example, limb shaking is typically triggered by diffuse hemispheric hypoperfusion caused by severe stenosis of the internal carotid artery [24, 25]. Similarly, in moyamoya disease, limb shaking and other involuntary movements are thought to be induced by intracranial major arterial occlusion [14, 26]. Indeed, in moyamoya patients with hemichorea, diffuse hemispheric hypoperfusion on the side opposite to that of the affected limbs has been observed in SPECT and PET images [9, 10, 12, 22, 27].

Another possible mechanism is perturbation of sex hormones [7], because hormonal changes have been reported to be involved in the pathophysiology of chorea (i.e., "chorea gravidarum" or estrogen-induced chorea [28, 29]). In a review of moyamoya disease and pregnancy, Komiyama and colleagues [30] suggested that this condition may appear or worsen during pregnancy. Gonzalez-Alegre et al. [7] also described a patient who developed chorea at the end of the first trimester of her pregnancy. Unno et al. [31] reported that the chorea observed in a pregnant girl completely subsided after abortion. These reports suggest that increased sex hormones during pregnancy may trigger chorea by enhancing the dopaminergic sensitivity of the basal ganglia. Oral contraceptive drugs may also be a risk factor for the development of chorea [32] or even moyamoya disease itself.

The third plausible mechanism is hyperthyroidism [33], which has also been implicated in the development of moyamoya disease itself [34]. Hyperthyroidism may be a predisposing factor for chorea [35, 36], presumably by modifying the functions of the basal ganglia through increasing the sensitivity of the dopaminergic receptors. Furthermore, thyroid hormones may also control the expression of the genes regulating the motor functions in the central nervous system.

Treatment

As is the case for involuntary movements associated with other conditions, haloperidol is very effective for controlling the choreic movements associated with moyamoya disease [15, 27]. Pavlakis et al. [4] reported a moyamoya patient with chorea who responded to steroid therapy. Direct and/or indirect [14] bypass surgeries have been suggested to be beneficial, via normalizing the cerebral hypoperfusion [37]. Although both are reported to be effective, more prompt effects can be expected following direct bypass with or without indirect bypass (within 2 days [22] to a few weeks [10]) than following indirect bypass alone (several months [37, 38]). The optimal revascularization procedure is selected according to the patient's age, symptoms, and findings on cerebral perfusion images.

Conclusion

Patients with moyamoya disease can present with various types of involuntary movements, especially chorea, as the initial symptom. Therefore, when such involuntary movements are observed, careful consideration should be given to excluding moyamoya disease. Although the underlying mechanism is still not fully understood, interruption of the basal ganglia–thalamocortical circuits by diffuse hemispheric hypoperfusion, rather than focal ischemia, seems to play a pivotal role. The predominance of the condition in females and the role of sex hormones remain to be elucidated.

References

1. Kudo T (1968) Spontaneous occlusion of circle of Willis. Neurology 18:485–496
2. Suzuki J, Takaku A (1969) Cerebrovascular "moyamoya" disease. Disease showing abnormal net-like vessels in base of brain. Arch Neurol 20:288–299
3. Maki Y, Enomoto T (1988) Moyamoya disease. Childs Nerv Syst 4:204–212
4. Pavlakis SG, Schneider S, Black K et al (1991) Steroid-responsive chorea in moyamoya disease. Mov Disord 6:347–349
5. Watanabe K, Negoro T, Maehara M et al (1990) Moyamoya disease presenting with chorea. Pediatr Neurol 6:40–42
6. Kuriyama S, Kusaka Y, Fujimura M et al (2008) Prevalence and clinicoepidemiological features of moyamoya disease in Japan: findings from a nationwide epidemiological survey. Stroke 39:42–47
7. Gonzalez-Alegre P, Ammache Z, Davis PH et al (2003) Moyamoya-induced paroxysmal dyskinesia. Mov Disord 18:1051–1056
8. Han SH, Kim YG, Cha SH et al (2000) Moyamoya disease presenting with singing induced chorea. J Neurol Neurosurg Psychiatry 69:833–834
9. Lyoo CH, Oh SH, Joo JY et al (2000) Hemidystonia and hemichoreoathetosis as an initial manifestation of moyamoya disease. Arch Neurol 57:1510–1512
10. Hong YH, Ahn TB, Oh CW et al (2002) Hemichorea as an initial manifestation of moyamoya disease: reversible striatal hypoperfusion demonstrated on single photon emission computed tomography. Mov Disord 17:1380–1383
11. Bakdash T, Cohen AR, Hempel JM et al (2002) Moyamoya, dystonia during hyperventilation, and antiphospholipid antibodies. Pediatr Neurol 26:157–160
12. Li JY, Lai PH, Peng NJ (2007) Moyamoya disease presenting with hemichoreoathetosis and hemidystonia. Mov Disord 22:1983–1984

13. Lyoo CH, Kim DJ, Chang H et al (2007) Moyamoya disease presenting with paroxysmal exercise-induced dyskinesia. Parkinsonism Relat Disord 13:446–468
14. Im SH, Oh CW, Kwon OK et al (2004) Involuntary movement induced by cerebral ischemia: pathogenesis and surgical outcome. J Neurosurg 100:877–882
15. Hama A, Furune S, Nomura K et al (2001) A case of unilateral moyamoya disease presenting with hemichorea. No To Hattatsu 33:166–171 (in Japanese)
16. Martin JP (1957) Hemichorea (hemiballismus) without lesions in the corpus Luysii. Brain 80:1–10
17. Bhatia KP, Marsden CD (1994) The behavioural and motor consequences of focal lesions of the basal ganglia in man. Brain 117 (Pt 4):859–876
18. Ikeda M, Tsukagoshi H (1991) Monochorea caused by a striatal lesion. Eur Neurol 31:257–258
19. Barinagarrementeria F, Vega F, DelBrutto OH (1989) Acute hemichorea due to infarction in the corona radiata. J Neurol 236:371–372
20. Ringelstein E, Stögbauer F (2001) Border zone infarcts. In: Bogousslavsky J, Caplan L (eds) Stroke syndromes. Cambridge University Press, Cambridge, pp 564–582
21. Kosakai A, Nogawa S, Tanahashi N et al (2002) Vascular hemichorea in a patient with a persistent primitive trigeminal artery and ipsilateral occlusion of the internal carotid artery: pathological significance of subcortical white matter lesions induced by hypoperfusion. JMDD 12:93–100 (in Japanese)
22. Zheng W, Wanibuchi M, Onda T et al (2006) A case of moyamoya disease presenting with chorea. Childs Nerv Syst 22:274–278
23. Alexander GE, Crutcher MD (1990) Functional architecture of basal ganglia circuits: neural substrates of parallel processing. Trends Neurosci 13:266–271
24. Baquis GD, Pessin MS, Scott RM (1985) Limb shaking – a carotid TIA. Stroke 16:444–448
25. Yanagihara T, Piepgras DG, Klass DW (1985) Repetitive involuntary movement associated with episodic cerebral ischemia. Ann Neurol 18:244–250
26. Kim HY, Chung CS, Lee J et al (2003) Hyperventilation-induced limb shaking TIA in moyamoya disease. Neurology 60:137–139
27. Miura T, Kobayashi M, Sonoo M et al (2002) An adult case of moyamoya disease presenting with transient hemichorea. Rinsho Shinkeigaku 42:45–47 (in Japanese)
28. Barber PV, Arnold AG, Evans G (1976) Recurrent hormone dependent chorea: effects of oestrogens and progestogens. Clin Endocrinol (Oxf) 5:291–293
29. Caviness JN, Muenter MD (1991) An unusual cause of recurrent chorea. Mov Disord 6:355–357
30. Komiyama M, Yasui T, Kitano S et al (1998) Moyamoya disease and pregnancy: case report and review of the literature. Neurosurgery 43:360–368
31. Unno S, Iijima M, Osawa M et al (2000) A case of chorea gravidarum with moyamoya disease. Rinsho Shinkeigaku 40:378–382 (in Japanese)
32. Leys D, Destee A, Petit H et al (1987) Chorea associated with oral contraception. J Neurol 235:46–48
33. Garcin B, Louissaint T, Hosseini H et al (2008) Reversible chorea in association with Graves' disease and moyamoya syndrome. Mov Disord 23:620–622
34. Sasaki T, Nogawa S, Amano T (2006) Co-morbidity of moyamoya disease with Grave's disease. Intern Med 45:649–653
35. Pozzan GB, Battistella PA, Rigon F et al (1992) Hyperthyroid-induced chorea in an adolescent girl. Brain Dev 14:126–127
36. Ristic AJ, Svetel M, Dragasevic N et al (2004) Bilateral chorea-ballism associated with hyperthyroidism. Mov Disord 19:982–983
37. Kamijo K, Matsui T (2008) Dramatic disappearance of moyamoya disease-induced chorea after indirect bypass surgery. Neurol Med Chir (Tokyo) 48:390–393
38. Kim YO, Kim TS, Woo YJ et al (2006) Moyamoya disease-induced hemichorea corrected by indirect bypass surgery. Pediatr Int 48:504–506

Progression of Moyamoya Disease

Kentaro Hayashi and Izumi Nagata

Introduction

Moyamoya disease is characterized by progressive stenosis of the terminal portion of the internal carotid artery (ICA) and its main branches [1]. The disease associated with the development of dilated, fragile collateral vessels at the base of the brain, which are termed moyamoya vessels [1]. Regardless of the course, moyamoya disease inevitably progresses in the majority of patients.

Angiographical Progression

Angiographically, moyamoya disease progress along with the six-stages introduced by Suzuki [1]. Firstly, stenosis appears in the terminal portion of the ICA and the proximal portion of the anterior cerebral artery (ACA) and middle cerebral artery bilaterally. Development of an extensive collateral network at the base of the brain along with the classic "puff of smoke" appearance on angiography is seen in the intermediate stage. "Basal moyamoya" includes abnormal dilatation of the perforating arteries, such as the lenticulostriate artery and the thalamo-perforating artery, in the basal ganglia and thalamus. The occlusive process also involves the posterior circulation, including the basilar and posterior cerebral arteries. Total occlusion of the ICA terminal results in disappearance of "basal moyamoya," and simultaneous development of other collateral circulation is observed in the advanced stage. "Ethmoidal moyamoya" involves dilation of the anterior and posterior ethmoidal arteries, which also function as a collateral pathway, mainly from the ophthalmic artery to the ACA branches [2]. Finally, the collateral flow from the dural arteries to pial

K. Hayashi (✉) and I. Nagata
Department of Neurosurgery, Nagasaki University School of Medicine,
1-7-1 Sakamoto, Nagasaki-city 852-8501, Japan
e-mail: kenkuni@net.nagasaki-u.ac.jp

B.-K. Cho and T. Tominaga (eds.), *Moyamoya Disease Update*,
DOI 10.1007/978-4-431-99703-0_19, © Springer 2010

arteries develops and this pathway is known as "vault moyamoya" [2]. Most of the patients present with intermediate stages and are treated promptly; therefore, the advanced stage is nowadays rarely seen [3].

Age and Progression

The incidence peaks in two age groups: children who are approximately 5 years of age and adults in their mid-40s [2]. Whether there are any differences in etiology or other characteristics between pediatric and adult moyamoya disease except for the age of onset is unclear. Despite the progressive nature of the occlusive lesions in pediatric patients, the prevalence of the progression in adult patients is undetermined. Occlusive lesions in the carotid terminal commonly worsen in pediatric patients and carry high morbidity and mortality [4] (Fig. 19.1). The disease progresses along with the angiographic stage until adolescence, but almost stabilizes by the age of 20 years [5, 6]. In some cases, the first symptoms appear in adulthood [7]. Disease progression in adult-onset moyamoya disease was previously believed to be very rare. However, increasing evidence suggests that a substantial number of the patients with adult-onset moyamoya disease also presented progression of steno-occlusive lesions and that disease progression occurs in 10–20% of patients [8, 9] (Fig. 2).

Unilateral to Bilateral

The official diagnosis criteria of the Research Committee on Spontaneous Occlusion of the Circle of Willis (Moyamoya Disease) classified that definite cases of moyamoya disease are diagnosed in patients with bilateral lesion, whereas patients with unilateral lesion are diagnosed as probable cases [10]. Progression of carotid arterial systems is not always symmetrical. Bilateral lesions are likely to develop within 1–2 years in young children with unilateral evidence of moyamoya disease, whereas lesions in adults tend to remain unilateral [11–14]. Furthermore, unilateral patients with contralateral equivocal arterial stenotic changes are at an increased risk of progression [15]. Based on these results, the diagnosis criteria were modified in 1988 as follows: pediatric unilateral lesion with contralateral stenosis is sufficient to be definite moyamoya disease. Patients with adult-onset unilateral lesion tend not to progress to bilateral, and this condition is influenced with other etiology, i.e., arteriosclerosis. Therefore, they are distinguished from moyamoya disease. However, they should be carefully followed-up to monitor potential progression to bilateral lesion since the incidence of progression to bilateral disease might be higher than previously thought [8, 16–18].

Those Who Are Likely to Progress

Incidence of disease progression is higher in female patients than in male patients [11]. Contralateral abnormalities seen on initial imaging, i.e., equivocal arterial stenotic changes, congenital cardiac anomalies, previous cranial irradiation, Asian ethnic origin, and familial moyamoya disease are associated with an increased risk of disease progression [15, 19].

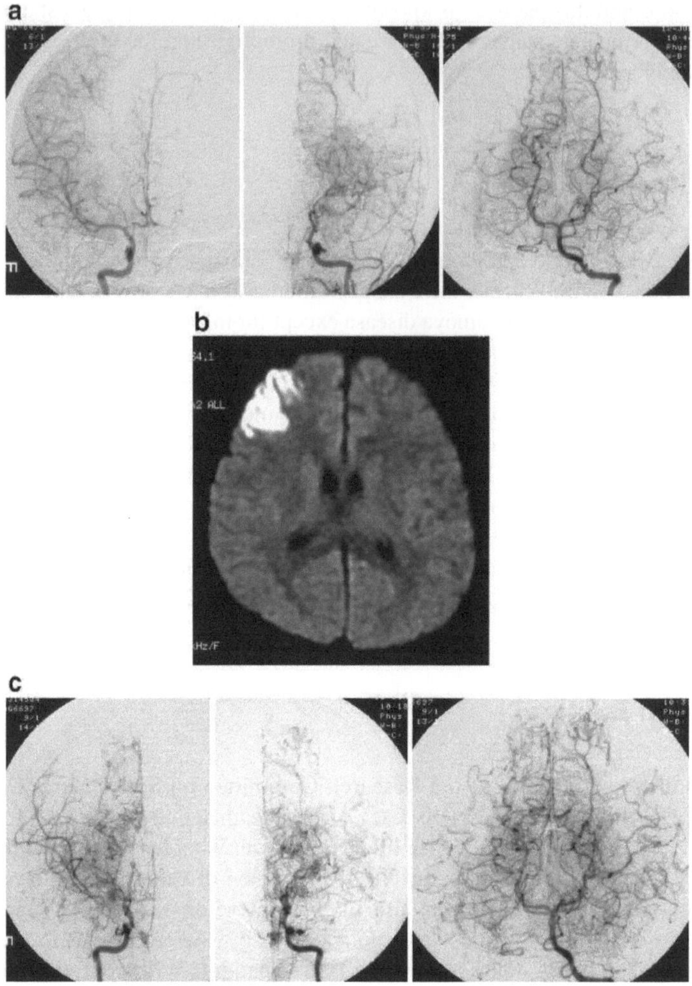

Fig. 1 Typical progression of moyamoya disease in a 3-year-old boy, who presented with transient ischemic attack. Angiography showed occlusion of the terminal portion of the left internal carotid artery (ICA) and stenosis of the proximal portion of the right anterior cerebral artery (ACA). Moyamoya vessels were seen on the left side (**a**). One year later, he developed left hemiparesis and MRI diffusion-weighted image revealed fresh infarction in the right frontal lobe (**b**). Angiography demonstrated high-grade stenosis in the terminal portion of the right ICA. Moyamoya vessels were seen in bilaterally. Collateral flow from posterior cerebral arteries was developed (**c**)

Mechanism of Progression

Levels of many growth factors, enzymes, and other peptides, including basic fibroblast growth factor, transforming growth factor-β1, hepatocyte growth factor, vascular endothelial growth factor, matrix metalloproteinase, intracellular adhesion molecule, and hypoxia-inducible factor-1α, have been reported to be increased in association of with fibrocellular thickening of the intima or neovascularization, and may be related to the disease progression [20–23].

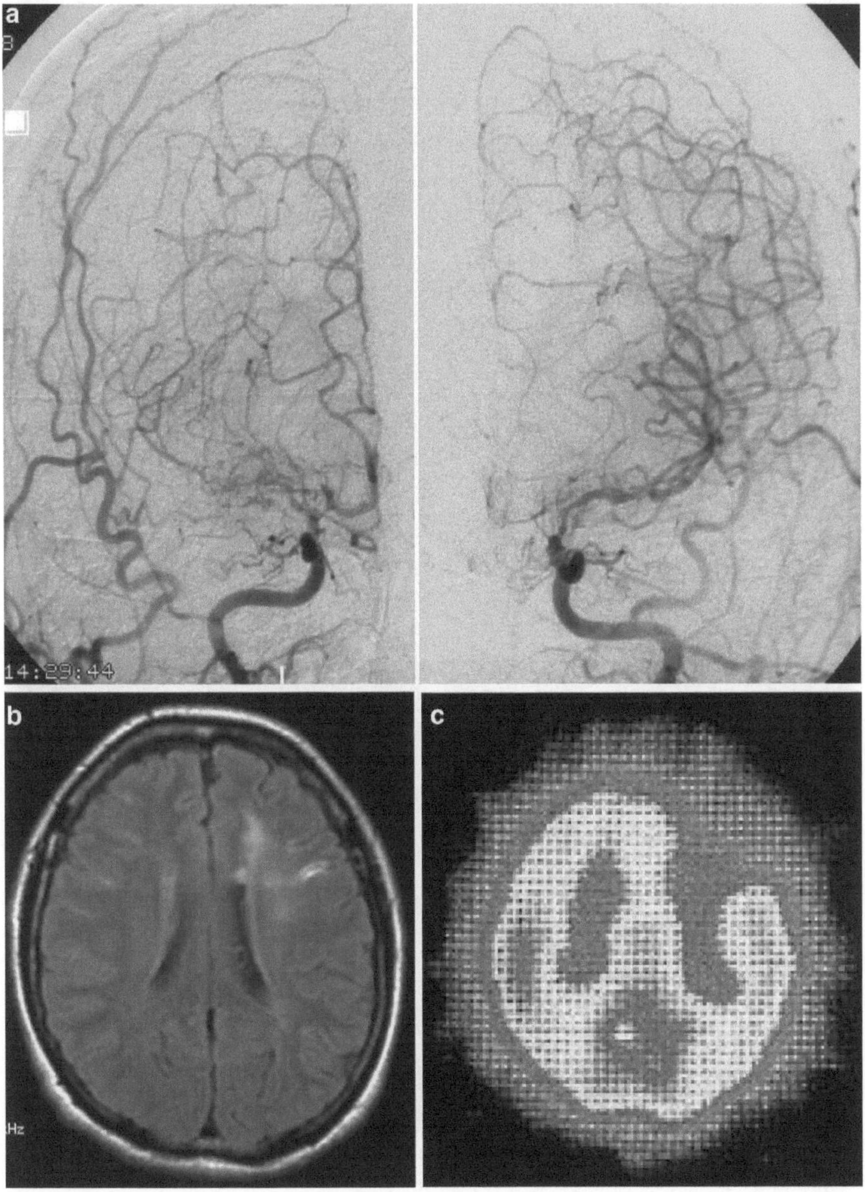

Fig. 2 Progression of moyamoya disease in a 40-year-old woman, who was diagnosed incidentally. Angiography demonstrated high-grade stenosis of the terminal portion of the bilateral ICA. Moyamoya vessels were seen on the right side (**a**). MRI fluid-attenuated inversion recovery (FLAIR) image showed ischemic lesion in the left frontal deep white matter (**b**). Left frontal hyoperfusion was revealed by single photon emission tomography (**c**). Four years later, she experienced transient ischemic attack and angiography revealed occlusion of the right ACA and left ICA. Moyamoya vessels were seen especially on the left side (**d**). MRI FLAIR image showed widespread left frontal infarction (**e**) and cerebral blood flow was impaired in the bilateral frontal region (**f**)

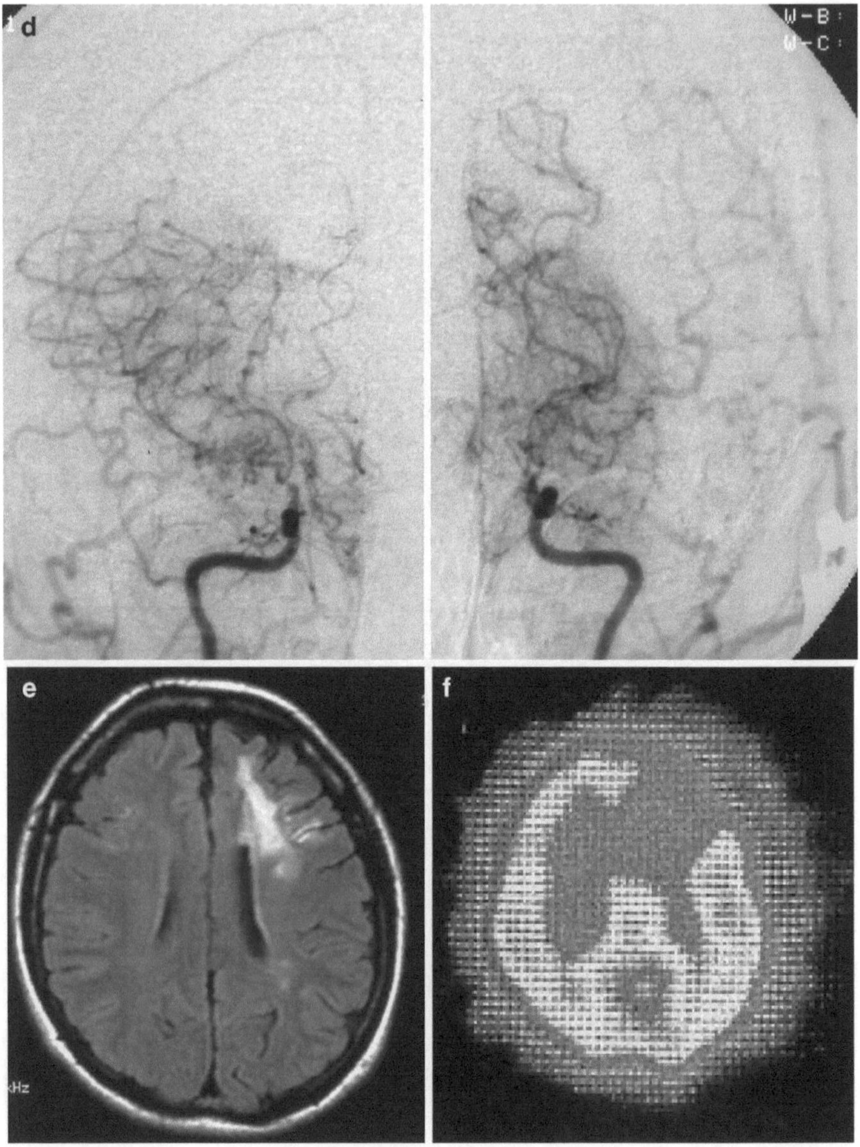

Fig. 2 (continued)

Progression of Clinical Sign

The clinical features of moyamoya disease differ substantially between children and adults. Most pediatric patients have ischemic attacks, whereas adult patients can have ischemic attacks, intracranial bleeding, or both [2]. The angiographic stage in patients with hemorrhagic onset is not significantly different from those with ischemic onset [3]. Moyamoya disease usually causes some cerebral ischemia in the territory of the ICA, particularly in the frontal lobe [21, 22]. Therefore, most patients with moyamoya disease present with focal neurological signs, such as dysarthria, aphasia, or hemiparesis. In the cases of poor development of these collateral circulations, a high tendency of mental retardation is noted [6]. There are two main causes of intracranial bleeding in moyamoya disease: rupture of dilated, fragile moyamoya vessels or rupture of saccular aneurysm in the circle of Willis [24]. Rebleeding is the most important factor in the poor outcomes of patients with hemorrhagic moyamoya disease and occurs at an increased rate when patients reach the age of 46–55 years [25]. Since asymptomatic moyamoya disease is not a silent disorder and might potentially cause ischemic or hemorrhagic stroke, careful follow-up is warranted by routine radiological study [26].

Imaging Studies to Detect Progression

MRI, including T2-weighted and fluid-attenuated inversion recovery image, is useful to identify the ischemic and hemorrhagic lesions in the brain. An acute infarct is more likely to be detected with the use of diffusion-weighted image. Magnetic resonance angiography (MRA) is also useful to follow-up the progression of moyamoya disease in a noninvasive way. Regarding cerebral circulation analysis, pediatric patients have lower cerebral blood flow, particularly after ischemic stroke, and the distribution typically shows posterior dominance [27]. Cerebrovascular reactivity to acetazolamide or carbon dioxide is widely impaired in the territory of the ICA [28]. Cerebral hemodynamics and metabolism can change substantially after effective surgical revascularization [28].

Influence of Bypass Surgery to Progression

No medical treatment has been used to prevent progression of moyamoya disease. Bypass surgery is considered to be effective for improving cerebral blood flow and metabolism and preventing progression. The incidence of ischemic attack rapidly decreases after bypass surgery and rebleeding might also be reduced. Moyamoya vessels start to regress after bypass surgery, and the deep temporal artery and the middle meningeal artery increase their calibers and can be identified by MRA [29]. Stenotic change in the carotid terminal quickly progress after surgery [30].

Conclusions

Regardless of the course, moyamoya disease inevitably progresses in the majority of patients. Once a patient manifests the progression of cerebrovascular occlusive lesion or ischemic symptoms, bypass surgery should be performed for the affected hemisphere after the confirmation of the flow compromise.

References

1. Suzuki J, Takaku A (1969) Cerebrovascular "moyamoya" disease. Disease showing abnormal net-like vessels in base of brain. Arch Neurol 20:288–299
2. Suzuki J, Kodama N (1983) Moyamoya disease-a review. Stroke 14:104–109
3. Houkin K, Yoshimoto T, Kuroda S et al (1996) Angiographic analysis of moyamoya disease-how does moyamoya disease progress? Neurol Med Chir (Tokyo) 36:783–788
4. Kim SK, Seol HJ, Cho BK et al (2004) Moyamoya disease among young patients: its aggressive clinical course and the role of active surgical treatment. Neurosurgery 54:840–846
5. Ezura M, Yoshimoto T, Fujiwara S et al (1995) Clinical and angiographic follow-up of childhood-onset moyamoya disease. Childs Nerv Syst 11:591–594
6. Takahashi A, Fujiwara S, Suzuki J (1986) Long-term follow-up angiography of moyamoya disease-cases followed from childhood to adolescence. No Shinkei Geka 14:23–29
7. Tomida M, Muraki M, Yamasaki K (2000) Angiographically verified progression of moyamoya disease in an adult. Case report. J Neurosurg 93:1055–1057
8. Kuroda S, Ishikawa T, Houkin K et al (2005) Incidence and clinical features of disease progression in adult moyamoya disease. Stroke 36:2148–2153
9. Narisawa A, Fujimura M, Tominaga T (2009) Efficacy of the revascularization surgery for adult-onset moyamoya disease with the progression of cerebrovascular lesions. Clin Neurol Neurosurg 111:123–126
10. Fukui M (1997) Guidelines for the diagnosis and treatment of spontaneous occlusion of the circle of Willis ('moyamoya' disease). Research Committee on Spontaneous Occlusion of the Circle of Willis (Moyamoya Disease) of the Ministry of Health and Welfare, Japan. Clin Neurol Neurosurg 2(99 Suppl):S238–S240
11. Kawano T, Fukui M, Hashimoto N et al (1994) Follow-up study of patients with "unilateral" moyamoya disease. Neurol Med Chir (Tokyo) 34:744–747
12. Kurose K, Kishi H, Nishijima Y (1991) Moyamoya disease developing from bilateral moyamoya disease. Neurol Med Chir (Tokyo) 31:597–599
13. Matsushima T, Take S, Fujii K et al (1988) A case of moyamoya disease with progressive involvement from unilateral to bilateral. Surg Neurol 30:471–475
14. Seol HJ, Wang KC, Kim SK et al (2006) Unilateral (probable) moyamoya disease: long-term follow-up of seven cases. Childs Nerv Syst 22:145–150
15. Kelly ME, Bell-Stephens TE, Marks MP et al (2006) Progression of unilateral moyamoya disease: a clinical series. Cerebrovasc Dis 22:109–115
16. Kagawa R, Okada Y, Moritake K et al (2004) Magnetic resonance angiography demonstrating adult moyamoya disease progressing from unilateral to bilateral involvement. Neurol Med Chir (Tokyo) 44:183–186
17. Murphy MJ (1980) Progressive vascular changes in moyamoya syndrome. Stroke 11:656–658
18. Wanifuchi H, Takeshita M, Aoki N (1996) Adult moyamoya disease progressing from unilateral to bilateral involvement. Neurol Med Chir (Tokyo) 36:87–90
19. Smith ER, Scott RM (2008) Progression of disease in unilateral moyamoya syndrome. Neurosurg Focus 24:E17
20. Houkin K, Abe H, Yoshimoto T et al (1996) Is "unilateral" moyamoya disease different from moyamoya disease? J Neurosurg 85:772–776
21. Kuroda S, Houkin K (2008) Moyamoya disease: current concepts and future perspectives. Lancet Neurol 7:1056–1066
22. Scott RM, Smith ER (2009) Moyamoya disease and moyamoya syndrome. N Engl J Med 360:1226–1237
23. Takagi Y, Kikuta K, Nozaki K et al (2007) Expression of hypoxia-inducing factor-1 alpha and endoglin in intimal hyperplasia of the middle cerebral artery of patients with Moyamoya disease. Neurosurgery 60:338–345
24. Kawaguchi S, Sakaki T, Morimoto T et al (1996) Characteristics of intracranial aneurysms associated with moyamoya disease. A review of 111 cases. Acta Neurochir (Wien) 138:1287–1294
25. Morioka M, Hamada J, Todaka T et al (2003) High-risk age for rebleeding in patients with hemorrhagic moyamoya disease: long-term follow-up study. Neurosurgery 52:1049–1055

26. Yamada M, Fujii K, Fukui M (2005) Clinical features and outcomes in patients with asymptomatic moyamoya disease – from the results of nation-wide questionnaire survey. No Shinkei Geka 33:337–342
27. Kuroda S, Ishikawa T, Houkin K et al (2002) Clinical significance of posterior cerebral artery stenosis/occlusion in moyamoya disease. No Shinkei Geka 30:1295–300
28. Honda M, Ezaki Y, Kitagawa N et al (2006) Quantification of the regional cerebral blood flow and vascular reserve in moyamoya disease using split-dose iodoamphetamine I 123 single-photon emission computed tomography. Surg Neurol 66:155–159
29. Honda M, Kitagawa N, Tsutsumi K et al (2005) Magnetic resonance angiography evaluation of external carotid artery tributaries in moyamoya disease. Surg Neurol 64:325–330
30. Houkin K, Nakayama N, Kuroda S et al (2004) How does angiogenesis develop in pediatric moyamoya disease after surgery? A prospective study with MR angiography. Childs Nerv Syst 20:734–741

Systemic Arterial Involvement in Moyamoya Disease

Hae Il Cheong and Yong Choi

Introduction

Moyamoya disease is a rare cerebrovascular occlusive disorder that is characterized by stenosis or occlusion of the distal internal carotid or proximal anterior or middle cerebral arteries, which causes the formation of multiple tiny collateral vascular networks (moyamoya vessels) at the base of the brain [1–3]. While this disorder commonly occurs alone (moyamoya disease), it occasionally occurs with well-recognized associated conditions including sickle cell disease, neurofibromatosis type I, cranial therapeutic irradiation, and Down syndrome (moyamoya syndrome) [4].

In addition to typical intracranial vascular lesions associated with moyamoya disease, steno-occlusive lesions of extracranial vessels including renal, coronary, pulmonary, mesenteric, and peripheral arteries have also been reported [5–31]. Among these extracranial arteries, moyamoya disease most commonly impacts the renal artery [12–31].

Prevalence of Renal Arterial Involvement in Moyamoya Disease

Although many studies have documented renal arterial involvement in patients with moyamoya disease [29–31], most of those papers were case reports, and there have been only three relatively large-scale systematic studies of renal arterial involvement in patients with moyamoya disease [29–31] (Table 1).

The first study was conducted by Choi et al. in 1997 [29], who performed a retrospective analysis of 72 Korean children with moyamoya disease and found that 6 (8.3%) of them had

H.I. Cheong (✉) and Y. Choi
Department of Pediatrics, Seoul National University Children's Hospital, 101, Daehang-ro, Jongno-gu, Seoul 110-769, Republic of Korea
Kidney Research Institute, Medical Research Center, Seoul National University College of Medicine, 103 Daehang-ro, Jongno-gu, Seoul 110-799, Republic of Korea
e-mail: cheonghi@snu.ac.kr

H.I. Cheong
Research Center for Rare Disease, Seoul National University Hospital, 101 Daehang-ro, Jongno-gu, Seoul 110-769, Republic of Korea

B.-K. Cho and T. Tominaga (eds.), *Moyamoya Disease Update*,
DOI 10.1007/978-4-431-99703-0_20, © Springer 2010

Table 1 Three large studies of renal arterial involvement in patients with moyamoya disease

Study	Subjects			Renal arterial lesion	Renovascular hypertension
	Nationality	Age	Number of patients		
Choi et al. [30]	Korean	children	72	stenosis in 6 (8.3%)	6 (8.3%)
Yamada et al. [31]	Japanese	all age	86	stenosis in 6 (7.0%) aneurysm in 1 (1.2%)	2 (2.3%)
Togao et al. [32]	Japanese	all age	73	stenosis in 4 (5.5%)	2 (2.7%)

renal artery stenosis and renovascular hypertension. The mean ages at the onset of the initial neurologic symptoms and at the detection of hypertension were 3.33 years (range, 0.75–7.08) and 7.87 years (range, 4.33–12.25), respectively. Renal arteriography revealed bilateral lesions in three of the patients and unilateral lesions in the other three patients. In addition to the renal artery, the superior mesenteric artery was also involved in one case and the external iliac artery was involved in another case. Abdominal bruit was audible in two patients. Basal plasma renin activity was elevated in all six cases. Renal ultrasonography and a captopril technetium 99 m-labeled dimercaptosuccinic acid renal scan revealed abnormal findings in four of five and in three of four available studies, respectively. However, both imaging studies only revealed abnormal findings in the more severely affected kidneys, even in cases of bilateral renal artery stenosis. In all six cases, the stenotic lesion was located in the proximal portion of the renal artery. Two patients were treated with antihypertensive drugs alone, while percutaneous transluminal balloon angioplasty of the stenotic renal arteries was performed in four cases. Balloon angioplasty was successful (normal blood pressure without further antihypertensive drug) in only one case and partially successful (normal blood pressure with antihypertensive drugs) in another case. In the remaining two cases, the catheter could not be introduced through the stenotic segment of the renal artery. One patient underwent autotransplantation of the left kidney after angioplasty failure, and the renal artery specimen obtained during the autotransplantation revealed intimal fibroplasias.

In 2000, Yamada et al. [30] analyzed the cerebral angiography and abdominal aortography findings, which were prospectively performed in 86 consecutive Japanese patients of all ages with idiopathic moyamoya disease. They found renal arterial lesions in seven patients (8.1%, 2 children and 5 young adults), stenosis in six patients (7.0%), and a small saccular aneurysm in one patient (1.2%). Two patients (2.3%) with marked renal artery stenosis presented with renovascular hypertension, which was successfully treated by balloon angioplasty in both cases. There was no significant correlation between the presence of renal arterial lesions and the gender or age of the patient, or the cerebral angiographic findings.

In 2004, Togao et al. [31] performed another large-scale study of renal and abdominal arterial involvement in moyamoya disease. They retrospectively reviewed the abdominal angiography of 73 Japanese patients of all ages with idiopathic moyamoya disease and found unilateral renal artery stenosis in four (5.5%) patients, including a moderate degree of stenosis in three patients and mild stenosis in one patient. In the three patients with moderate stenosis, the renal artery stenosis was located in the proximal region of the main branch. Two patients (3%) with moderate stenosis of the unilateral renal artery had renovascular hypertension. No statistically significant differences were observed in age, sex, and the cerebral angiographic stage of patients with and without renal artery stenosis. Additionally, no stenosis or occlusions were found in other extracranial arteries.

Radiologic and Pathologic Findings of Renal Arteries Involved in Moyamoya Disease

In most cases of moyamoya disease, in which the renal artery was involved, renal artery stenosis tended to involve the proximal one-third of the main branch [15,17,21,29,31]. Differential diagnosis of renal artery stenosis and/or renovascular hypertension includes atherosclerosis, Takayasu's arteritis, and fibromuscular dysplasia. Renal arterial lesions in fibromuscular dysplasia usually involve relatively distal segment of the main branch with a typical string-of-beads appearance. However, atherosclerosis and Takayasu's arteritis often involve the proximal region of the renal artery, which would make it difficult to differentiate them from moyamoya disease based on angiographic appearance alone [32,33].

Although the definitive cause and pathogenesis of moyamoya disease remain unclear, pathologic studies of the steno-occlusive lesions of the cerebral vessels typically reveal fibrous thickening of the intima with a small amount of lipid deposition. Inflammatory cell infiltration is not noted in the vascular walls, and the internal elastic lamina is well preserved [3,34]. Ikeda [7] conducted careful histopathologic examination and morphologic analysis of extracranial vessels in 13 autopsy cases of moyamoya disease and found similar findings of intimal fibrous thickening in the extracranial vessels. Taken together, these findings suggest that moyamoya disease is likely to have systemic factors as well as focal etiologic factors, and that the former factors may be responsible for extracranial vascular change. In addition, several other studies have reported intimal thickening of the extracranial vessels of patients with moyamoya disease, and this thickening has been found to be advanced relative to their ages [5,12,15,20,24,29] (Fig. 1).

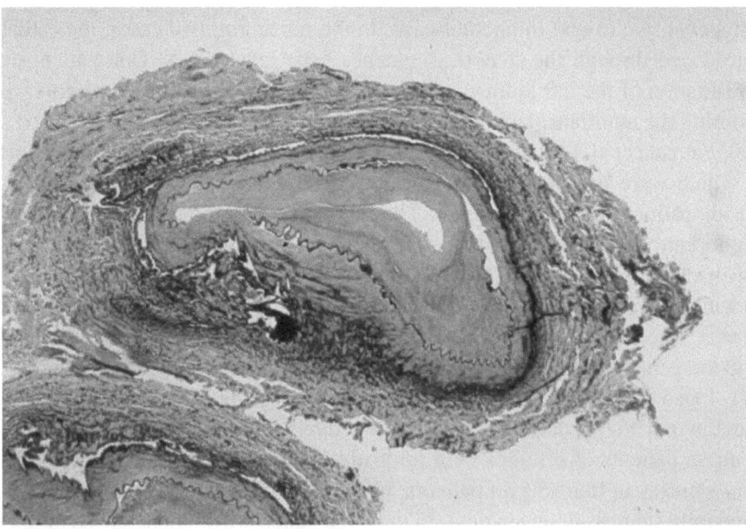

Fig. 1 Light microscopic evaluation (×10) of elastic staining of the renal artery, which was obtained during renal autotransplantation. A cross-section of the renal artery shows markedly thickened intimal tissue along the inner side of internal elastic lamina (From [29], with permission)

Treatment of Renovascular Hypertension in Moyamoya Disease

In addition to antihypertensive medication, renal artery stenosis with renovascular hypertension can be treated with balloon angioplasty [16,29,30], stent implantation [26], or renal autotransplantation [17,21,29] (Fig. 2). Although balloon angioplasty is a common modality for the treatment of renovascular hypertension, the effectiveness of balloon angioplasty for the treatment of renal artery stenosis in moyamoya disease varies [31]. It is known that bilateral involvement in renal artery stenosis is generally more common during childhood [35,36]. In fact, in a review conducted by Nakano et al. [19], five of seven children with renovascular hypertension associated with moyamoya disease had bilateral renal artery stenosis, and three of six pediatric cases in a Korean study [29] revealed bilateral renal arterial involvement. Thus, prior to vascular intervention therapy, angiography of both side renal arteries should be conducted. In addition, control of blood pressure in some patients with moyamoya disease prior to restoration of the cerebral blood flow may aggravate cerebral ischemic attacks [29]. Therefore, it may be desirable to defer procedures for the definitive treatment of hypertension such as renal balloon angioplasty and autotransplantation until after the restoration of cerebral blood flow,

Transient and mild hypertension may easily be overlooked in patients with moyamoya disease. This is because most patients have obvious neurologic symptoms, and it is well known that cerebral ischemia can cause transient high blood pressure. In fact, in a Korean study [29], 9 (12.5%) of 72 patients had transient hypertension, which abated spontaneously within 2 weeks of the transient ischemic attacks. Furthermore, three additional patients in that study who had intermittent hypertension became normotensive within a month of encephaloduroarteriosynangiosis. As a result, hypertension in patients with moyamoya disease does not always suggest the presence of renal arterial lesion. Nevertheless, some patients with renal arterial lesions remain normotensive; therefore, abdominal aortography including renal angiography is recommended in all patients with moyamoya disease regardless of accompanying hypertension. Conversely, screening of the cerebral artery may be necessary in some patients with

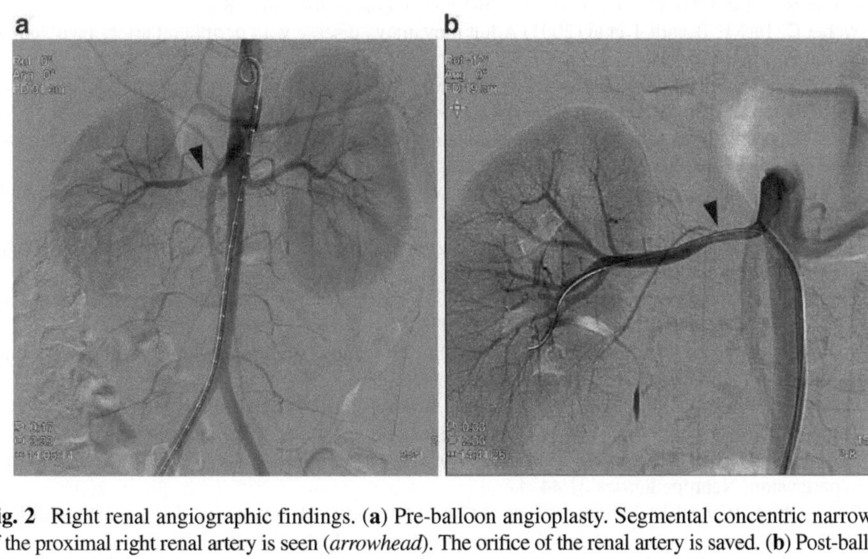

Fig. 2 Right renal angiographic findings. (**a**) Pre-balloon angioplasty. Segmental concentric narrowing of the proximal right renal artery is seen (*arrowhead*). The orifice of the renal artery is saved. (**b**) Post-balloon angioplasty. The stenotic segment of renal artery is moderately dilated after the balloon angioplasty (*arrowhead*)

renovascular hypertension because patients with moyamoya disease occasionally present with renovascular hypertension as the first symptom [21].

Other Extracranial Artery Involvement in Moyamoya Disease

In addition to the renal artery, the coronary [10,23], pulmonary [5,7,8,11], superior mesenteric [8,21,29], pancreatic [7], iliac [29], and peripheral [6,9] arteries have also been reported to be involved in moyamoya disease. However, there have been no reports of the prevalence of the involvement of major abdominal vessels except for the renal artery, and involvement of abdominal vessels other than the renal artery are considered less common.

References

1. Suzuki J, Takaku A (1969) Cerebrovascular "moyamoya" disease: disease showing abnormal net-like vessels in base of brain. Arch Neurol 20:288–299
2. Suzuki J, Kodama N (1983) Moyamoya disease: a review. Stroke 14:104–109
3. Nishimoto A, Takeuchi S (1968) Abnormal cerebrovascular network related to the internal carotid arteries. J Neurosurg 29:255–260
4. Scott RM, Smith ER (2009) Moyamoya disease and moyamoya syndrome. N Engl J Med 360: 1226–1237
5. Kapusta L, Daniëls O, Renier WO (1990) Moyamoya syndrome and primary pulmonary hypertension in childhood. Neuropediatrics 21:162–163
6. Goldenberg HJ (1974) "Moyamoya" associated with peripheral vascular occlusive disease. Arch Dis Child 49:964–966
7. Ikeda E (1991) Systemic vascular changes in spontaneous occlusion of the circle of Willis. Stroke 22:1358–1362
8. De Vries RR, Nikkels PG, van der Laag J et al (2003) Moyamoya and extracranial vascular involvement: fibromuscular dysplasia? A report of two children. Neuropediatrics 34:318–321
9. Weber C, Tatò F, Brandl T et al (2001) Adult moyamoya disease with peripheral artery involvement. J Vasc Surg 34:943–946
10. Komiyama M, Nishikawa M, Yasui T et al (2001) Moyamoya disease and coronary artery disease – case report. Neurol Med Chir (Tokyo) 41:37–41
11. Ou P, Dupont P, Bonnet D (2006) Fibromuscular dysplasia as the substrate for systemic and pulmonary hypertension in the setting of Moya-Moya disease. Cardiol Young 16:495–497
12. Godin M, Helias A, Tadie M et al (1978) Moyamoya syndrome and renal artery stenosis. Kidney Int 15:450
13. Ellison PH, Largent JA, Popp AJ (1981) Moya-moya disease associated with renal artery stenosis. Arch Neurol 38:467
14. Terasawa K, Yamaguchi Y, Ishihara O et al (1983) Moya-moya disease associated with fibromuscular dysplasia of renal artery. No To Hattatsu 15:350–355
15. Yamashita M, Tanaka K, Kishikawa T et al (1984) Moyamoya disease associated with renovascular hypertension. Hum Pathol 15:191–193
16. Halley SE, White WB, Ramsby GR et al (1988) Renovascular hypertension in moyamoya syndrome. Therapeutic response to percutaneous transluminal angioplasty. Am J Hypertens 1:348–352
17. Jansen JN, Donker AJ, Luth WJ et al (1990) Moyamoya disease associated with renovascular hypertension. Neuropediatrics 21:44–47
18. Rupprecht T, Wenzel D, Schmitzer E et al (1992) Diagnosis of moyamoya disease with additional renal artery stenosis by colour coded Doppler sonography. Pediatr Radiol 22:527–528
19. Nakano T, Azuma E, Ido M et al (1993) Moyamoya disease associated with bilateral renal artery stenosis. Acta Paediatr Jpn 35:354–357

20. Van der Vliet JA, Zeilstra DJ, Van Roye SF et al (1994) Renal artery stenosis in moyamoya syndrome. J Cardiovasc Surg (Torino) 35:441–443
21. Shoskes DA, Novick AC (1995) Surgical treatment of renovascular hypertension in moyamoya disease: case report and review of the literature. J Urol 153:450–452
22. Takagi Y, Hashimoto N, Goto Y (1997) Haemodynamic ischaemia in paediatric moyamoya disease associated with renovascular hypertension. Acta Neurochir (Wien) 139:257–258
23. Akasaki T, Kagiyama S, Omae T et al (1998) Asymptomatic moyamoya disease associated with coronary and renal artery stenosis – a case report. Jpn Circ J 62:136–138
24. Kuwayama F, Hamasaki Y, Shinagawa T et al (2001) Moyamoya disease complicated with renal artery stenosis and nephrotic syndrome: reversal of nephrotic syndrome after nephrectomy. J Pediatr 138:418–420
25. Caldarelli M, Di Rocco C, Gaglini P (2001) Surgical treatment of moyamoya disease in pediatric age. J Neurosurg Sci 45:83–91
26. Hoshino Y, Nakano A, Oguri M et al (2001) Intravascular ultrasound detects coarctation of the renal artery in a patient with Moyamoya disease. Hypertens Res 24:283–287
27. Fuchs FD, Francesconi CR, Caramori PR et al (2001) Moyamoya disease associated with renovascular disease in a young African-Brazilian patient. J Hum Hypertens 15:499–501
28. Kaczorowska M, Jóźwiak S, Litwin M et al (2005) Moyamoya disease associated with stenosis of extracranial arteries: a case report and review of the literature. Neurol Neurochir Pol 39:242–246
29. Choi Y, Kang BC, Kim KJ et al (1997) Renovascular hypertension in children with moyamoya disease. J Pediatr 131:258–263
30. Yamada I, Himeno Y, Matsushima Y et al (2000) Renal artery lesions in patients with moyamoya disease. Angiographic findings. Stroke 31:733–737
31. Togao O, Mihara F, Yoshiura T et al (2004) Prevalence of stenoocclusive lesions in the renal and abdominal arteries in moyamoya disease. Am J Radiol 183:119–122
32. Safian RD, Textor SC (2001) Renal artery stenosis. N Engl J Med 344:431–442
33. Castellote E, Romero R, Bonet J et al (1995) Takayasu's arteritis as a cause of renovascular hypertension in a non-Asian population. J Hum Hypertens 9:841–845
34. Hosoda Y (1984) Pathology of so-called "spontaneous occlusion of the circle of Willis." Pathol Annu 2:221–244
35. Deal JE, Snell MF, Barratt TM et al (1992) Renovascular disease in childhood. J Pediatr 121:378–384
36. Ellis D, Shapiro R, Scantleburg VP et al (1995) Evaluation and management of bilateral renal artery stenosis in children: a case series and review. Pediatr Nephrol 9:259–267

Associated Neurosurgical Diseases

Miki Fujimura and Teiji Tominaga

Introduction

Moyamoya disease is a chronic, occlusive cerebrovascular disease with unknown etiology, characterized by bilateral steno-occlusive changes at the terminal portion of the internal carotid artery and an abnormal vascular network at the base of the brain [1]. The association of moyamoya disease with further neurosurgical diseases, such as cerebral aneurysms [2–5], brain tumors, cervical carotid artery stenosis, and cerebrovascular malformations, has been described previously [6–11]. It is well known that moyamoya disease is frequently associated with intracranial aneurysms located within the abnormal basal network or the circle of Willis, which are explained by the intrinsic pathology of moyamoya disease, such as hemodynamic stress and fragile structure of the collateral vessels [2–5]. On the other hand, the association with atherosclerotic cervical carotid artery stenosis or with brain tumors leads to the diagnosis of akin moyamoya disease (quasi-moyamoya disease) according to the diagnostic criteria of the Research Committee on Spontaneous Occlusion of the Circle of Willis, of the Ministry of Health, Labor, and Welfare, Tokyo, Japan. The coincidence of moyamoya disease with cerebral vascular malformations including arteriovenous malformation [6,7], cerebral cavernous malformation [8–10], and venous malformation [10] has been reported in the literature. A rare association of with dural arteriovenous fistula is also demonstrated [11]. In this chapter, we especially focus on the association of moyamoya disease with further cerebrovascular disease based on our experience.

M. Fujimura (✉)
Department of Neurosurgery, Kohnan Hospital, 4-20-1 Nagamachi-minami, Taihaku-ku, Sendai, 982-8523, Japan
e-mail: fujimur@kohnan-sendai.or.jp

T. Tominaga
Department of Neurosurgery, Tohoku University Graduate School of Medicine, Sendai, Japan

B.-K. Cho and T. Tominaga (eds.), *Moyamoya Disease Update*,
DOI 10.1007/978-4-431-99703-0_21, © Springer 2010

Akin Moyamoya Disease (Quasi-Moyamoya Disease)

Atherosclerosis is one of the most common causes of akin moyamoya disease, which may be diagnosed by the detection of atherosclerotic cervical carotid artery stenosis in association with moyamoya disease. Regardless of the associated diseases, extracranial–intracranial revascularization surgery is the optimal treatment for the patients with ischemic symptom. A 52-year-old man, with a past history of hypertension and diabetes, presented with minor completed stroke on the left hemisphere and was admitted to our clinic. Bilateral carotid angiogram satisfied the diagnostic criteria of moyamoya disease (Fig. 1a, b), while his cervical carotid artery showed apparent atherosclerotic stenosis (Fig. 1c) bilaterally. *N*-isopropyl-*p*-[^{123}I]iodoamphetamine single-photon emission computed tomography demonstrated significant hemodynamic compromise of the affected hemisphre (Fig. 2). We performed superficial temporal artery-middle cerebral artery (STA-MCA) anastomosis with pial synangiosis [12] on the left hemisphere, which resolved his hemodynamic compromise. Postoperative course was uneventful, and magnetic resonance angiography after surgery showed a thick high signal of STA (arrow in Fig. 3). The patient has not suffered a cerebrovascular event during the follow-up period of 5 months.

Association with Vascular Malformations: Arteriovenous Malformation

Moyamoya disease can be associated with cerebral vascular malformations such as arteriovenous malformation [6,7], cerebral cavernous malformation [8–10], and venous malformation [10]. A 25-year-old man visited our clinic due to a syncope attack, and was found by magnetic resonance imaging/angiography to have right frontal arteriovenous malformation in association with moyamoya disease (Fig. 4). He had not previously suffered cerebral ischemic symptom. Bilateral carotid angiogram demonstrated steno-occlusive changes at the terminal portion of

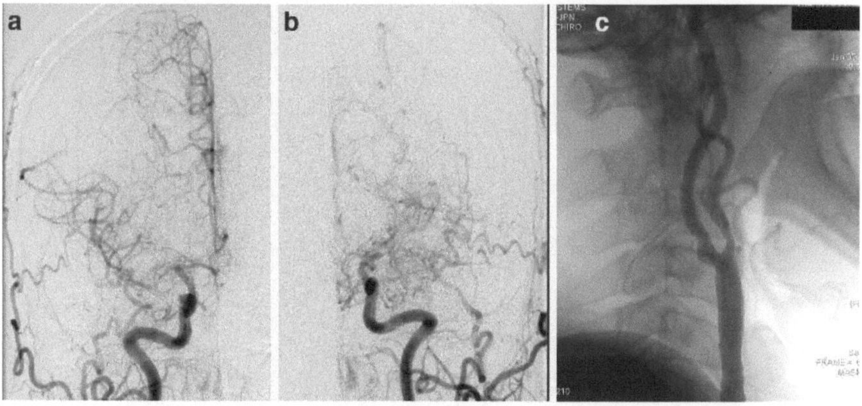

Fig. 1 A 52-year-old man with minor completed stroke on the left hemisphere. Carotid angiogram demonstrating steno-occlusive changes at the terminal portion of the bilateral internal carotid arteries and the development of moyamoya vessels (**a**, **b**). Cervical carotid artery showing apparent atherosclerotic stenosis bilaterally (**c**), leading to the diagnosis of akin moyamoya disease

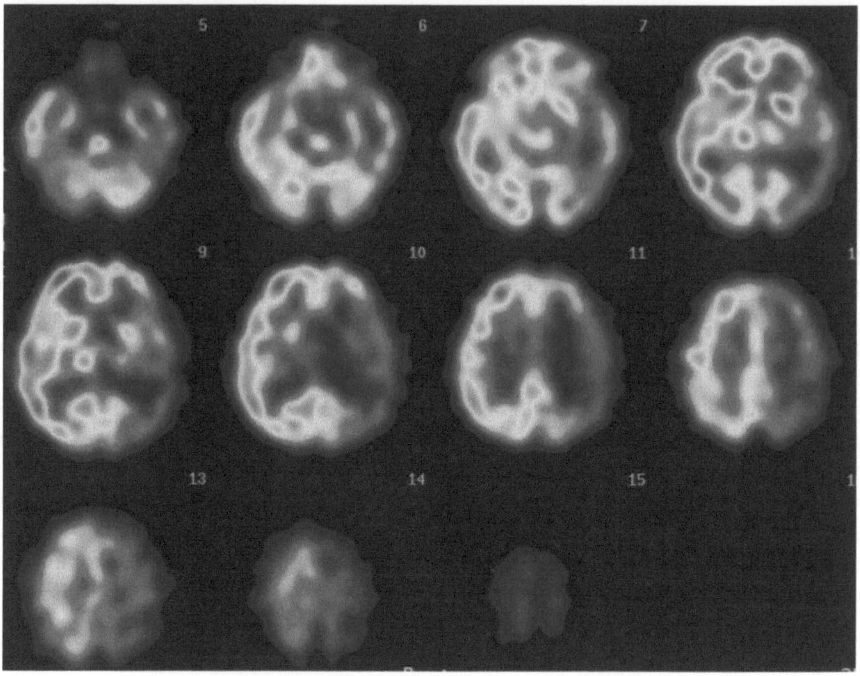

Fig. 2 Preoperative *N*-isopropyl-*p*-[123I]iodoamphetamine single-photon emission computed tomography demonstrating significant hemodynamic compromise on the symptomatic hemisphere

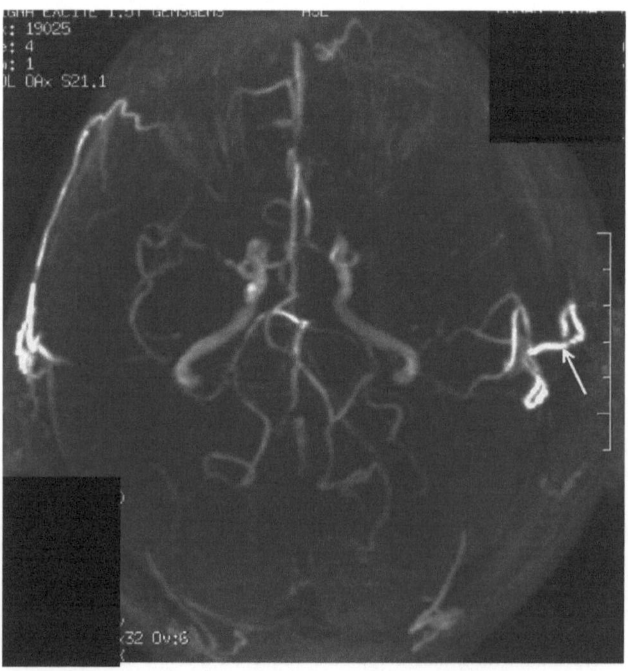

Fig. 3 Postoperative magnetic resonance angiography showing apparently patent STA-MCA bypass with peripheral branches of middle cerebral artery

internal carotid arteries with abnormal vascular network at the base of the brain (Fig. 5), indicating stage III moyamoya disease by Suzuki's classification [1]. Right frontal arteriovenous malformation was also demonstrated in the feeding arteries from the branch of anterior cerebral artery and a part of the abnormal vascular network. There was a single drainer to the superior sagittal sinus via the cortical vein (Fig. 5). Since he was diagnosed with asymptomatic, unruptured arteriovenous malformation and single-photon emission computed tomography failed to detect any hemodynamic compromise, we conservatively followed him up every 6 months with outpatient magnetic resonance imaging. Regarding the management of arteriovenous malformation in association with moyamoya disease, Seol and colleagues reported the efficacy of gamma knife radiosurgery [7]. Radiosurgical obliteration of arteriovenous malformation may be beneficial to reduce the risk of revascularization surgery for moyamoya disease.

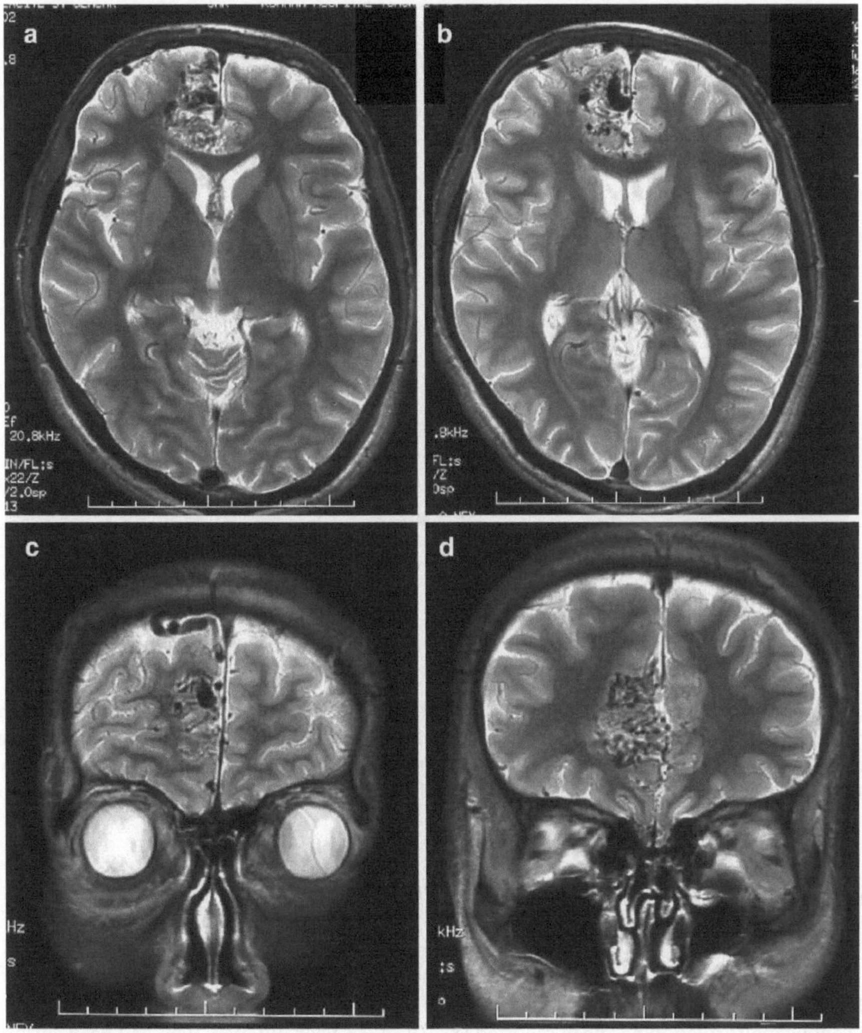

Fig. 4 A 25-year-old man incidentally found to have moyamoya syndrome associated arteriovenous malformation. Axial (**a**, **b**) and coronal view (**c**, **d**) of the T2-weighted magnetic resonance imaging demonstrating the presence of nidus in right frontal lobe

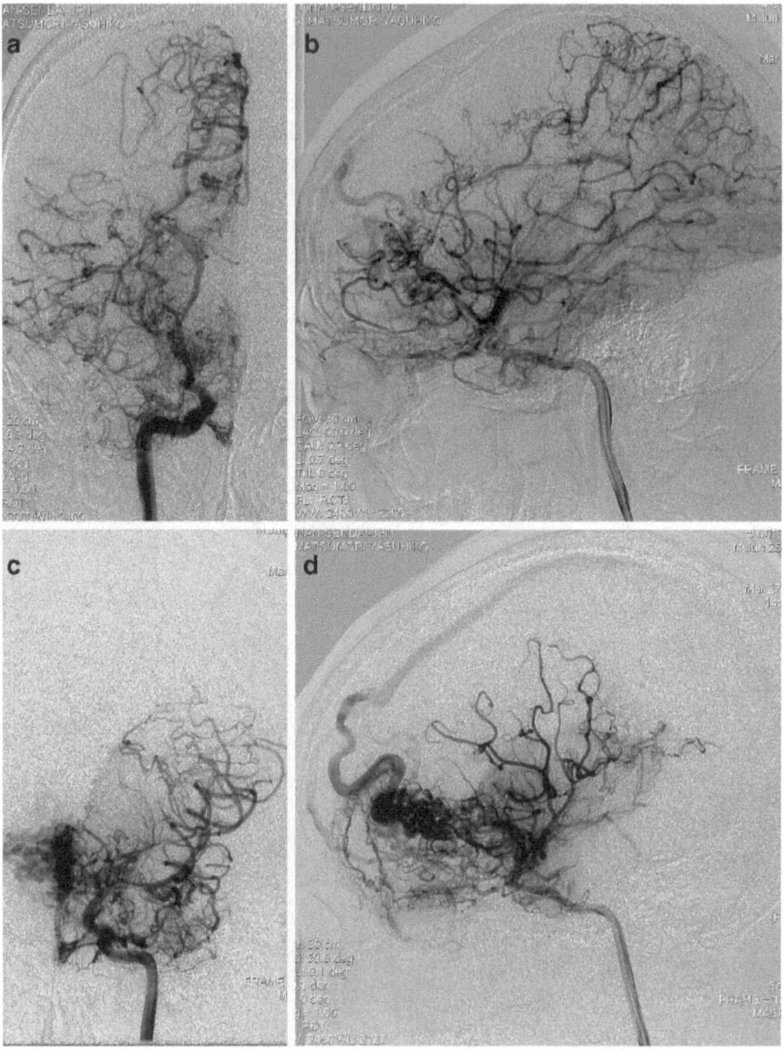

Fig. 5 *Right* (**a**) AP view, (**b**) lateral view, and *left* (**c**) AP view, (**d**) lateral view carotid angiogram demonstrating steno-occlusive changes at the terminal portion of internal carotid arteries with abnormal vascular network at the base of the brain. Right frontal arteriovenous malformation was also demonstrated with the feeding arteries from the branch of anterior cerebral artery and a part of the abnormal vascular network

Association with Cavernous Malformation and Venous Malformation

The rare association of moyamoya disease with cerebral/cerebellar cavernous malformations and venous malformation has been reported [8–10]. A 33-year-old man, who had been suffering from moyamoya syndrome with transient ischemic attack during the past 3 years, was admitted to our hospital due to crescendo transient ischemic attacks. Magnetic resonance angiography and carotid angiogram showed apparent progression of the steno-occlusive changes bilaterally

(Fig. 6a, b). We therefore planned surgical revascularization on the symptomatic side. At the time of readmission for surgery, magnetic resonance imaging and cerebral angiogram revealed de novo cavernous malformation (arrow in Fig. 6d) and a newly formed venous malformation (arrow in Fig. 6c, e). One month later, STA-MCA anastomosis with pial synangiosis was performed without complications. De novo formation of cerebellar cavenous malformation [8,9] and venous malformation [9] in patients with moyamoya disease gives rise to particular interest since they may suggest a common biological background between moyamoya disease and such vascular malformations [13,14].

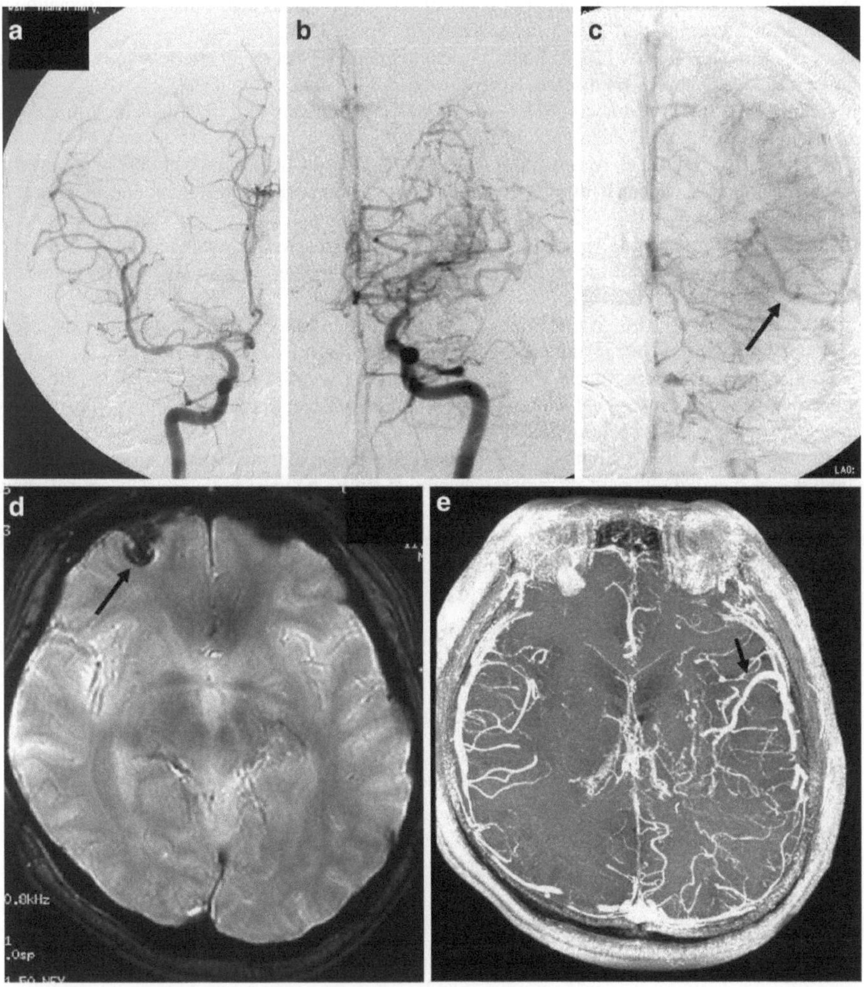

Fig. 6 *Right* (**a**) and *left* (**b, c**) carotid angiogram after progression showing the progression of stenosis in the right middle cerebral artery (**a**), the occlusion of the left middle cerebral artery with moyamoya vessels (**b**), as well as the newly formed left venous malformation (*arrow* in (**c**)). (**d**) T2*-weighted (MR) imaging shows the hypointense right frontal lesion, suggesting cerebral cavernous malformation (*arrow*). (**e**) A susceptibility-weighted minimal intensity projection image also shows the characteristic caput medusae appearance of the venous malformation with enlarged medullary veins and dilated veins in the sylvian fissure (*arrow*)

References

1. Suzuki J, Takaku A (1969) Cerebrovascular 'moyamoya' disease. Disease showing abnormal net-like vessels in base of brain. Arch Neurol 20:288–299
2. Adams HP Jr, Kassell NF, Wisoff HS et al (1979) Intracranial saccular aneurysm and moyamoya disease. Stroke 10:174–179
3. Konishi Y, Kadowaki C, Hara M et al (1985) Aneurysm associated with moyamoya disease. Neurosurgery 16:484–491
4. Kuroda S, Houkin K, Kamiyama H et al (2001) Effects of surgical revascularization on peripheral artery aneurysms in moyamoya disease: report of three cases. Neurosurgery 49:463–467
5. Kodama N, Sato M, Sasaki T (1996) Treatment of ruptured cerebral aneurysm in moyamoya disease. Surg Neurol 46:62–66
6. Nakashima T, Nakayama N, Furuichi M et al (1998) Arteriovenous malformation in association with moyamoya disease. Report of two cases. Neurosurg Focus 15:e6
7. Seol HJ, Kim DG, Oh CW (2002) Radiosurgical treatment of a cerebral arteriovenous malformation in a patient with moyamoya disease. Neurosurgery 51:478–481
8. Kerchner GA, Smith W, Lawton MT et al (2006) Co-occurrence of a cavernous malformation and contralateral moyamoya. Neurology 66:1601–1602
9. Korematsu K, Yoshioka S, Maruyama T et al (2007) De novo appearance of cerebellar cavernous malformation in a patient with moyamoya disease: case report and review of the literature. Clin Neurol Neurosurg 109:708–712
10. Januschek E, Fujimura M, Mugikura S et al (2008) Progressive moyamoya syndrome associated with de novo formation of the ipsilateral venous and contralateral cavernous malformations: case report. Surg Neurol 69:423–427
11. Killory BD, Gonzalez LF, Wait SD et al (2008) Simultaneous unilateral moyamoya disease and ipsilateral dural arteriovenous fistula: case report. Neurosurgery 62:1375–1376
12. Fujimura M, Mugikura S, Kaneta T et al (2009) Incidence and risk factors for symptomatic cerebral hyperperfusion after superficial temporal artery-middle cerebral artery anastomosis in patients with moyamoya disease. Surg Neurol 71:442–447
13. Fujimura M, Watanabe M, Shimizu H et al (2007) Expression of matrix metalloproteinase and tissue inhibitor of metalloproteinase in cerebral cavernous malformations: immunihistochemical analysis of MMP-2, -9, and TIMP-2. Acta Neurochir (Wien) 149:179–183
14. Fujimura M, Watanabe M, Narisawa A et al (2009) Increased expression of serum matrix metalloproteinase-9 in patients with moyamoya disease. Surg Neurol 72:476–480

Part VII
Diagnostic Evaluation I: Morphological Imaging

Overview of Image Diagnosis of Moyamoya Disease

Kiyohiro Houkin, Satoshi Iihoshi, and Takeshi Mikami

Digital Subtraction Angiography

As mentioned in the Introduction, when the original concept of moyamoya disease is reviewed, digital subtraction angiography (DSA) is still the most reliable diagnostic modality. However, as mentioned in the following sections, as far as the depiction of the steno-occlusive change of the Willis ring is concerned, other modalities such as magnetic resonance angiography (MRA) and 3-dimensional computed tomography angiography (3D-CTA) with best quality is quite compatible with DSA. However, the depiction of the moyamoya vessels and the collateral circulation is not always clear in MRA and magnetic resonance imaging (MRI). In addition, 3D-CTA essentially depicts the morphological aspect of vasculature that is not necessarily identical to the true circulation of the blood flow. In addition, the collateral circulation such as (1) basal moyamoya, and (2) transdural anastomosis of the meningeal artery including the vault moyamoya and ethmoidal moyamoya is not well demonstrated in other modalities (Figs. 1 and 2).

In addition, as is well known, a micro-aneurysm is supposed to be the cause of the intra-cerebral and intra-ventricular hemorrhage. The diagnosis of this small micro-aneurysm is not always possible with other modalities except for DSA (Fig. 3).

CT Scan

CT scan is the most convenient radiological modality that is available in most hospitals and can be used even at midnight without any specific support. Therefore, it is conceivable that CT scan is used as the first diagnostic tool in most cases. However, it is well known that CT scan cannot offer any diagnostic information on moyamoya disease. It must be kept in mind that you can miss the right diagnosis of moyamoya disease if you depend on the CT scan. In advanced stages, cerebral infarction and unusual cerebral atrophy are well recognized even in CT scan (Fig. 4).

K. Houkin (✉), S. Iihoshi, and T. Mikami
Department of Neurosurgery, Sapporo Medical University, Sapporo 060-8556, Japan
e-mail: houkin@sapmed.ac.jp

B.-K. Cho and T. Tominaga (eds.), *Moyamoya Disease Update*,
DOI 10.1007/978-4-431-99703-0_22, © Springer 2010

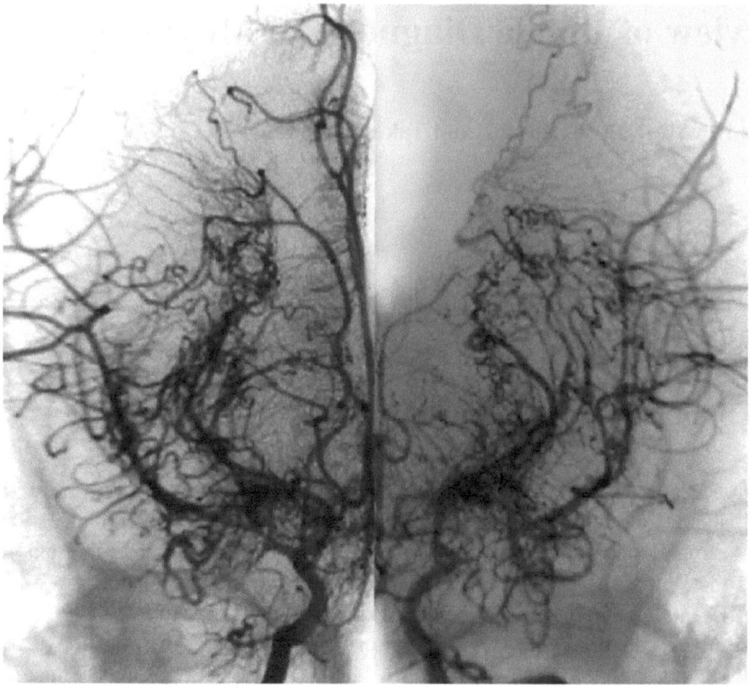

Fig. 1 A 7-year-old girl. Anterior–posterior views of the bilateral carotid angiography are overlapped. The terminal portion of the bilateral carotid artery shows stenotic change and development of the moyamoya vessels in the basal ganglia

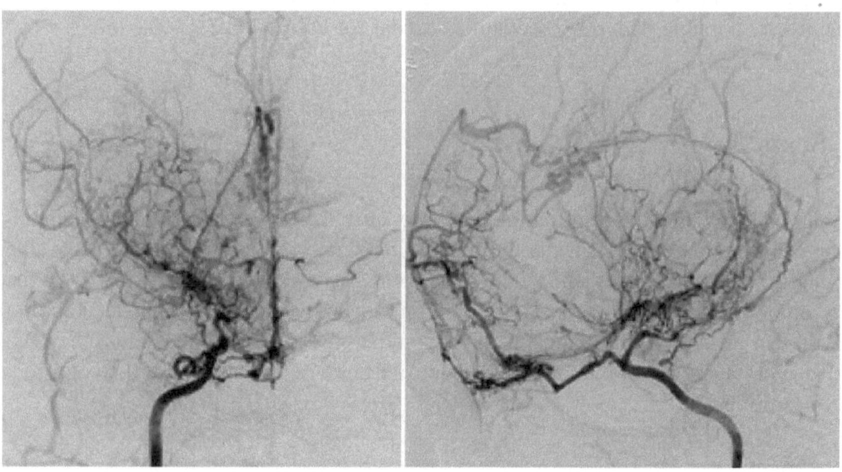

Fig. 2 Adult moyamoya patient. Collateral circulation such as ethmoidal moyamoya, basal, moyamoya, and trans-pial anastomosis is well demonstrated in digital subtraction angiography (DSA)

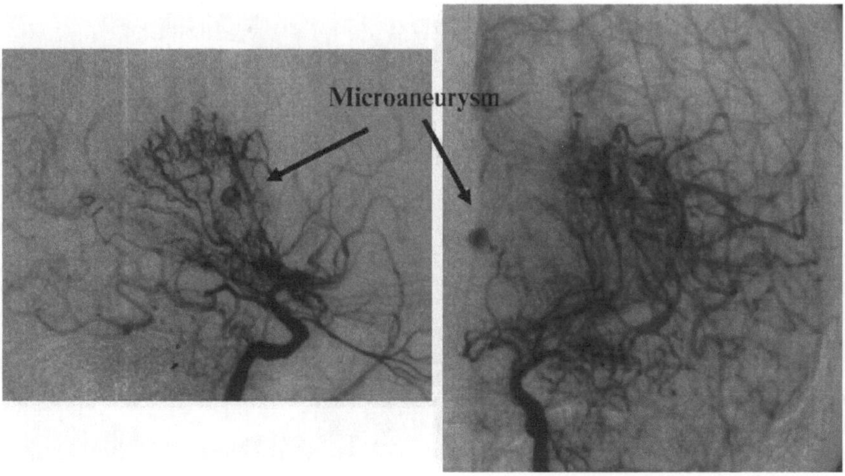

Fig. 3 Microaneurysm is well shown in DSA

However, in CT scan, the steno-occlusive change and development of moyamoya vessels are not depicted since the vasculature system such as the circle of Willis ring shows nonspecific density. Enhanced CT scan may reveal the steno-occlusive change and development of moyamoya vessels. In any case, if there is a possibility of moyamoya disease in the present/past history and family history, normal CT scan is not enough to exclude moyamoya disease and further examination such as high resolution MRI/MRA is recommended. Moreover, intractable headache seen in pediatric patients should also be checked with MRI to exclude this disease.

On the other hand, plain CT scan is still the most reliable modality for the diagnosis of a hemorrhagic event. In moyamoya disease, the most frequent hemorrhage is seen as the intra-ventricular hemorrhage and the intra-cerebral hemorrhage (Fig. 5). In all cases of supra-tentorial intra-cerebral hemorrhage seen in CT scan, hemorrhage due to moyamoya disease must be kept in mind as the differential diagnosis.

Magnetic Resonance Image

The guidelines for the diagnosis of moyamoya disease in Japan by the Japanese Ministry of Health and Welfare has introduced MRI and MRA as a noninvasive diagnostic modality [4–6]. MRI/MRA has been acknowledged as a reliable diagnostic tool with high sensitivity and specificity as a result of the remarkable development of MR imaging technology [7–11]. However, it must be recognized that the quality of MRI/MRA is strongly dependent on the machine's magnetic resonance, in particular, on the strength of the static magnetic field. In other words, it must be kept in mind that images obtained using a 1.5 or more Tesla machine is the minimum requirement for the proper reliable diagnosis of moyamoya disease.

The steno-occlusive change of the circle of Willis is well disclosed in axial T2-weighted images at the level of basal cistern (David star level) (Fig. 6).

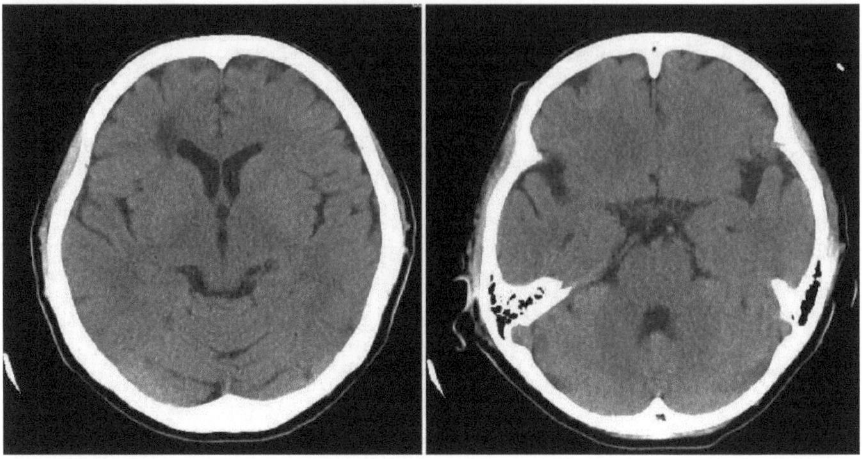

Fig. 4 *Left* Small asymptomatic infarction is seen in the right frontal lobe but this infarction is not specific to moyamoya disease. *Right* CT scan at the level of the Willis ring. No abnormality is seen

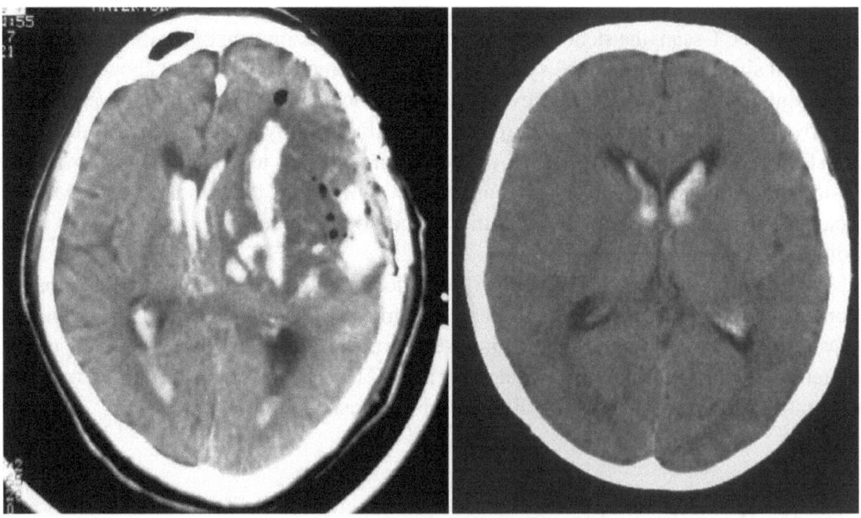

Fig. 5 *Left* Intra-cerebral hemorrhage. *Right* Intra-ventricular hemorrhage

In the guideline, more than two signal voids suggesting these moyamoya vessels must be confirmed in MRI at the level of basal ganglia (Fig. 7).

In general, these signal voids are not always well seen in T2-weighted images. As reported, T1-weighted coronal image and T2-reversed image and 3-Tesla images are more sensitive for revealing the moyamoya vessels (Fig. 8).

In addition, a contemporary sequence of T2*-weighted images can reveal the micro-silent hemorrhage in moyamoya patients (Fig. 9). Susceptibility-weighted image (SWI) may also be very sensitive to these small hemorrhages that are not well shown in CT scan.

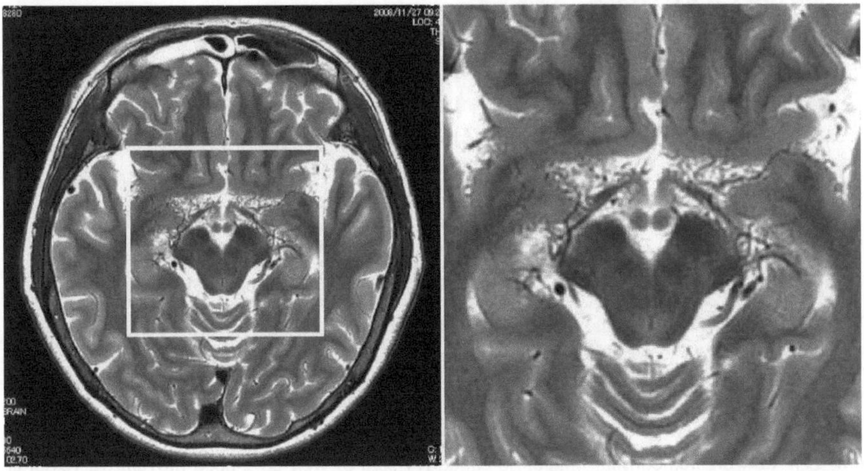

Fig. 6 *Left* Whole image of T2 weighted MRI at the level of basal cistern. *Right* Enlarged image of the left image. The horizontal portion of middle cerebral artery is not identified. On the other hand, small characteristic signal voids suggesting moyamoya vessels are well depicted

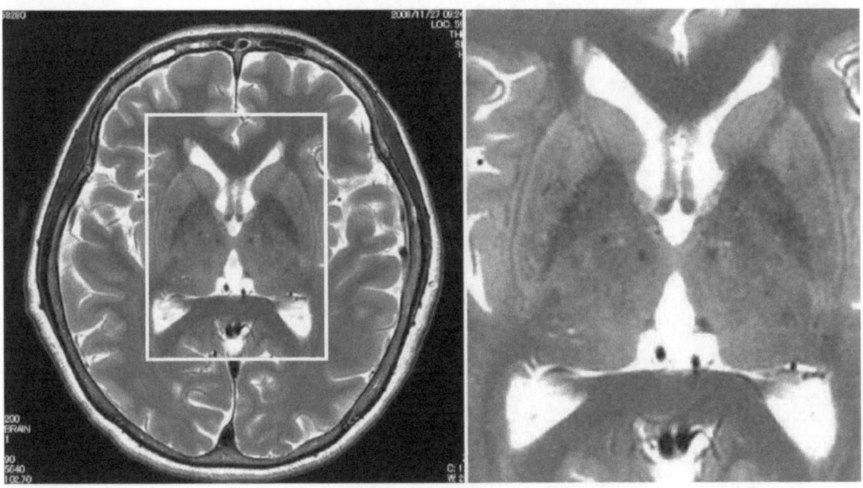

Fig. 7 *Left* Whole T2-weighted image at the level of basal ganglia. *Right* Small signal voids are well confirmed

Magnetic Resonance Angiography

MRA is becoming the practical substitute for DSA in the diagnosis of moyamoya disease. In particular, the rapid spread of the high Tesla machines has accelerated the diagnosis using MR. MRA is a noninvasive modality and it can reveal the typical change of moyamoya disease in many cases (Fig. 10).

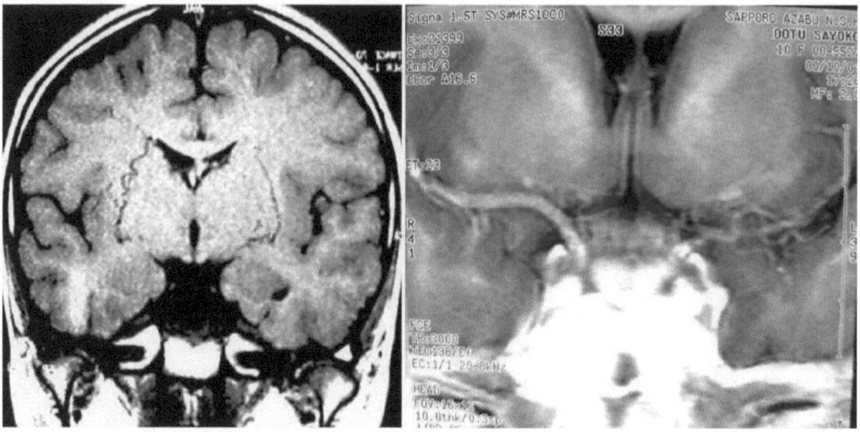

Fig. 8 *Left* T1-weighted coronal image. So-called ivy sign of well-developed moyamoya vessel at the level of basal ganglia is clearly shown. *Right* Reversed heavily T2-weighted image clearly shows steno-occlusive change of the middle cerebral artery

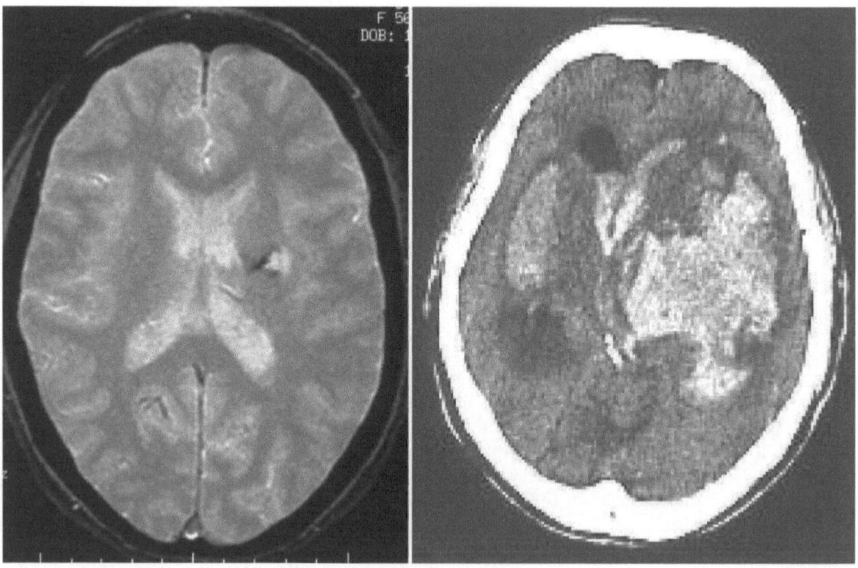

Fig. 9 *Left* T2*-weighted image of symptomatic moyamoya patient. Deposition of hemosiderin suggesting the small old hemorrhage is seen in the left basal ganglia. *Right-* Same patient conservatively observed more than 2 years. Severe fatal intra-cerebral hemorrhage occurred

However, in many cases, these typical changes are not always observed. Moyamoya vessels are occasionally underestimated in MRA. On the other hand, steno-occlusive changes are often over-estimated in MRA (Figs. 11 and 12).

It is well known that moyamoya disease is a dynamically changing disease and that these changes range from a very early stage of mild stenosis in the intracranial artery without moyamoya vessels to an end stage with the occlusion of the carotid fork and remarkable development of collateral circulation [12–14]. Suzuki's staging is based on these particular changes observed in moyamoya disease [13]. As far as its staging is concerned, conventional angiography is still the gold standard. However, very high resolution MRA can offer a novel classification based on MRA scoring. The detail of this score is well described by Houkin et al [15]. In addition, it is well known that MRA is a useful modality with which to follow the drastic change after surgical treatment [16].

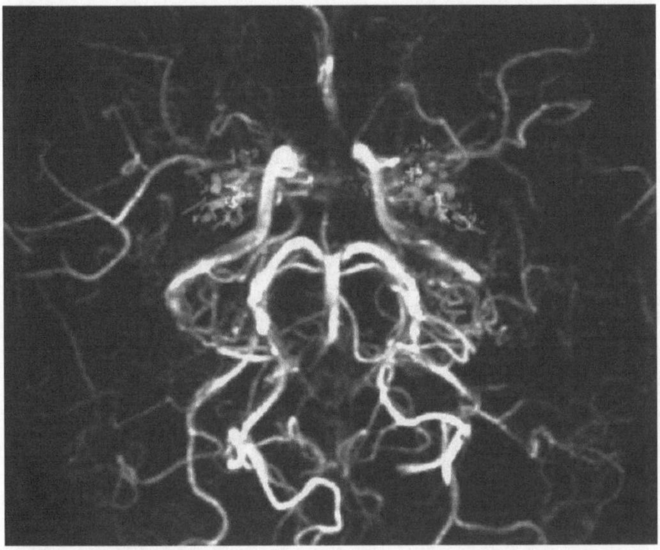

Fig. 10 Steno-occlusive change and basal moyamoya vessels are clearly shown

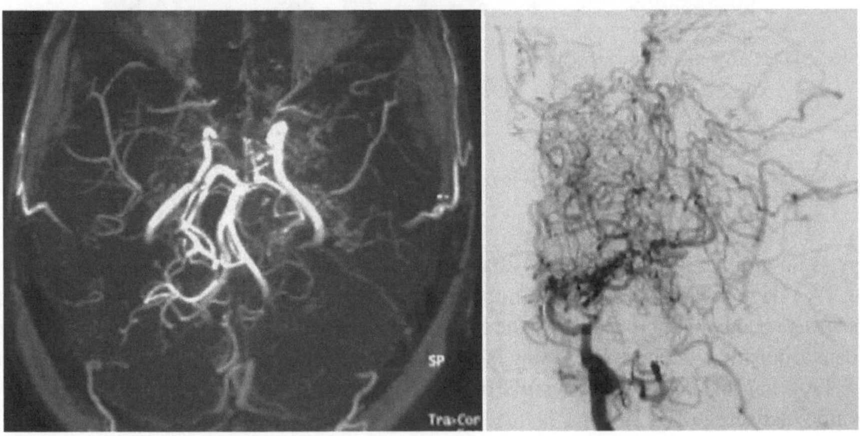

Fig. 11 MRA (*left*) reveals steno-occlusive change of the circle of Willis. However, the moyamoya vessels are not well demonstrated compared to the conventional angiography (*right*)

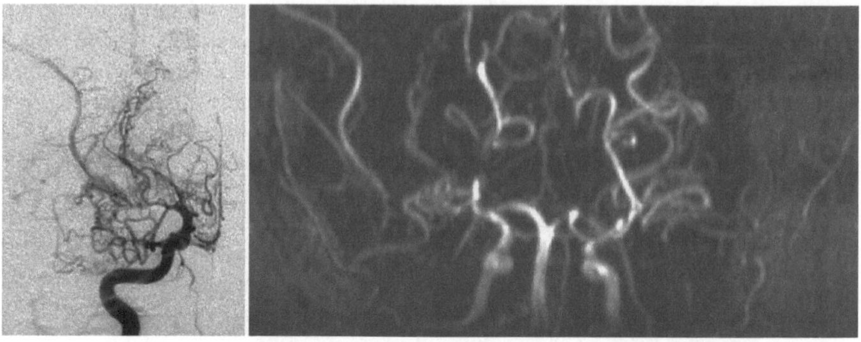

Fig. 12 In conventional angiography (*left*), the horizontal portion of the right middle cerebral artery (MCA) shows severe stenosis but is not completely occluded

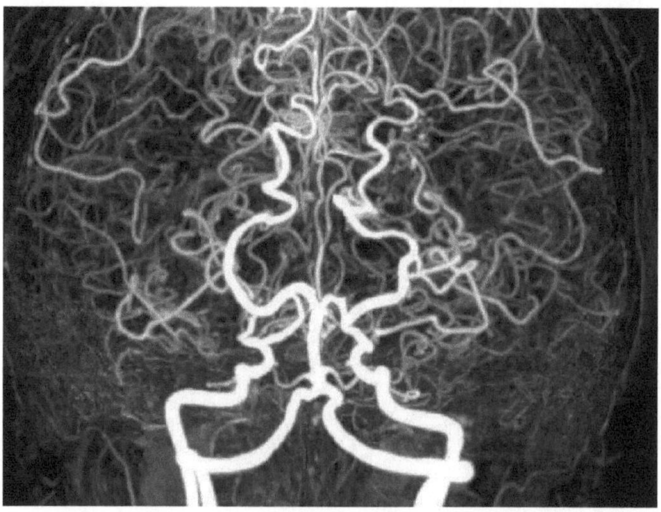

Fig. 13 3D-CTA of moyamoya disease

3D-CTA

There is no guideline on the diagnosis based on 3D-CTA. As is seen in MRA, the quality of 3D-CTA images is dependent on both the machine specification and also on the technique of post-data acquisition procedure by the image technologist. Therefore, the standardization of the data acquisition and post-processing is indispensable. However, contemporary sophisticated 3D-CTA imaging is quite powerful for the confirmation of the basic change seen in moyamoya disease (Fig. 13).

Acknowledgment This work was supported in part by a grant from the Research Committee on Spontaneous Occlusion of the Circle of Willis sponsored by the Ministry of Health and Welfare of Japan.

References

1. Suzuki J, Takaku A (1969) Cerebrovascular "moyamoya" disease. Disease showing abnormal net-like vessels in base of brain. Arch Neurol 20:288–299
2. Suzuki J, Kodama N (1983) Moyamoya disease – a review. Stroke 14:104–109
3. Suzuki J, Kodama N (1971) Cerebrovascular "Moyamoya" disease. 2. Collateral routes to forebrain via ethmoid sinus and superior nasal meatus. Angiology 22:223–236
4. Fukui M (1997) Current state of study on moyamoya disease in Japan. Surg Neurol 47:138–143
5. Fukui M (1997) Guidelines for the diagnosis and treatment of spontaneous occlusion of the circle of Willis ('moyamoya' disease). Research Committee on Spontaneous Occlusion of the Circle of Willis (Moyamoya Disease) of the Ministry of Health and Welfare, Japan. Clin Neurol Neurosurg 99:S238–S240
6. Houkin K, Aoki T, Takahashi A et al (1994) Diagnosis of moyamoya disease with magnetic resonance angiography. Stroke 25:2159–2164
7. Yamada I, Suzuki S, Matsushima Y (1995) Moyamoya disease: comparison of assessment with MR angiography and MR imaging versus conventional angiography. Radiology 196:211–218
8. Kikuchi M, Asato M, Sugahara S (1996) Evaluation of surgically formed collateral circulation in moyamoya disease with 3D-CT angiography: comparison with MR angiography and X-ray angiography. Neuropediatrics 27:45–49
9. Hasuo K, Mihara F, Matsushima T (1998) MRI and MR angiography in moyamoya disease. J Magn Reson Imaging 8:762–766
10. Shirane R, Mikawa S, Ebina T (1999) A case of adult moyamoya disease showing progressive angiopathy on cerebral angiography. Clin Neurol Neurosurg 101:210–214
11. Takanashi JI, Sugita K, Niimi H (1998) Evaluation of magnetic resonance angiography with selective maximum intensity projection in patients with childhood moyamoya disease. Eur J Paediatr Neurol 2:83–89
12. Aoki S, Yoshikawa T, Hori M et al (2000) Two-dimensional thick-slice MR digital subtraction angiography for assessment of cerebrovascular occlusive diseases. Eur Radiol 10:1858–1864
13. Thibaud C, Garnier-Viarouge MP, De Kersaint-Gilly A et al (2001) Moyamoya disease: importance of the MRI-MRA combination and difficulties in management and follow-up in 7 cases. J Neuroradiol 28:84–91
14. Yamada I, Nakagawa T, Matsushima Y et al (2001) High-resolution turbo magnetic resonance angiography for diagnosis of Moyamoya disease. Stroke 32:1825–1831
15. Houkin K, Nakayama N, Kuroda S, et al (2005) Novel magnetic resonance angiography stage grading for moyamoya disease. Cerebrovasc Dis 20:347–354
16. Houkin K, Nakayama N, Kuroda S, et al (2004) How does angiogenesis develop in pediatric moyamoya disease after surgery ? A prospective study with MR angiography. Childs Nerv Syst 20:734–741

Preoperative and Postoperative MRA

Takeshi Mikami, Satoshi Iihoshi, and Kiyohiro Houkin

Diagnostic Criteria for Moyamoya Disease with MRA

Magnetic resonance angiography (MRA) has opened the door to noninvasive evaluation of the intracranial major arteries. The contemporary MRA can clearly disclose the major intracranial arteries and has become an indispensable modality for the management of cerebrovascular stroke. Based on this dramatic technical evolution, since 1994 new diagnostic guidelines for moyamoya disease have included good MRA as the definitive diagnostic technique for moyamoya disease [1–4]. Nowadays, MRA can be an alternative to conventional angiography in moyamoya disease, and has been acknowledged as a reliable diagnostic tool with high sensitivity and specificity as a result of the remarkable development of MR imaging technology [5–13]. Moreover, MRA is useful not only for the diagnosis but also for follow-up of moyamoya disease in a noninvasive way.

In accordance with the guidelines of the Research Committee for Diagnosis of Moyamoya Disease in Japan [1, 3, 14], cerebral angiography is not mandatory if MRI and MRA show all the following findings:

1. Stenosis or occlusion of the terminal portion of the internal carotid artery (ICA) or at the proximal part of the anterior cerebral artery (ACA) and middle cerebral artery (MCA) on MRA
2. An abnormal vascular network seen in the basal ganglia with MRA (more than two signal voids being apparent)
3. Bilateral presentation of the above two findings

In order to understand the background of this minor revision of the diagnostic criteria in Japan, knowledge of the social system of financially supporting patients with moyamoya disease in Japan is required. Patients with moyamoya disease who meet the diagnostic criteria set by the Research Committee can receive full payment of their medical costs from the government. The diagnostic criteria have to be strict to eliminate doubtful cases. After the nationwide study led by this Committee, MRA that meets the conditions set by the committee was accepted into the diagnostic criteria.

T. Mikami (✉), S. Iihoshi, and K. Houkin
Department of Neurosurgery, Sapporo Medical University, S-1, W-16, chuoku, Sapporo 060-8543, Japan
e-mail: tmikami@sapmed.ac.jp

B.-K. Cho and T. Tominaga (eds.), *Moyamoya Disease Update*,
DOI 10.1007/978-4-431-99703-0_23, © Springer 2010

Quality of MRA for the Diagnosis of Moyamoya Disease

Based on the recent advanced technology, 3-dimensional time-of-flight (3D TOF) MRA is supposed to be superior to 3-dimensional phase contrast (3D PC) MRA for routine examinations or screening examinations because TOF MRA has excellent spatial resolution [15]. Despite these advantages, MRA with the TOF technique has the disadvantage of false negative findings, particularly in the detection of slow flow. 3D PC MRA is occasionally useful to detect small moyamoya vessels that are barely depicted in 3D TOF MRA. 3D TOF MRA does not clearly reflect the collateral pathway formed at the periphery [3, 5]. However, the poor spatial resolution and long data acquisition time of the 3D PC technique is a practical limitation for considering MRA for evaluation of the staging or postoperative follow-up of moyamoya disease.

The quality of MRA largely depends on the strength of the static magnetic field. The new criteria of the Research Committee recommended MRA with a 1.5 T machine. A 3.0 T MRA produces the highest quality (Fig. 1). MRA machines with 1.0 or 0.5 T static magnetic fields can reveal a possible diagnosis of moyamoya disease, but in most cases an MRA from a 1.0 or 0.5 T machine is not always diagnostic [3, 5, 7, 16].

As for the possibility of false positive findings, overestimation of accuracy and spatial resolution should always be taken into account because of the imaging quality of MRA. Probable causes of overestimation are considered as follows [17–22]:

1. Lamina flow of carotid siphon and carotid fork
2. Phase dispersion by disturbed flow at stenotic lesion
3. Degradation of flow contrast by degradation of flow rate at stenotic lesion

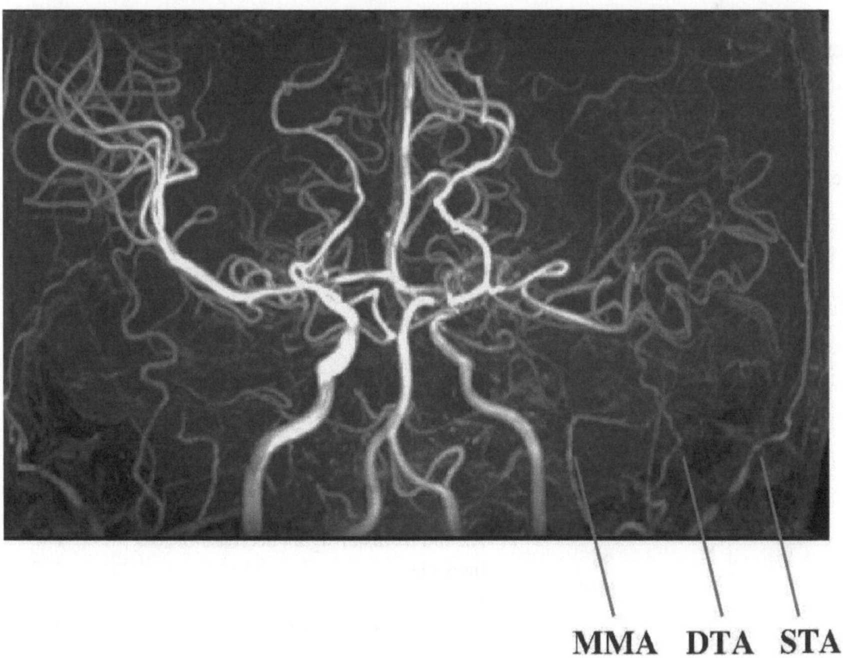

Fig. 1 Demonstrative case of 3.0 T MRA showing the superficial temporal artery (STA), the temporal muscle (DTA), and the dura mater (MMA)

Especially both in the early and the end stages of moyamoya disease, diagnosis by means of MRA should be carefully evaluated since in these stages typical findings of steno-occlusive change and the development of moyamoya vessels are not always demonstrated.

Novel Staging of Moyamoya Disease

It is well known that moyamoya disease is a dynamically changing disease and that these changes are observed angiographically, ranging from a very early stage of equivocal mild stenotic change in the intracranial artery without moyamoya vessels to an end stage with the occlusion of the carotid fork and remarkable development of collateral circulation [22–24]. Dynamic changes that drastically modify the angiographical findings include development of moyamoya vessels and collateral anastomosis, which follows the initial steno-occlusive change of the carotid fork [22]. Suzuki's staging is well recognized as the standard angiographical staging based on these particular changes observed in moyamoya disease [23]. Therefore, as far as its staging is concerned, conventional angiography is still the gold standard. Houkin et al. have proposed the following grading system of MRA in moyamoya disease [25]: MRA scores are assigned on the basis of the severity of the occlusive changes in the ICA, of the horizontal portions of the MCA, ACA, and posterior cerebral artery, and of the flow signals of the distal branches of these arteries. MRA scores correlated well with the six-stage classification on cerebral angiography, with a high sensitivity and specificity.

MRA Score

Depending on the severity of its steno-occlusive change, a point was assigned to each of the ICA, the MCA, the ACA, and the posterior cerebral artery (PCA; Table 1).

Table 1 Summary of the MRA score

ICA	
Normal	0
Stenosis of C1	1
Discontinuity of C1 signal	2
Invisible	3
MCA	
Normal	0
Stenosis of M1	1
Discontinuity of M1 signal	2
Invisible	3
ACA	
Normal A2 and its distal	0
A2 and its distal signal decrease or loss	1
Invisible	2
PCA	
Normal P2 and its distal	0
P2 and its distal signal decrease or loss	1
Invisible	2
Total	0–10

1. ICA (Figs. 2 and 3)

The intracranial portion of the ICA was evaluated. The extracranial portion, including the cavernous portion, was excluded from this evaluation because it does not show specific findings in moyamoya disease. Scores are assigned to the ICA depending on the severity of the steno-occlusive change of the horizontal portion of the MCA (M1) and the visibility of its distal branches.

Point 0: Normal or minimum equivocal change of the ICA

Point 1: Stenosis was apparent at the intracranial carotid artery (C1 portion, distal to the posterior communicating artery)

Point 2: Signal decrease or loss of the C1 portion.

Point 3. Intracranial ICA is not depicted.

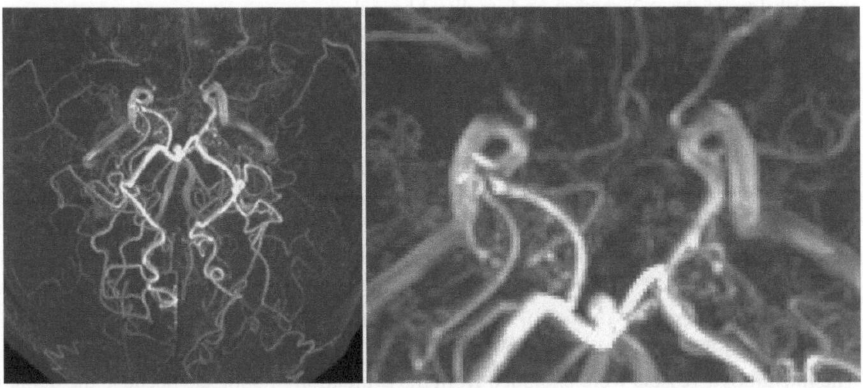

Fig. 2 Demonstrative case of the MRA grade. In this case, MRA grades are bilaterally 3 (MR score 6; ICA2, MCA3, ACA1, PCA0)

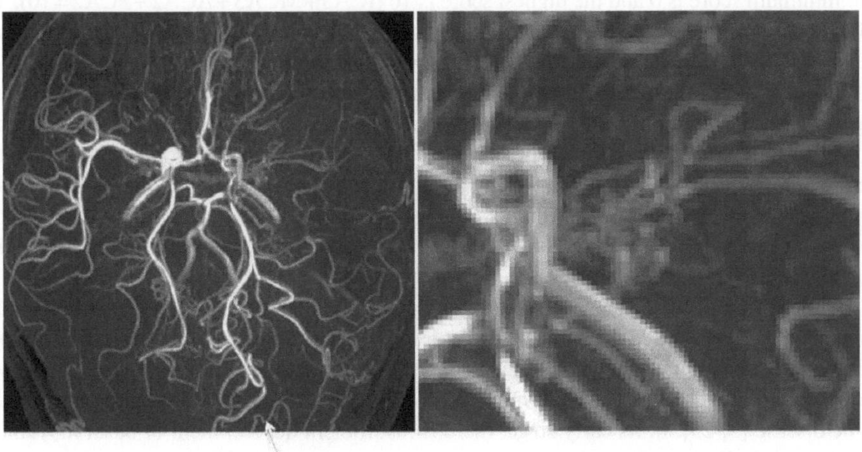

Fig. 3 Demonstrative case of the MRA grade. In this case, MRA grades are 3 for the left side (MR score 5; ICA 1, MCA 3, ACA 0, PCA 1)

2. MCA (Figs. 2 and 3)

Scores were assigned to the MCA depending on the severity of the steno-occlusive change of the horizontal portion of the MCA (M1) and the visibility of its distal branches.

Point 0: Normal or minimum equivocal change of the horizontal portion of the MCA (M1 portion), including its wall irregularity.

Point 1: Stenosis of the horizontal portion of the MCA with normal or equivocal signal reduction of its distal branches.

Point 2: Signal decrease or loss of the horizontal portion of the MCA with obvious signal reduction of its distal branches.

Point 3: Most of the MCA territory is not depicted.

3. ACA (Figs. 2 and 3)

It is well known that the horizontal portion of the ACA (A1) is often hypoplastic on the basis of its reciprocal relationship to the other side of A1. Therefore, the ACA was evaluated based on the visibility of the A2 portion and its distal branches.

Point 0: Normal signal intensity of the A2 and its distal branches.

Point 1: Signal decrease or loss of the A2 and its distal branches.

Point 2: Most of the ACA is not depicted.

4. PCA (Fig. 3)

Scores were assigned to the PCA depending on the visibility of the ambient segment (P2) and its distal branches because the first segment of the PCA is occasionally hypoplastic as a normal variation.

Point 1: The signal of P2 and its distal branches is normal or equivocally stenotic.

Point 2: Signal decrease or loss of P2 and its distal branches diminishes.

Point 3: Most of the PCA is not depicted.

The moyamoya vessels were excluded from the evaluation of subjects because the depiction of these small vessels is not always constant. In addition, it is well known that its development is not related to the severity of this disease since the moyamoya vessels regress as the disease progresses, once they are formed.

The MRA score was defined as the total points of the four main cerebral arteries. The minimum score is 0 and the highest score is 10 (ICA3 + MCA3 + ACA2 + PCA2 = 10). The MRA score was classified into four grades for more convenient evaluation of the progress of the disease (MRA grades 1–4).

With this grading system, a good correlation was revealed between the conventional angiographical stage and this MRA score, and this novel MRA grading revealed a good sensitivity and specificity compatible with the conventional staging. For the establishment of the novel MRA scoring system for the staging of moyamoya disease, both the limitations and advantages of this particular modality and the features of moyamoya disease described above have to be carefully considered. As expected, the most controversial point in terms of MRA scoring is whether the development of moyamoya vessels should be considered.

The detection of well-developed basal moyamoya vessels is not always difficult using the contemporary high Tesla MR machine. Therefore, it is quite practical to evaluate the development of basal moyamoya vessels and include this factor into the scoring system. However, it is well known that the development of basal moyamoya vessels is not linearly correlated to the staging of the disease [3, 23]. In its early stage, there is insufficient development of basal moyamoya vessels, and similarly, in its end stage, basal moyamoya vessels vanish due to the development of transdural collateral circulation such as the vault moyamoya vessels [22–24]. Therefore, the scoring based on the development of moyamoya vessels is not always a good parameter for evaluating the stage of the disease. The evaluation of moyamoya vessels is indispensable for the primary diagnosis of the disease using MRA. However, once it is diagnosed, the evaluation of its steno-occlusive change is more practical for its staging.

It is true that careful observation of the signal intensity of main branches by an imaging condition is required to apply this MRA score because overestimation of the stenosis and occlusion are occasionally observed on MRA, as reported in numerous papers. In this MRA scoring method, this overestimation is also considered.

Suzuki's angiographical staging does not necessarily relate to the clinical severity and cerebral blood flow. This point is also considered in this MRA scoring method.

Postoperative MRA

Prominent neovascularization is known to develop in patients with moyamoya disease after surgical revascularization. Two different processes of neovascularization take place following bypass surgery in patients with moyamoya disease: angiogenesis induced by the indirect bypass and revascularization through direct bypass. It appears that neovascularization induces the disappearance of the moyamoya vessels and progression of the ICA to steno-occlusive change. As a result, surgical treatment apparently seems to accelerate the upgrading of the angiographical stage. This process is, however, hypothesized from the fragmentary information obtained by conventional angiography performed after surgery [26–32]. Indeed, the accurate longitudinal changes taking place after surgery have not been fully elucidated since conventional angiography is invasive and frequent repetition of this procedure is not practical, especially in pediatric cases. Its noninvasive nature is ideal for the diagnosis of this pediatric cerebrovascular disease. In addition, recent advances have enabled reliable visualization of fine moyamoya vessels and steno-occlusive changes in the circle of Willis, identification of which are essential for the diagnosis of moyamoya disease [3, 7, 16, 33, 34]. MRA is also a practical means for longitudinal observation of postoperative angiographical changes. Serial postoperative MRA examinations have shown how neovascularization occurs between the donor tissue and brain after surgery [35]. Figure 4 shows typical changes as follows:

1. Disappearance or reduction of moyamoya vessels. These changes were recognized on MRA within 1 month of surgery. This change gradually increased on the follow-up MRA
2. Progression of the steno-occlusive change. This change was confirmed more than 3 months after surgery following confirmation of neovascularization through the direct and indirect bypass on MRA
3. STA signal (direct revascularization) increase. Signal intensity increase of the STA was confirmed 1 month after surgery or later
4. DTA/MMA signal (angiogenesis through indirect neovascularization) increase. The signal intensity of the DTA/MMA increased within 3 months. Once this signal intensity increase has been observed, it seems to become gradually more obvious on MRAs up to 6 months later

The timings when the changes described above have also been investigated by Houkin et al. [35]. There is a reciprocal relationship between neovascularization and the regression of moyamoya vessels. The appearance of angiogenesis around the anastomosized part [29] through the temporal muscle (DTA) and dura mater (MMA) is the most important point on MRA 3 months after surgery. The mechanism of the angiogenesis through the indirect encephalosynangiosis is still unknown. The basic FGF might have some role [36, 37]. It is conceivable that some angiogenetic factors including basic FGF may play an important role in the induction of angiogenesis through the temporal muscle and dura mater.

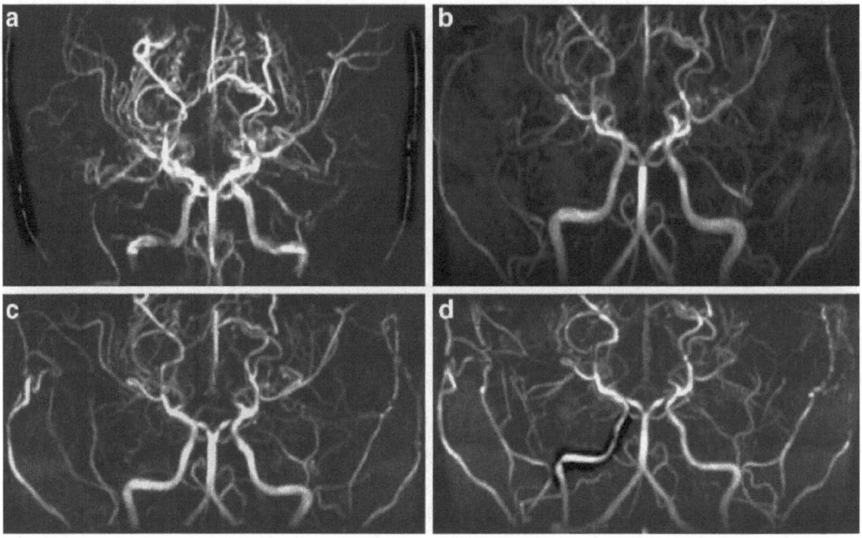

Fig. 4 (**a**)–(**d**) Sequential follow-up MRAs. (**a**) Preoperative MRA shows basal moyamoya vessels. (**b**) MRA 1 month after surgery demonstrates the reduction of moyamoya vessels and the STA signal increase is shown. (**c**) MRA 3 months after surgery reveals DTA/MMA signal increase shown in addition to the STA signal increase. (**d**) MRA 6 months after surgery more obviously shows the increase in the DTA/MMA signal and progression of the steno-occlusive change in ICA (bilateral sides) and the MCA (left side)

References

1. Fukui M (1997) Guidelines for the diagnosis and treatment of spontaneous occlusion of the circle of Willis ('moyamoya' disease). Research Committee on Spontaneous Occlusion of the Circle of Willis (Moyamoya Disease) of the Ministry of Health and Welfare, Japan. Clin Neurol Neurosurg 99 Suppl 2:S238–240
2. Numaguchi Y, Gonzalez CF, Davis PC et al (1997) Moyamoya disease in the United States. Clin Neurol Neurosurg 99 Suppl 2:S26–30
3. Houkin K, Aoki T, Takahashi A et al (1994) Diagnosis of moyamoya disease with magnetic resonance angiography. Stroke 25:2159–2164
4. Yamada I, Matsushima Y, Suzuki S (1992) Moyamoya disease: diagnosis with three-dimensional time-of-flight MR angiography. Radiology 184:773–778
5. Yamada I, Suzuki S, Matsushima Y (1995) Moyamoya disease: comparison of assessment with MR angiography and MR imaging versus conventional angiography. Radiology 196:211–218
6. Kikuchi M, Asato M, Sugahara S (1996) Evaluation of surgically formed collateral circulation in moyamoya disease with 3D-CT angiography: comparison with MR angiography and X-ray angiography. Neuropediatrics 27:45–49
7. Hasuo K, Mihara F, Matsushima T (1998) MRI and MR angiography in moyamoya disease. J Magn Reson Imaging 8:762–766
8. Shirane R, Mikawa S, Ebina T (1999) A case of adult moyamoya disease showing progressive angiopathy on cerebral angiography. Clin Neurol Neurosurg 101:210–214
9. Takanashi JI, Sugita K, Niimi H (1998) Evaluation of magnetic resonance angiography with selective maximum intensity projection in patients with childhood moyamoya disease. Eur J Paediatr Neurol 2:83–89
10. Aoki S, Yoshikawa T, Hori M et al (2000) Two-dimensional thick-slice MR digital subtraction angiography for assessment of cerebrovascular occlusive diseases. Eur Radiol 10:1858–1864
11. Thibaud C, Garnier-Viarouge MP, De Kersaint-Gilly A et al (2001) Moyamoya disease: importance of the MRI-MRA combination and difficulties in management and follow-up in 7 cases. J Neuroradiol 28:84–91

12. Yamada I, Nakagawa T, Matsushima Y et al (2001) High-resolution turbo magnetic resonance angiography for diagnosis of moyamoya disease. Stroke 32:1825–1831
13. Kuroda S, Houkin K (2008) Moyamoya disease: current concepts and future perspectives. Lancet Neurol 11:1056–1066
14. Fukui M (1997) Current state of study on moyamoya disease in Japan. Surg Neurol 47:138–143
15. Houkin K (2001) Magnetic resonance image (MRI) and CT scan diagosis. In: Ikezaki K, Loftus CM (eds) Moyamoya disease. AANS, Rolling Meadows, IL
16. Houkin K, Tanaka N, Takahashi A et al (1994) Familial occurrence of moyamoya disease. Magnetic resonance angiography as a screening test for high-risk subjects. Childs Nerv Syst 10:421–425
17. Anderson CM, Saloner D, Tsuruda JS et al (1990) Artifacts in maximum-intensity-projection display of MR angiograms. AJR Am J Roentgenol 154:623–629
18. Creasy JL, Price RR, Presbrey T et al (1990) Gadolinium-enhanced MR angiography. Radiology 175:280–283
19. Marchal G, Bosmans H, Van Fraeyenhoven L et al (1990) Intracranial vascular lesions: optimization and clinical evaluation of three-dimensional time-of-flight MR angiography. Radiology 175:443–448
20. Motomiya M, Karino T (1984) Flow patterns in the human carotid artery bifurcation. Stroke 15:50–56
21. Ruggieri PM, Laub GA, Masaryk TJ et al (1989) Intracranial circulation: pulse-sequence considerations in three-dimensional (volume) MR angiography. Radiology 171:785–791
22. Suzuki J, Takaku A (1969) Cerebrovascular "moyamoya" disease. Disease showing abnormal net-like vessels in base of brain. Arch Neurol 20:288–299
23. Suzuki J, Kodama N (1983) Moyamoya disease – a review. Stroke 14:104–109
24. Suzuki J, Kodama N (1971) Cerebrovascular "Moyamoya" disease. 2. Collateral routes to forebrain via ethmoid sinus and superior nasal meatus. Angiology 22:223–236
25. Houkin K, Nakayama N, Kuroda S et al (2005) Novel magnetic resonance angiography stage grading for moyamoya disease. Cerebrovasc Dis 20:347–354
26. Asfora WT, West M, McClarty B (1993) Angiography of encephalomyosynangiosis and superficial temporal artery to middle cerebral artery anastomosis in moyamoya disease. Am J Neuroradiol 14:29–30
27. Eller TW, Pasternak JF (1987) Revascularization for moyamoya disease: five-year follow-up. Surg Neurol 28:463–467
28. Houkin K, Kamiyama H, Abe H et al (1996) Surgical therapy for adult moyamoya disease. Can surgical revascularization prevent the recurrence of intracerebral hemorrhage? Stroke 27:1342–1346
29. Kinugasa K, Mandai S, Kamata I et al (1993) Surgical treatment of moyamoya disease: operative technique for encephalo-duro-arterio-myo-synangiosis, its follow-up, clinical results, and angiograms. Neurosurgery 32:527–531
30. Matsushima T, Inoue T, Suzuki SO et al (1992) Surgical treatment of moyamoya disease in pediatric patients – comparison between the results of indirect and direct revascularization procedures. Neurosurgery 31:401–405
31. Sakamoto H, Kitano S, Yasui T et al (1997) Direct extracranial–intracranial bypass for children with moyamoya disease. Clin Neurol Neurosurg 99 Suppl 2:S128–133
32. Suzuki R, Matsushima Y, Takada Y et al (1989) Changes in cerebral hemodynamics following encephalo-duro-arterio-synangiosis (EDAS) in young patients with moyamoya disease. Surg Neurol 31:343–349
33. Aoki T, Matsuzawa H, Houkin K et al (1993) Usefulness and limitation of MR imaging and MR angiography in diagnosis of juvenile moyamoya disease. No Shinkei Geka 21:305–311
34. Yamada I, Matsushima Y, Suzuki S (1992) Moyamoya disease: diagnosis with three-dimensional time-of-flight MR angiography. Radiology 184:773–778
35. Houkin K, Nakayama N, Kuroda S et al (2004) How does angiogenesis develop in pediatric moyamoya disease after surgery? A prospective study with MR angiography. Childs Nerv Syst 20:734–741
36. Takahashi A, Sawamura Y, Houkin K et al (1993) The cerebrospinal fluid in patients with moyamoya disease (spontaneous occlusion of the circle of Willis) contains high level of basic fibroblast growth factor. Neurosci Lett 160:214–216
37. Yoshimoto T, Houkin K, Takahashi A et al (1996) Angiogenic factors in moyamoya disease. Stroke 27:2160–2165

Diagnostic Evaluation: Morphological Imaging MRI

Kazuhiko Nishino, Takatoshi Sorimachi, and Yukihiko Fujii

Introduction

The recent advent of magnetic resonance imaging (MRI) and magnetic resonance angiography (MRA) has contributed significantly to the diagnosis of moyamoya disease. According to the guidelines for the diagnosis and treatment of spontaneous occlusion of the circle of Willis, i.e., moyamoya disease, cerebral angiography is not mandatory, if MRI and MRA identify all the findings required for diagnosis [1].

This section will present the latest knowledge concerning MRI/MRA findings of moyamoya disease and their contribution to the management of this entity.

Importance of MRI/MRA for the Management of Moyamoya Disease

Early Diagnosis

Even for asymptomatic patients with early-stage moyamoya disease, MRA can identify slight stenotic changes in the internal carotid artery (ICA). Although the natural course of asymptomatic moyamoya disease is not fully understood, a recent multicenter survey revealed that asymptomatic cases are not a silent disorder [2]. However, it is unreasonable with regard to the cost-benefit ratio to perform random MRA screenings because moyamoya disease is a rare entity [3–5]. At present, it seems justified to perform MRA for asymptomatic patients who have a family history of moyamoya disease, or pediatric patients who have recurring headache despite the absence of abnormal findings on computed tomography (CT).

K. Nishino (✉), T. Sorimachi, and Y. Fujii
Department of Neurosurgery, Brain Research Institute, University of Niigata, 757 Asahimachi-dori 1, Chuo-ku, Niigata 951-8585, Japan
e-mail: nishino@bri.niigata-u.ac.jp

B.-K. Cho and T. Tominaga (eds.), *Moyamoya Disease Update*,
DOI 10.1007/978-4-431-99703-0_24,

If a symptomatic patient remains undiagnosed and untreated, it results in irreversible neurological deficit, especially in pediatric patients [6–8]. Therefore, MRI/MRA must be performed without hesitation in pediatric patients with ischemic stroke or transient ischemic attack (TIA).

Evaluation of Treatment Strategies

Once a patient has been diagnosed with moyamoya disease, the patient should undergo further MR analysis to assess the present condition. First, it is important to evaluate the degree of disease progression, regardless of whether or not surgery is planned. An MRA can be employed to determine the disease stage, which was previously decided by conventional angiography [9]. Second, an evaluation of parenchymal damage by MRI is also essential to predict the outcome and to determine appropriate surgical strategies. Third, a hemodynamic study is required before surgery. Although existing modalities are reliable, recent MRI techniques can be utilized to roughly assess the cerebral hemodynamics without exposure to ionizing radiation [10–14]. Finally, several findings seen on MRI/MRA indicate an increased risk for future stroke including infarction and hemorrhage. Accordingly, such findings should be taken into consideration when determining treatment strategies.

Follow-Up

After surgery, it is essential to evaluate the development of a collateral pathway via the external carotid artery (ECA) system and subsequent changes occurring in intracranial arteries. Although MRA is inferior in spatial resolution to angiography, it is capable of demonstrating the serial morphological changes that responded to surgery in a noninvasive way.

Steno-occlusive lesions in intracranial arteries frequently progress naturally in pediatric patients [15–17]. In addition, a recent report showed that the incidence of disease progression in adult patients is much higher than previously recognized [18–20]. Hence, careful MRA follow-up is essential in nonoperated cases.

Morphological Evaluation

MRI

Although MRI in asymptomatic cases as well as in cases with TIA frequently discloses no abnormality, old ischemic or hemorrhagic lesions are occasionally detected in the brain parenchyma. These ischemic lesions are commonly seen in anterior or posterior watershed zones [21], showing bilateral hemispheric distribution. To detect such lesions, T2-weighted and fluid-attenuated inversion recovery (FLAIR) imaging is useful. As the disease progresses, steno-occlusive changes in the ICA and its tributaries can be detected as a decrease in the diameter of flow void in T2-weighted images, whereas the posterior cerebral artery (PCA) shows a marked increase in diameter (Fig. 1a). Around this stage, moyamoya vessels can be

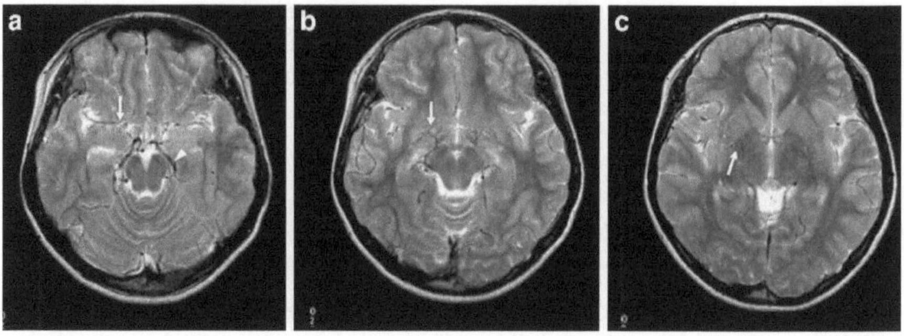

Fig. 1 Typical findings of moyamoya disease with T2-weighted magnetic resonance imaging (MRI) includes the disappearance of the flow void signal of the terminal portion of the internal carotid artery (ICA; *arrow*), the reciprocal dilatation of the posterior cerebral artery (PCA; *arrowhead*) (**a**), and the development of many tiny flow voids (moyamoya vessels) in the basal cistern (*arrow*) (**b**) and basal ganglia (*arrow*) (**c**)

seen in basal cistern or basal ganglia, and the abnormal fine vessels are clearly depicted as numerous flow voids in T2-weighted images (Fig. 1b, c).

Leptomeningeal enhancement (ivy sign) on contrast-enhanced T1-weighted images is a characteristic MRI finding of moyamoya disease (Fig. 2, upper row) [22, 23], and FLAIR images can also reveal the ivy sign without the use of contrast media (Fig. 2, lower row) [23, 24]. The ivy sign is due to an engorged pial network via a leptomeningeal anastomosis, which diminishes after bypass surgery with the development of new transdural collateral vessels [22–24]. However, subarachnoid hemorrhage (SAH), meningitis, and spontaneous intracranial hypotension [25, 26] should be considered when the ivy sign is identified.

Recent reports showing T2*-weighted images reveal that asymptomatic microbleeds occur in 15–56% of moyamoya disease patients [27–29]. Although the clinical implications of the microbleeds have yet to be understood, the presence of multiple microbleeds might be a predictor of subsequent hemorrhagic stroke.

Recent development of high field MRI has made it possible to reveal brain vessel microstructure in moyamoya disease. Coworkers at our institution observed transverse lines (medullary streaks) in white matter using 3-Tesla MRI T2-reversed imaging (Fig. 3) and concluded that the increase in medullary streak diameters observed in patients with moyamoya disease represent vessels dilated due to cerebral hypoperfusion [30].

Once ischemic stroke occurs, diffusion-weighted (DW) imaging is useful to localize ischemic lesions, which are depicted as high intensity areas in the early acute phase (Fig. 4). The main cause of intracranial hemorrhage is rupture of dilated, fragile moyamoya vessels, resulting in intraventricular hemorrhage or intracerebral hematoma (ICH) [31–34]. Although CT is usually superior to MRI for detecting acute ICH, the ICH commonly shows high intensity on T2-weighted images in the early acute phase, and high intensity accompanied by a low intensity rim on DW images. Rupture of a saccular aneurysm around the circle of Willis causes SAH [34, 35]. For detecting SAH in the acute phase, FLAIR imaging is sensitive [36, 37]. In addition, T2*-weighted images are also helpful in detecting SAH in the subacute and chronic phases, which are generally unclear on CT [37].

Longstanding brain ischemia results in brain atrophy, which is usually seen in the frontal lobe in the early stage but becomes diffused with progression of the disease [21].

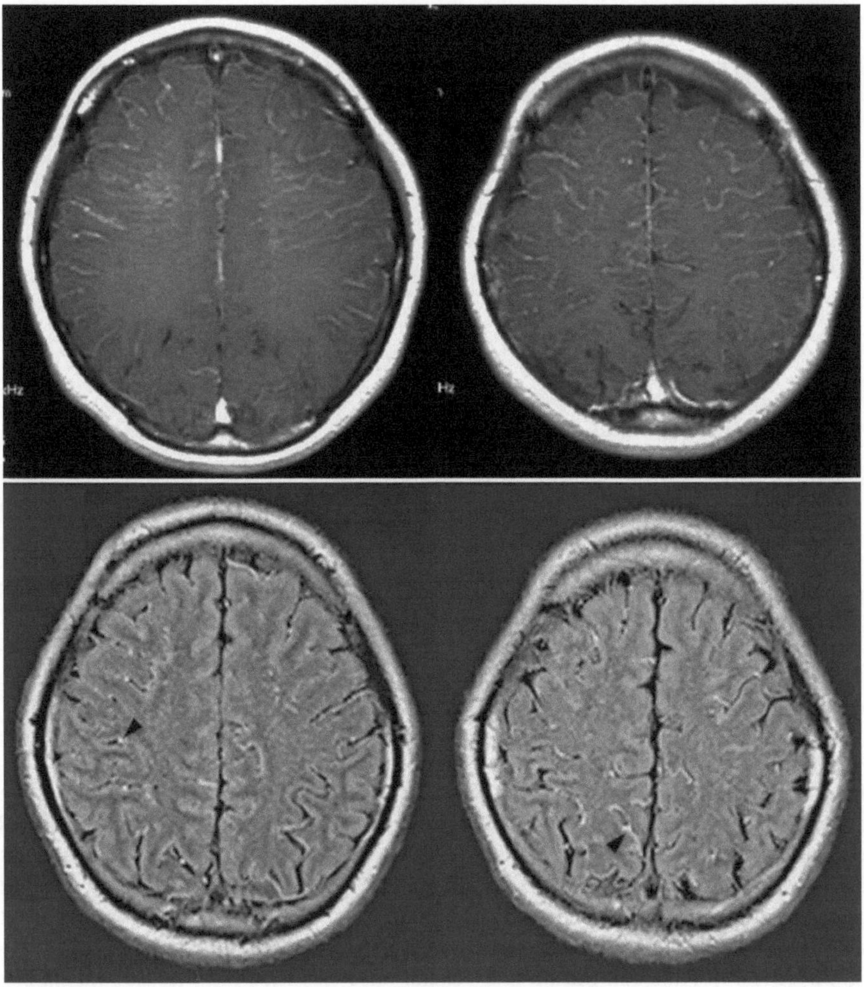

Fig. 2 Ivy sign. Contrast-enhanced T1-weighted MRI shows diffuse leptomeningeal enhancement (*upper row*). Ivy sign can be identified with fluid-attenuated inversion recovery (FLAIR) images (*arrowheads*; *lower row*)

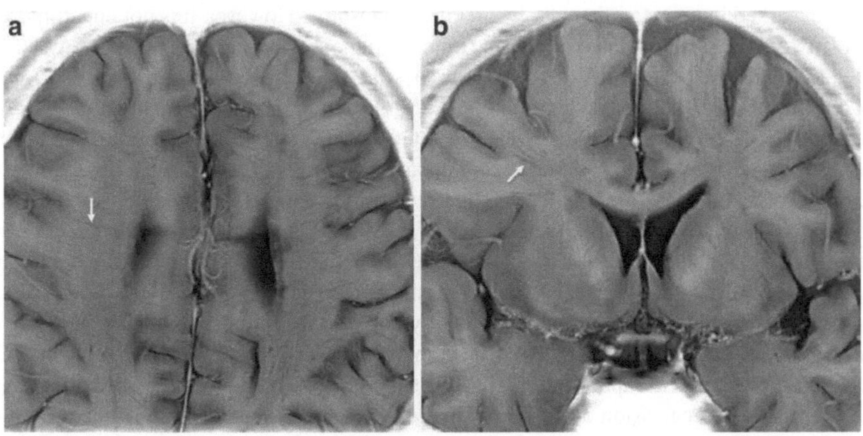

Fig. 3 T2-reversed 3-Tesla MRI in a moyamoya disease patients ((**a**) axial, (**b**) coronal view) shows transverse lines (medullary streaks) that likely represent vessels dilated due to cerebral hypoperfusion

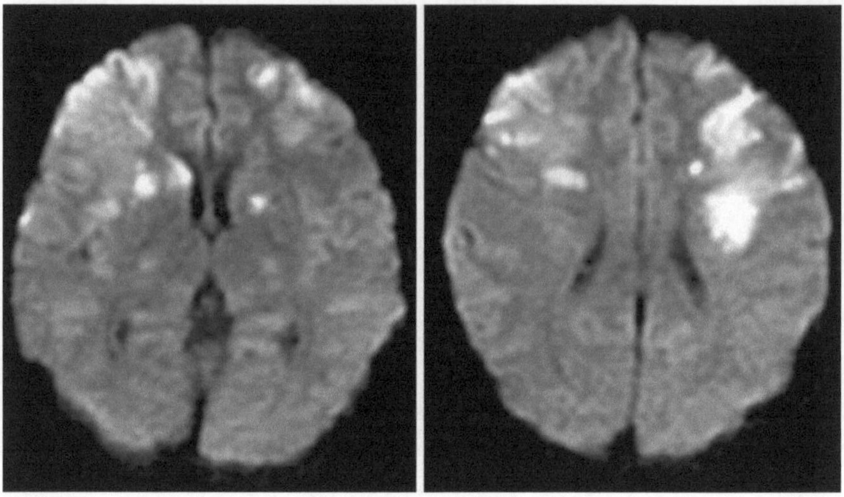

Fig. 4 Diffusion-weighted (DW) MRI obtained 4 h after ischemic stroke in a moyamoya disease patient reveals the ischemic lesions as a high intensity area in early acute phase

MRA

MRA is the most useful modality to diagnose early-stage moyamoya disease, irrespective of the type of acquisition techniques including 3D time-of-flight MRA, phase contrast MRA, and contrast-enhanced MRA [38, 39]. In the very early stage, MRA shows slight stenosis of the ICA terminal portion (Fig. 5a). As the disease progresses, MRA discloses the typical findings of moyamoya disease including the steno-occlusive change in the ICA and its tributaries, the development of moyamoya vessels, and an increase in the diameter of the ECA system (Fig. 5b) [21, 40]. Although Suzuki and Takaku once classified this disease into six stages based on angiographic findings [41], a novel grading of MRA findings correlates well with angiographic staging [9]. Interestingly, the disease stage does not always correlate with the severity of clinical symptoms, i.e., it is not rare that a patient in an advanced stage remains asymptomatic (Fig. 5b). In cases of advanced stage moyamoya disease, the PCA frequently shows a marked increase in diameter in a reciprocal fashion. However, it is not uncommon for the PCA to have steno-occlusive changes (Fig. 6). Some reports suggested that PCA stenosis correlates with the occurrence of cerebral infarction [42–44]. Moyamoya vessels originate not only from the ICA but also from the PCA. Some authors have reported that the MRA in hemorrhagic cases shows marked dilatation of choroidal arteries or posterior pericallosal arteries, compared to that in patients experiencing an ischemic event [45, 46]. In addition, the dilatation of thalamoperforating arteries is commonly seen, especially in cases with ICH (Fig. 7). Accordingly, these findings on MRA might be a predictor of hemorrhagic events. Another cause of hemorrhage is saccular aneurysms on the circle of Willis, which occur quite often at the basilar artery [3, 34] and can be easily detected by MRA.

MRA is also the most appropriate modality for postoperative follow-up because of its noninvasiveness. After surgery, MRA can demonstrate not only the development of ECA, including the superior temporal artery (STA), deep temporal artery, and middle meningeal artery, but also the regression of moyamoya vessels or progression of stenotic changes in the ICA [47–49] (Fig. 8).

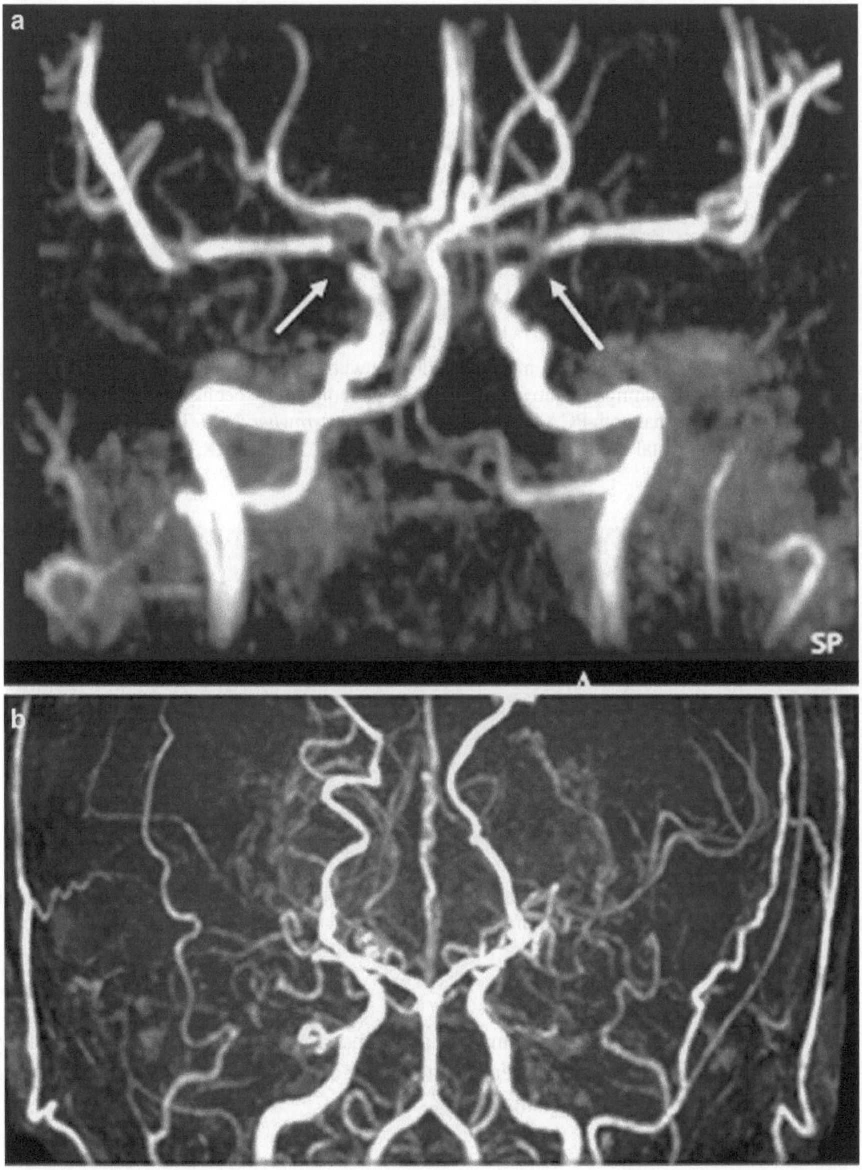

Fig. 5 MR angiography (MRA) of two cases with asymptomatic moyamoya disease. (**a**) MRA of a 20-year-old woman with a family history of moyamoya disease shows slight stenotic change of the terminal portion of bilateral ICA (*arrow*). (**b**) MRA of 52-year-old-woman who never had neurological symptoms ever reveals moyamoya disease in a more advanced stage

The development of MR technology has become available for MRA on 3-Tesla MR systems [50, 51]. 3-Tesla MRA depicts moyamoya vessels more clearly than 1.5-Tesla MRA. In addition, distal branches of intracranial arteries can be clearly visualized by using 3-Tesla MRA (Fig. 6b, c). However, even though the high field MRA was employed, it seems difficult to identify collateral circulation in peripheral regions including a leptomeningeal

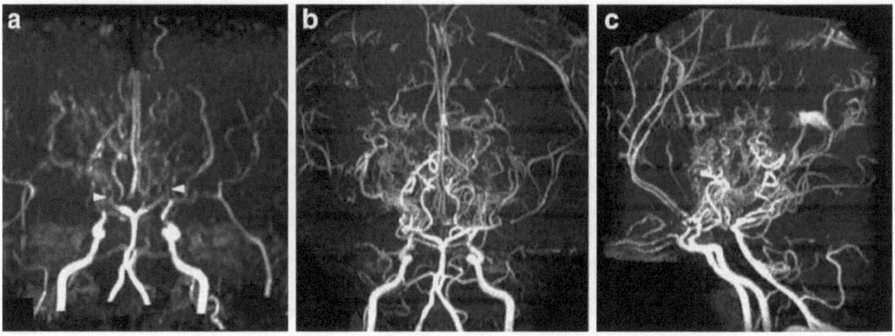

Fig. 6 MRA of a 23-year-old man with moyamoya disease who suffered from ischemic stroke. 1.5-Tesla MRA (**a**) shows typical findings of moyamoya disease including ICA occlusion and development of moyamoya vessels. Note that both PCA show stenotic changes (*arrowheads*). 3-Tesla MRA (**b**, **c**) depicts moyamoya vessels and distal cortical arteries more clearly than 1.5-Tesla MRA

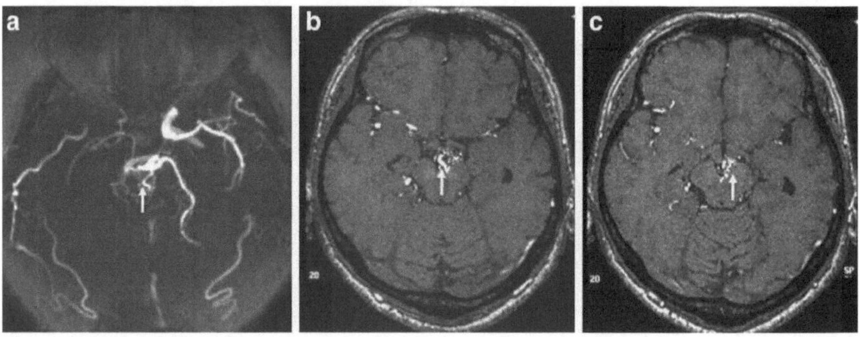

Fig. 7 MRA (**a**) and source images (**b**, **c**) of a 56-year-old woman with moyamoya disease. Thalamoperforating arteries originating from the basilar artery show marked enlargement (*arrow*). The patient later suffered from thalamic hemorrhage

anastomosis on the cortical surface or a transdural anastomosis via a vault or ethmoidal moyamoya. Furthermore, it is also difficult to ascertain the detailed course of STA which is important information for harvesting STA for direct bypass.

Hemodynamic Evaluation

It is well known that positron emission tomography and single photon emission CT are reliable tools for evaluating cerebral hemodynamics and metabolism. However, recent adjunctive MRI techniques can be utilized to roughly assess the cerebral hemodynamics in moyamoya disease. Perfusion-weighted MRI can reveal the mean transit time (MTT), time to peak enhancement (TTP), and cerebral blood volume. Recent reports showed that the MTT positively correlates with the degree of ICA stenosis, and that changes in TTP after bypass surgery correlate with clinical outcome [10–12]. An emerging technique for the assessment of cerebral vascular resistance (CVR) is blood oxygen-level dependent MRI [13, 14]. CVR

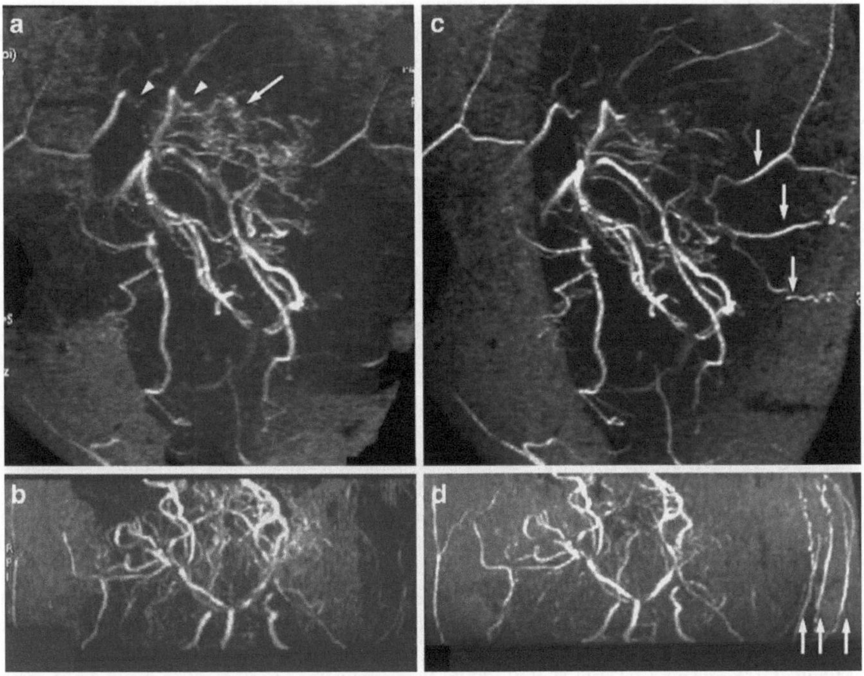

Fig. 8 Preoperative MRA (infero-lateral view (**a**), coronal view (**b**)) shows occlusion in the terminal of bilateral ICA (*arrowheads*) and development of moyamoya vessels (*arrow*). MRA (infero-lateral view (**c**), coronal view (**d**)) obtained 4 months after combined bypass surgery reveals an increase in the diameter of the superficial temporal artery and deep temporal arteries (*arrows*) as well as the remission of moyamoya vessels

mapping can be obtained by rapidly manipulating end-tidal PCO_2 between a hypercapnic and hypocapnic state (30–50 mmHg), and the map is capable of revealing the presence and spatial extent of exhausted autoregulation [13].

Conclusions

Early diagnosis and appropriate treatment are crucial to improve the long-term outcome for cases with moyamoya disease. Although the imaging quality of MRI/MRA is still inferior to the existing modalities in some aspects, future progress of the technology will increase the role of MRI/MRA in the management of moyamoya disease.

References

1. Fukui M (1997) Guidelines for the diagnosis and treatment of spontaneous occlusion of the circle of Willis (moyamoya disease) of the Ministry of Health and Welfare, Japan. Clin Neurol Neurosurg 99:238–240

2. Kuroda S, Hashimoto N, Yoshimoto T et al (2007) Radiological findings, clinical course, and outcome in asymptomatic moyamoya disease: results of multicenter survey in Japan. Stroke 38:1430–1435
3. Kuroda S, Houkin K (2008) Moyamoya disease: current concept and future perspectives. Lancet Neurol 7:1056–1066
4. Kuriyama S, Kusaka Y, Fujimura M et al (2008) Prevalence and clinicoepidemiological features of moyamoya disease in Japan: Findings from a nationwide epidemiological survey. Stroke 39:42–47
5. Baba T, Houkin K, Kuroda S (2007) Novel epidemiological features of moyamoya disease. J Neurol Neurosurg Psychiatry 79:900–904
6. Kurokawa T, Tomita S, Ueda K et al (1985) Prognosis of occlusive disease of the circle of Willis (moyamoya disease) in children. Pediatr Neurol 1:274–277
7. Imaizumi T, Hayashi K, Saito K et al (1998) Long-term outcome of pediatric moyamoya disease monitored to adulthood. Pediatr Neurol 18:321–325
8. Imaizumi C, Imaizumi T, Osawa M et al (1999) Serial intelligence test scores in pediatric moyamoya disease. Neuropediatrics 30:294–299
9. Houkin K, Nakayama N, Kuroda S et al (2005) Novel magnetic resonance angiography stage grading for moyamoya disease. Cerebrovasc Dis 20:347–354
10. Lee SK, Kim DI, Jeong EK et al (2003) Postoperative evaluation of moyamoya disease with perfusion-weighted MR imaging: initial experience. Am J Neuroradiol 24:741–747
11. Togao O, Mihara F, Yoshiura T et al (2006) Cerebral hemodynamics in moyamoya disease: correlation between perfusion-weighted MR imaging and cerebral angiography. Am J Neuroradiol 27:391–397
12. Yun TJ, Cheon JE, Na DG et al (2009) Childhood moyamoya disease: quantitative evaluation of perfusion MR imaging: correlation with clinical outcome after revascularization surgery. Radiology 251:216–223
13. Mikulis DJ, Krolczyk G, Desal H et al (2005) Preoperative and postoperative mapping of cerebrovascular reactivity in moyamoya disease by using blood oxygen level-dependent magnetic resonance imaging. J Neurosurg 103:347–355
14. Bacigaluppi S, Dehdashti AR, Agid R et al (2009) The contribution of imaging in diagnosis, preoperative assessment, and follow-up of moyamoya disease. Neurorsurg Focus 26:E3
15. Takahashi A, Fujiwara S, Suzuki J (1986) Long-term followup angiography of moyamoya disease-cases followed from childhood to adolescence. No Shinkei Geka 14:23–29
16. Ezura M, Yoshimoto T, Fujiwara S et al (1995) Clinical and angiographic follow-up of childhood-onset moyamoya disease. Childs Nerv Syst 11:591–594
17. Kim SK, Seol HJ, Cho BK et al (2004) Moyamoya disease among young patients: its clinical course and the role of active surgical treatment. Neurosurgery 54:840–844
18. Smith ER, Scott RM (2008) Progression of disease in unilateral moyamoya disease. Neurosurg Focus 24:E17
19. Kelly ME, Bell-Stephens TE, Marks MP (2006) Progression of unilateral moyamoya disease: a clinical series. Cerebrovasc Dis 22:109–115
20. Kuroda S, Ishikawa T, Houkin K et al (2005) Incidence and clinical features of disease progression in adult moyamoya disease. Stroke 36:2148–2153
21. Hasuo K, Mihara F, Matsushima T (1998) MRI and MR angiography in moyamoya disease. J Magn Reson Imaging 8:762–766
22. Maeda M, Tsuchida C (1999) "Ivy sign" on fluid-attenuated inversion-recovery images in childhood moyamoya disease. Am J Neuroradiol 20:1836–1838
23. Yoon HK, Shin HJ, Chang YW (2002) "Ivy sign" in childhood moyamoya disease: depiction on FLAIR and contrast-enhanced T1-weighted MR images. Radiology 223:384–389
24. Fujiwara H, Momoshima S, Kuribayashi S (2005) Leptomeningeal high signal intensity (ivy sign) on fluid-attenuated inversion-recovery (FLAIR) MR images in moyamoya disease. Eur J Radiol 55:224–230
25. Maeda M, Yagishita A, Yamamoto T et al (2003) Abnormal hyperintensity within the subarachnoid space evaluated by fluid-attenuated inversion-recovery MR imaging: a spectrum of central nervous system disease. Eur Radiol 13 (4 Suppl):L192–L201
26. Tosaka M, Sato N, Fujimaki H et al (2008) Diffuse pachymeningeal hyperintensity and subdural effusion/hematoma detected by fluid-attenuated inversion recovery MR imaging in patient with spontaneous intracranial hypotension. Am J Neuroradiol 29:1164–1170

27. Ishikawa T, Kuroda S, Nakayama N et al (2005) Prevalence of asymptomatic microbleeds in patients with moyamoya disease. Neurol Med Chir 45:495–500
28. Kikuta K, Takagi Y, Nozaki K et al (2005) Asymptomatic microbleeds in moyamoya disease: T2*-weighted gradient-echo magnetic resonance imaging study. J Neurosurg 102:470–475
29. Kikuta K, Takagi Y, Nozaki K et al (2008) The presence of multiple microbleeds as a predictor of subsequent cerebral hemorrhage in patients with moyamoya disease. Neurosurgery 62:104–110
30. Harada A, Fujii Y, Yoneoka Y et al (2001) High-field magnetic resonance imaging in patients with moyamoya disease. J Neurosurg 94:233–237
31. Gravel JH, Levine M, Hollis P et al (1989) Moyamoya-like disease associated with a lenticulostriate region aneurysm. J Neurosurg 70:802–803
32. Lee JK, Lee KH, Kim SH et al (2001) Distal anterior choroidal artery aneurysm in a patient with moyamoya disease: case report. Neurosurgery 48:222–225
33. Iwama T, Morimoto M, Hashimoto N et al (1997) Mechanism of intracranial rebleeding in moyamoya disease. Clin Neurol Neurosurg 99:S187–S190
34. Kawaguchi S, Sakaki T, Morimoto T et al (1996) Characteristics of intracranial aneurysms associated with moyamoya disease. A review of 111 cases. Acta Neurochir (Wien) 138:1287–1294
35. Iwama T, Todaka T, Hashimoto N (1997) Direct surgery for major artery aneurysm associated with moyamoya disease. Clin Neurol Neurosurg 99:S191–S193
36. Wiesmann M, Mayer TE, Madele R et al (2002) Detection of hyperacute subarachnoid hemorrhage of the brain by using magnetic resonance imaging. J Neurosurg 96:684–689
37. Yuank MK, Lai PH, Chen JY et al (2005) Detection of subarachnoid hemorrhage at acute and subacute/chronic stages: comparison of four magnetic resonance imaging pulse sequences and computed tomography. J Clin Med Assoc 68:131–137
38. Özsarlak Ö, Van Goethem JW, Parizel PM (2004) MR angiography of the intracranial vessels: technical aspects and clinical applications. Neuroradiology 46:955–972
39. Tsuchiya K, Fujikawa A, Tateishi H et al (2005) Postoperative assessment of extracranial-intracranial bypass by time-resolved 3D contrast-enhanced MR angiography using parallel imaging. Am J Neuroradiol 26:2243–2247
40. Houkin K, Aoki T, Takahashi A et al (1994) Diagnosis of moyamoya disease with magnetic resonance angiography. Stroke 25:2159–2164
41. Suzuki J, Takaku A (1969) Cerebrovascular "moyamoya disease". Disease showing abnormal net-like vessels in base of the brain. Arch Neurol 20:288–299
42. Kuroda S, Ishikawa T, Houkin K et al (2002) Clinical significance of posterior cerebral artery stenosis/occlusion in moyamoya disease. No Shinkei Geka 30:1295–1300
43. Mugikura S, Takahashi S, Higano S et al (1999) The relationship between cerebral infarction and angiographic characteristics in childhood moyamoya disease. Am J Neuroradiol 20:336–343
44. Yamada I, Himeno Y, Suzuki S et al (1995) Posterior circulation in moyamoya disease: angiographic study. Radiology 197:239–246
45. Irikura K, Miyasaka Y, Tanaka R et al (1996) A source of haemorrhage in adult patients with moyamoya disease: the significance of tributaries from the choroidal artery. Acta Neurochir (Wien) 138:1282–1286
46. Morioka M, Hamada J, Kawano T et al (2003) Angiographic dilatation and branch extension of the anterior choroidal and posterior communicating arteries are predictors of hemorrhage in adult moyamoya patients. Stroke 34:90–95
47. Honda M, Kitagawa N, Tsutsumi K et al (2005) Magnetic resonance angiography evaluation of external carotid artery tributaries in moyamoya disease. Surg Neurol 64:325–330
48. Houkin K, Nakayama N, Kuroda S et al (2004) How does angiogenesis develop in pediatric moyamoya disease after surgery? Childs Nerv Syst 20:734–741
49. Yoon HK, Shin HJ, Lee M et al (2000) MR angiography of moyamoya disease before and after encephaloduroarteriosynangiosis. Am J Radiol 174:195–200
50. Fushimi Y, Miki Y, Kikuta K et al (2006) Comparison of 3.0- and 1.5-T three-dimensional time-of-flight MR angiography on moyamoya disease: preliminary experience. Radiology 239:232–237
51. Tomasian A, Salamon N, Lohan DG et al (2008) Supraaortic arteries: contrast material doze reduction at 3.0-T high spatial resolution MR angiography-Feasibility study. Radiology 249:980–990

Part VIII
Diagnostic Evaluation II: Functional Imaging

Functional Neuroimagings "Overview"

Jyoji Nakagawara

Introduction

Moyamoya disease is characterized by progressive vascular occlusion of the circle of the Willis accompanied by dilated perforating arteries, which are so-called moyamoya vessels, in the regions of basal ganglia and thalami [1]. These findings was defined by cerebral angiography and also classified into the Suzuki's angiographical stages. More recently, the stage of moyamoya disease using magnetic resonance angiography (MRA) was proposed as a less invasive assessment [2]. However, cerebral angiography and/or MRA cannot evaluate cerebral hemodynamics in patients with moyamoya disease, which should be assessed by functional neuroimagings such as ^{15}O-positron emission tomography (^{15}O-PET), single photon emission computed tomography (SPECT), and perfusion magnetic resonance imaging/computed tomography (MRI/CT).

These functional neuroimagings have been performed mainly to investigate the severity of hemodynamic cerebral ischemia using cerebral blood flow (CBF), cerebrovascular reserve, and oxygen metabolism in the affected territories. These parameters measured by functional neuroimagings could be useful to evaluate the indication of surgical revascularization, the changes of hemodynamics after surgical revascularization, and the prediction of the clinical outcome. In general, most pediatric patients who usually suffered from recurrent TIA can show severe hemodynamic cerebral ischemia such as the misery perfusion [3–5] defined by PET; however, most adult patients who suffered from intracerebral hemorrhage or intraventriclar hemorrhage can occasionally show the misery perfusion. The misery perfusion is generally thought to be an impaired cerebral hemodynamics suitable for surgical revascularization [6, 7]. Definite diagnosis of the misery perfusion can be only established by ^{15}O-PET, and therefore alternative methods using CBF-SPECT or perfusion MRI/CT to examine cerebral hemodynamics corresponding to the misery perfusion have been developed in recent years. In this chapter, the characteristics of each functional neuroimaging on cerebral hemodynamics are summarized.

J. Nakagawara (✉)
Department of Neurosurgery, Nakamura Memorial Hospital,
South-1, West-14, Chuo-ku, Sapporo 060-8570, Japan
e-mail: george@med.nmh.or.jp

B.-K. Cho and T. Tominaga (eds.), *Moyamoya Disease Update*,
DOI 10.1007/978-4-431-99703-0_25, © Springer 2010

^{15}O-PET

With respect to evaluating the cerebral hemodynamic status in patients with moyamoya disease, assessment using ^{15}O-PET could be one of the gold standards in comparison with alternative assessments using CBF-SPECT or perfusion MRI/CT. Regional CBF (rCBF), regional oxygen extraction fraction (rOEF), and regional cerebral metabolic rate of oxygen ($rCMRO_2$) are measured using the ^{15}O-steady state methods with continuous infusion of $H_2{}^{15}O$ or inhalation of $C^{15}O_2$ and $^{15}O_2$ [3–5]. The regional cerebral blood volume (rCBV) is measured by a single inhalation of $C^{15}O$. The rOEF and $rCMRO_2$ values can be corrected for rCBV. The regional mean transit time (MTT) is calculated as the ratio of rCBV to rCBF (rCBV/rCBF). The quantitative data of each parameter in region of interest (ROI) are compared with control values from a normal database.

The severity of hemodynamic cerebral ischemia can be classified using lower limits of the vascular and metabolic reserve which is functioning as a compensatory system to preserve cerebral oxygen metabolism towards the reduction of cerebral perfusion pressure (CPP) associated with occlusive cerebrovascular lesions [8]. As shown in Fig. 1, Stage I ischemia is defined by the maintenance of CBF with decrease of vascular reserve towards reduced CPP, within the autoregulation of CBF. Stage II ischemia is defined by the decrease of CBF with loss of vascular reserve and the maintenance of $CMRO_2$ with increase of OEF, below the lower limit of the autoregulation of CBF.

Stage II ischemia corresponds to the misery perfusion which is usually observed in patients with moyamoya disease suffering from cerebral ischemia. The misery perfusion can be reversed by surgical revascularization such as direct bypass surgery, e.g., STA-MCA anastomosis, or indirect bypass surgery, such as EDAS, EMS, EDAMS, and others.

CBF-SPECT

^{123}I- or ^{99m}Tc-labeled radiotracers for measurement of CBF using SPECT have been developed in the last 20 years. *N*-isopropyl-*p*-^{123}I-iodoamphetamine (^{123}I-IMP), ^{99m}Tc-hexamethyl-propyleneamine-oxime (^{99m}Tc-HMPAO), and ^{99m}Tc-ethyl-cysteinate dimmer (^{99m}Tc-ECD) have become available for CBF-SPECT imaging (Table 1). Functional neuroimagings using these tracers can be useful to evaluate the indications of surgical revascularization, the changes of hemodynamics after surgical revascularization, and the predictions of the clinical outcome [9–13]. These radiotracers have a common character in the chemical microsphere which can be accumulated in the entire brain through the blood–brain barrier reflecting the distribution of regional CBF. However, different extraction and retention mechanisms in each tracer can result in differing distributions of tracers in the brain. ^{99m}Tc-labeled CBF tracers generally underestimate true CBF due to the limited first-pass extraction fraction, and especially cannot accurately reflect further increase of CBF in the high flow range produced by the activation test. Out of these radiotracers, the distribution of ^{123}I-IMP in the brain can be linearly corresponding to the distribution of true CBF [14] (Fig. 2).

Technical advances have made it easy to quantify regional CBF using the ^{123}I-IMP SPECT and autoradiography (ARG) method based on a 2-compartment model [15] (Fig. 3). In this method, arterial input function is determined by one-point arterial blood sampling. Quantitative analysis of CBF-SPECT such as the IMP-ARG method can progress to making criteria for the stratification of hemodynamic cerebral ischemia. However, the IMP-ARG method is not yet widely adopted for pediatric patients because of its invasiveness, e.g., arterial blood sampling, which may make the patients cry and alter the result of the measurements. Therefore, semiquantitative ROI analysis using the dominant cerebellar hemisphere as the reference [10], or statistical imaging analysis

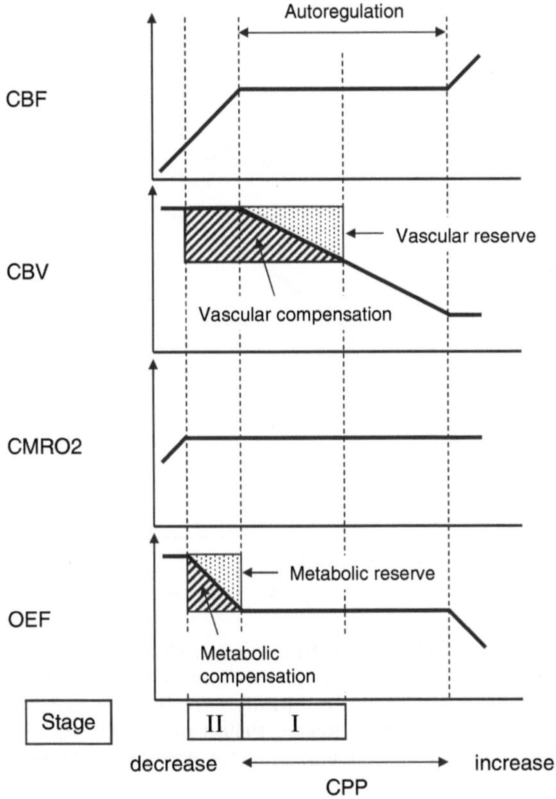

Fig. 1 Severity of hemodynamic cerebral ischemia can be classified using lower limits of vascular and metabolic reserve which function as a compensatory system to preserve cerebral oxygen metabolism towards the reduction of CPP. *CBF* cerebral blood flow, *CBV* cerebral blood volume, *$CMRO_2$* cerebral metabolic rate of oxygen, *OEF* oxygen extraction fraction, *CPP* cerebral perfusion pressure, *Stage I* maintenance of CBF and decrease of vascular reserve, *Stage II* decrease of CBF with loss of vascular reserve and maintenance of $CMRO_2$ with increase of OEF (decrease of metabolic reserve) (misery perfusion)

Table 1 Characteristics of CBF tracers for SPECT

Radiopharmaceuticals	IMP	HMPAO	ECD
Labeled nuclide	^{123}I	^{99m}Tc	^{99m}Tc
Type of injection	Labeled solution (LS)	Labeling kit	Labeling kit, LS
Injection amount	111~222 MBq	370~740 MBq	370~740 MBq
Stability	◎	○ (within 30 min)	◎ (over 30 min)
First-pass extraction	◎	○	○
Back diffusion	Little	Much	Moderate
Linearity to true CBF	◎	Δ	○
Wash-in to brain tissue	Gradually continue	Just after injection	Just after injection
Change of distribution	Observed (redistribution)	Rarely observed	Rarely observed
Influence of BBB disruptions	Influenced	Hyperfixation	Hypofixation
CBF quantification	Microsphere model 2-Compartment model	Patlak plot	Patlak Plot Microsphere model
Balloon occlusion test estimated	○	◎	◎
Acetazolamide-activation	◎		○
Emergency application	Difficult	Possible	Possible

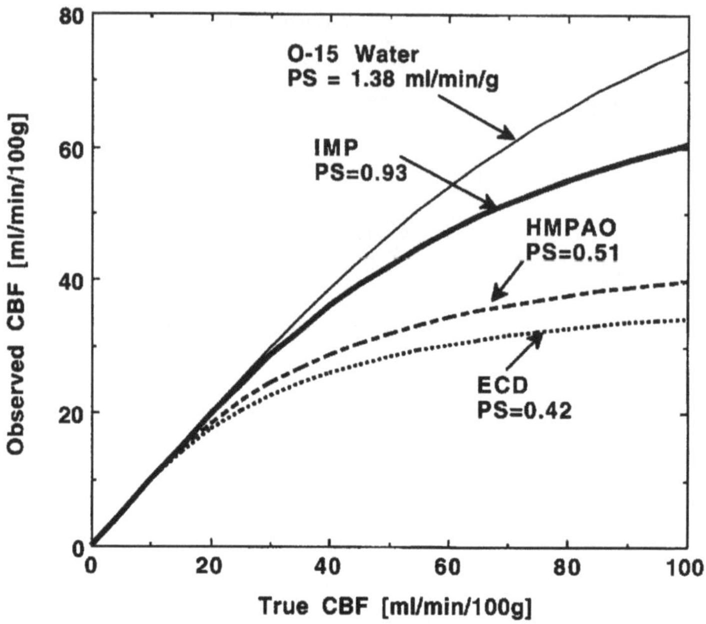

Fig. 2 Underestimation of observed CBF by rCBF tracer is produced due to the limited first-pass extraction fraction. The underestimation was estimated for four permeability-surface area product (PS) values, corresponding to four rCBF tracers of $H_2{}^{15}O$, ^{123}I-IMP, ^{99m}Tc-HMPAO, and ^{99m}Tc-ECD, respectively, according to the Renkin-Crone's equation (Renkin 1959; Crone 1963). PS values were obtained by Eichling et al. (1974) for $H_2{}^{15}O$ and by the Ehime group for other tracers (Murase et al. 1991) [14]

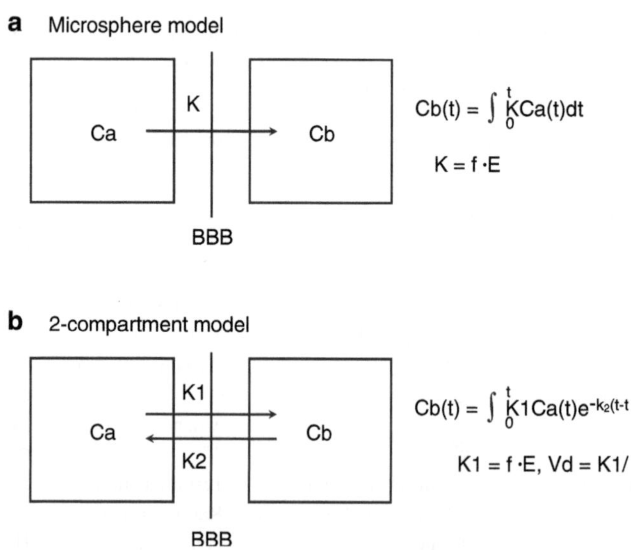

Fig. 3 Compartment models for the quantification of CBF using CBF tracer (chemical microsphere). (**a**) Microsphere model. (**b**) Two-compartment model. *BBB* blood–brain barrier, *K* (*K1*) rate constant of tracer from blood to brain, *k2* rate constant of tracer from brain to blood, *Vd* = *K1*/*k2* distribution volume, *f* cerebral blood flow (CBF), *Ca(t)* arterial input function at time *t*, *Cb(t)* radioactivity in the brain at time *t*, *E* first-pass extraction ($E = 1 - $ePS/f) (PS, permeability-surface area product)

such as 3-dimensional stereotactic surface projections (3D-SPP) [16] are accepted as an easy and less invasive method for pediatric patients.

Recently, both the dual-table ARG (DTARG) method [17] and segmental extraction estimation (SEE) analysis [18] have been developed. These methods could be clinically applied as newly standardized techniques to improve measurement accuracy and judgment accuracy for the stratification of hemodynamic cerebral ischemia.

Stratification of Hemodynamic Cerebral Ischemia Using IMP-ARG Method

Stratification of hemodynamic cerebral ischemia using the IMP-ARG method [15] could be established by both resting and acetazolamide-activated CBF quantification [19] (Fig. 4). The stage of hemodynamic cerebral ischemia can be stratified, as follows: Stage 0: vascular reserve [(acetazolamide-activated CBF-resting CBF)/resting CBF × 100%] is

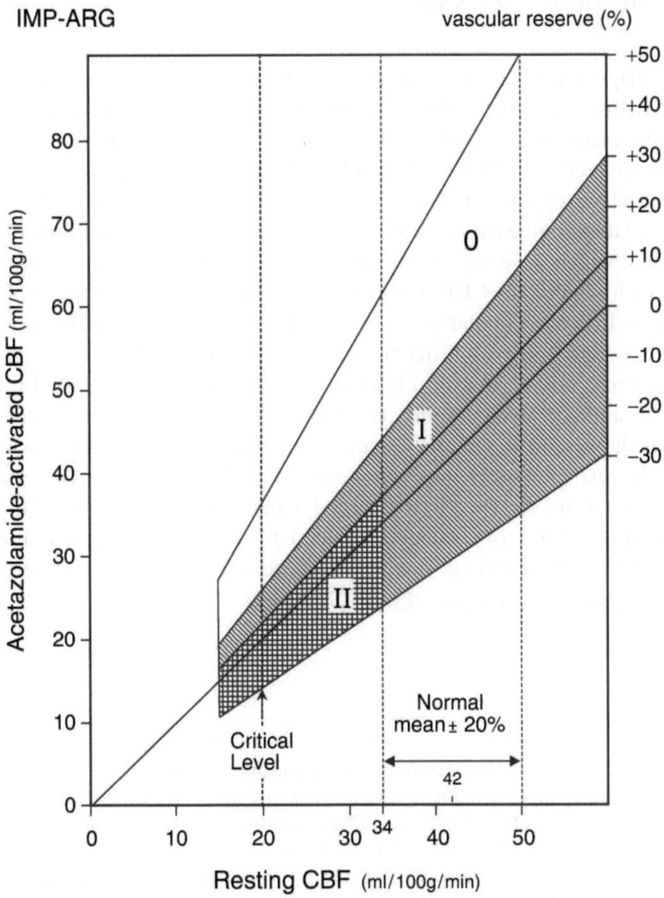

Fig. 4 Stratification of hemodynamic cerebral ischemia using quantified resting and acetazolamide-activated CBF-SPECT (the slope of the *oblique line* corresponds to the vascular reserve). *Stage 0* vascular reserve >30%, *Stage I* vascular reserve reduced from 10 to 30%, or vascular reserve <10% and resting CBF >80% of normal mean, *Stage II* vascular reserve <10% and resting CBF <80% of normal mean

preserved more than 30% (the oblique line slope corresponds to vascular reserve in Fig. 4); Stage I: vascular reserve is reduced from 10 to 30%, or vascular reserve is reduced less than 10% and resting CBF is preserved more than 80% of normal mean CBF; Stage II: vascular reserve is reduced less than 10% and resting CBF is reduced less than 80% of normal mean CBF.

Figure 5 shows quantification of CBF-SPECT in a pediatric patient with moyamoya disease before and after surgical revascularization. After the left STA-MCA bypass and EMS, preoperative Stage II ischemia in the left MCA territory was turned into postoperative Stage I ischemia.

A recent Japanese EC-IC Bypass Trial (JET Study) showed that the EC-IC Bypass was beneficial for stroke prevention in patients with Stage II hemodynamic cerebral ischemia [20]. Stage II hemodynamic cerebral ischemia defined by CBF-SPECT could be a surrogate marker of stroke recurrence.

Statistical Imaging Analysis Using 3-Dimensional Stereotactic Surface Projections (3D-SSP)

In statistical imaging analysis such as 3D-SSP [16], axial images of CBF-SPECT from subjects are transformed to the frame of Talairach's standard brain reference pixel by pixel, then the relative distribution of surface CBF from subjects is compared with the database from normal volunteers in which every pixel has both an average value and standard deviation (SD) normalized by specific brain territories. Differences between the subject's data and the normal database in each pixel are converted to Z-score as a multiple of SD, then the cluster of pixels, which have significant difference of Z-score > 2, can be identified as the specific area with significant CBF reduction on the stereotactic surface projections (total eight directions). In group comparisons between pediatric patients and the normal database using 3D-SSP, a statistically significant decrease of resting CBF was observed in widespread cortical areas on the anterior circulation of the pediatric patients. In a comparison between resting and acetazolamide-activated CBF distribution with a Z-score map in the same patient as the case in Fig. 5, the Z-score value in the cluster of pixels with a statistical difference on the resting Z-score map is augmented on the acetazolamide-activated Z-score map (Fig. 6). Therefore, the severity of hemodynamic cerebral ischemia can be classified by the combination of Z-score values estimated by resting and acetazolamide-activated Z-score maps (Table 2). Statistical imaging analysis using 3D-SSP can correspond to the stereotactic and qualitative analysis of CBF-SPECT.

Fig. 8 Assessment of hemodynamic cerebral ischemia using stereotactic extraction estimation (SEE) analysis for CBF-SPECT of a case in Fig. 5. From *upper* to *lower*, brain surface images of standardized brain MRI, resting CBF, acetazolamide-activated CBF, cerebrovascular reserve, and stage of hemodynamic ischemia are indicated. From *left* to *right*, eight directions (*Rt Lat, Lt Lat, Sup, Inf, Ant, Post, Rt Med, Lt Med*) of brain surface images are demonstrated. On the left lateral direction, decrease of resting and acetazolamide-activated CBF, reduction of cerebrovascular reserve less than 10% and mixed Stage I and II ischemia were demonstrated within the left MCA territory. On the right lateral direction, no increase of acetazolamide-activated CBF, reduction of cerebrovascular reserve, and Stage I ischemia were observed in the frontal lobe within the left MCA territory

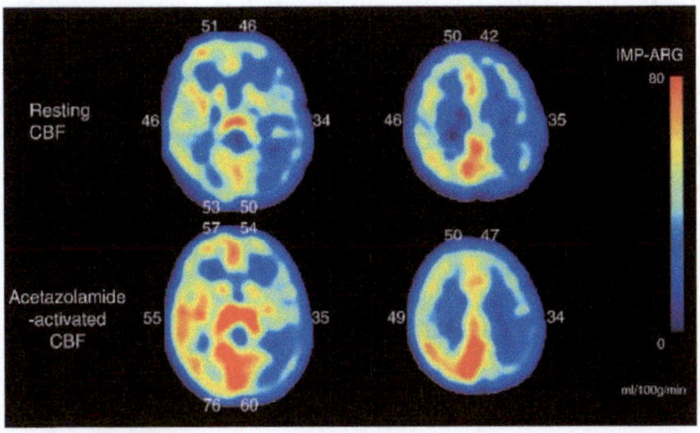

Fig. 5 Quantification of CBF-SPECT in a pediatric patient with moyamoya disease. (*Upper row*) resting CBF, (*lower row*) acetazolamide-activated CBF. A 7-year-old female, suffered from frequent TIA such as transient motor aphasia and bilateral hemiparesis. Initial EC-IC bypass surgery was scheduled for the left cerebral hemisphere based on severity of hemodynamic cerebral ischemia. Hemodynamic stage in the left MCA territory was estimated as Stage II based on the criterion of Fig. 4

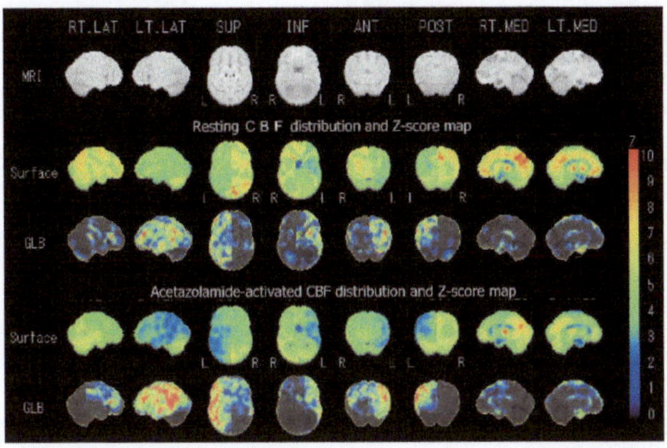

Fig. 6 Comparison between resting and acetazolamide-activated CBF distribution with a *Z*-score map using 3D-SSP in the same patient as a case in Fig. 5. From *upper* to *lower*, brain surface images of standardized brain (MRI), and 4 *Z*-score images normalized by global hemisphere (GLB), thalamus (TH), cerebellum (CBL), and pons (PNS). In a comparison between resting and acetazolamide-activated CBF distribution, a marked decrease of CBF in the left MCA territory and a mild decrease of CBF in the right frontal lobe were observed. On the other hand, in a comparison between resting and acetazolamide-activated *Z*-score maps, the *Z*-score value in the cluster of pixels with a statistical difference on the resting *Z*-score map is augmented on the acetazolamide-activated *Z*-score map

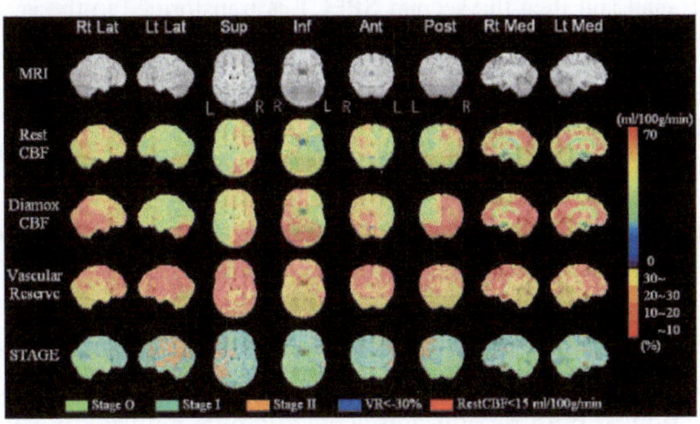

Table 2 Classification of severity of hemodynamic cerebral ischemia by the combination of *Z*-score values estimated by resting and acetazolamide-activated *Z*-score map

	Resting 3D-SSP	Acetazolamide-activated 3D-SSP
Normal	Z (rest) < 2	Z (acetazolamide) < 2
Mild	Z (rest) < 2	Z (acetazolamide) > Z (rest) + 2
Severe	Z (rest) > 2	Z (acetazolamide) > Z (rest) + 2

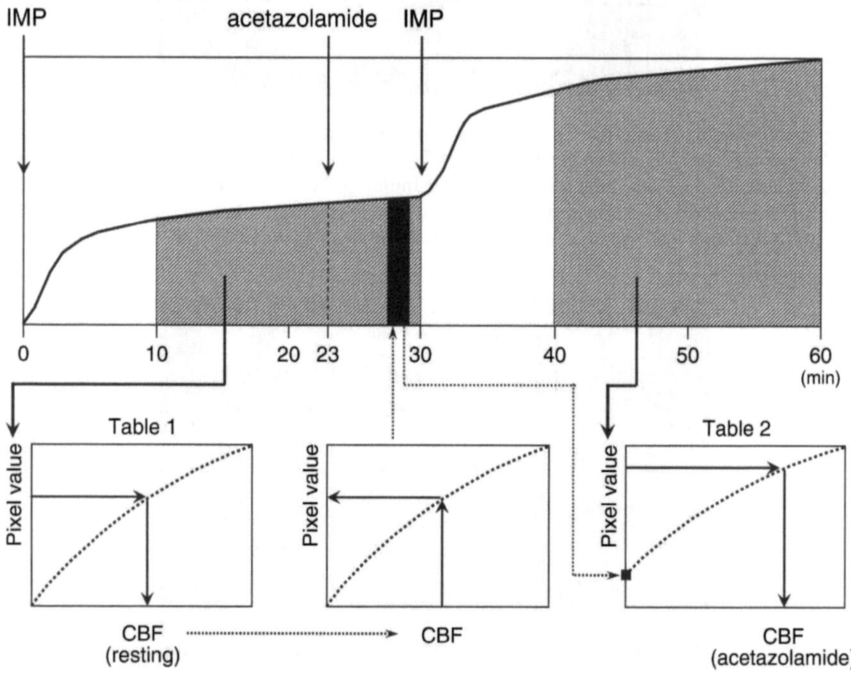

Fig. 7 Principle of dual-table ARG. In resting CBF quantification, a relationship between the pixel value of the first SPECT and resting CBF is calculated based on the two-compartment model to produce Table 1, and then the first SPECT is transformed to the resting CBF map pixel by pixel using the table look-up method in the same manner as the IMP-ARG method [15]. On the other hand, in acetazolamide-activated CBF quantification, the pixel value of the second SPECT is influenced by the background radioactivity of the first tracer injection. Therefore, a relationship between the pixel value of the second SPECT and the acetazolamide-activated CBF is calculated to make up Table 2 which consists of both a resting table and an acetazolamide-activated table (dual-table). Table 2 starts from the pixel value calculated from the resting CBF map and then the second SPECT is transformed to the acetazolamide-activated CBF map pixel by pixel using the table look-up method

Dual-Table ARG Method

Until now, stratification of hemodynamic cerebral ischemia has been defined using the IMP-ARG method; however, sufficient accuracy of vascular reserve using this method cannot yet be obtained. Especially, a measurement error can occur because of different arterial input functions associated with 2-day quantification of both resting and acetazolamide-activated CBF using the IMP-ARG method. On the other hand, the DTARG method [17] can provide same-day quantification of both resting and acetazolamide-activated CBF using a split dose of ^{123}I-IMP and common arterial input function (Fig. 7). Using the DTARG method, both resting and acetazolamide-activated CBF-SPECT can be serially quantified pixel by pixel to obtain high measurement accuracy on the vascular reserve.

Segmental Extraction Estimation

SEE analysis of hemodynamic cerebral ischemia has been developed to overcome the arbitrary estimation due to ROI analysis for quantified CBF-SPECT [18]. In this analysis, resting and acetazolamide-activated CBF-SPECT are stereotactically and quantitatively converted to brain surface CBF. The conversions are performed pixel by pixel on the frame of Talairach's standard brain reference which has been utilized in 3D-SSP analysis. Then, stereotactic estimations of cerebrovascular reserve and stereotactic stratification of hemodynamic cerebral ischemia (Stages 0–II) [19] can be completed pixel by pixel on the same frame (Fig. 8). SEE analysis for hemodynamic cerebral ischemia can correspond to the stereotactic and quantitative analysis of CBF-SPECT. As an advanced application of this analysis, the severity of hemodynamic cerebral ischemia can be estimated stereotactically using the identical template or segment on vascular territories for getting high judgment accuracy.

Perfusion MRI/CT

Just after intravenous infusion of contrast materials, time-intensity, or time-density curves obtained by rapid sequential MRI/CT can provide functional images of hemodynamic parameters [21]. Time-to-peak, MTT, and area under curve (AUC) are estimated from time-intensity or time-density curves. AUC corresponds to relative CBV, and AUT/MTT corresponds to relative CBF. Heterogeneity of the arrival time of contrast materials to regional brain tissue should be corrected in voxel level to obtain proper hemodynamic parameters. Quantification of hemodynamic parameters has been studied, but not yet established using a standardized analytic model. Concerning the diagnosis of perfusion state corresponding to the misery perfusion, perfusion MRI/CT has not sufficient accuracy to determine the thresholds for the stratification of hemodynamic cerebral ischemia. However, benefiting from the simultaneous estimation of hemodynamic parameters using perfusion MRI/CT, an affected area with decrease of CBF and increase of CBV associated with increase of MTT could suggest the presence of the misery perfusion.

Perfusion MRI combined with diffusion-weighted MRI can provide regional information of diffusion/perfusion mismatch corresponding to ischemic penumbra which is valuable for managing acute cerebral ischemia [22, 23]. Recently, a perfusion mismatch analyzer (PMA) has been developed by the ASIST Japan study to standardize the diagnostic ability of diffusion/perfusion mismatch by different MRI equipment [24]. Perfusion CT combined with reduction of CBV might also provide the same regional information as diffusion/perfusion mismatch on MRI.

References

1. Suzuki J, Takaku A (1969) Cerebrovascular "moyamoya" disease. Disease showing abnormal net-like vessels in base of brain. Arch Neurol 20: 288–299
2. Houkin K, Nakayama N, Kuroda S, et al (2005) Novel magnetic resonance angiography stage grading for moyamoya disease. Cerebrovasc Dis 20: 347–354

3. Ikezaki K, Matsushima T, Kuwabara Y, et al (1994) Cerebral circulation and oxygen metabolism in childhood moyamoya disease: a perioperative positron emission tomography study. J Neurosurg 81: 843–850
4. Kuwabara Y, Ichiya Y, Sasaki M, et al (1997) Cerebral hemodynamics and metabolism in moyamoya disease – a positron emission tomography study. Clin Neurol Neurosurg 99 Suppl 2: S74–78
5. Morimoto M, Iwama T, Hashimoto N, et al (1999) Efficacy of direct revascularization in adult moyamoya disease: haemodynamic evaluation by positron emission tomography. Acta Neurochir (Wien) 141: 377–384
6. Baron JC, Bousser MG, Rey A, et al (1981) Reversal of focal "misery perfusion syndrome" by extra- intracranial arterial bypass in hemodynamic cerebral ischemia: a case study with ^{15}O positron emission tomography. Stroke 12: 454–459
7. Samson Y, Baron JC, Bousser MG, et al (1985) Effects of extra-intracranial arterial bypass on cerebral blood flow and oxygen metabolism in humans. Stroke 16: 609–616
8. Powers WJ, Grubb RL Jr, Raichle ME (1984) Physiological responses to focal cerebral ischemia in humans. Ann Neurol 16: 546–552
9. Touho H, Karasawa J, Ohnishi H, et al (1996) Preoperative and postoperative evaluation of cerebral perfusion and vasodilatory capacity with ^{99m}Tc-HMPAO SPECT and acetazolamide in childhood moyamoya disease. Stroke 27: 282–289
10. Saito N, Nakagawara J, Nakamura H, et al (2004) Assessment of cerebral hemodynamics in childhood moyamoya disease using a quantitative and a semiquantitative IMP-SPECT study. Ann Nucl Med 18: 323–331
11. So Y, Lee HY, Kim SK, et al (2005) Prediction of the clinical outcome of pediatric moyamoya disease with postoperative basal/acetazolamide stress brain perfusion SPECT after revascularization surgery. Stroke 36: 1485–1489
12. Kuroda S, Ishikawa T, Houkin K, et al (2005) Incidence and clinical features of disease progression in adult moyamoya disease. Stroke 36: 2148–2153
13. Fujimura M, Kaneta T, Mugikura S, et al (2007) Temporary neurologic deterioration due to cerebral hyperperfusion after superficial temporal artery–middle cerebral artery anastomosis in patients with adult-onset moyamoya disease. Surg Neurol 67: 273–282
14. Iida H, Akutsu T, Endo K, et al (1996) A multicenter validation of regional cerebral blood flow quantitation using [^{123}I] iodoamphetamine and single photon emission computed tomography. J Cereb Blood Flow Metab 16: 781–793
15. Iida H, Itoh H, Nakazawa M, et al (1994) Quantitative mapping of regional cerebral blood flow using iodine-123-IMP and SPECT. J Nucl Med 35: 2019–2030
16. Minoshima S, Frey KA, Koeppe RA, et al (1995) A diagnostic approach in Alzheimer's disease using three-dimensional stereotactic surface projections of fluorine-18-FDG PET. J Nucl Med 36: 1238–1248
17. Kim KM, Watabe H, Hayashi T, et al (2006) Quantitative mapping of basal and vasareactive cerebral blood flow using split-dose ^{123}I-iodoamphetamine and single photon emission computed tomography. Neuroimage 33: 1126–1135
18. Mizumura S, Nakagawara J, Takahashi M, et al (2004) Three-dimensional display in staging hemodynamic brain ischemia for JET study: objective evaluation using SEE analysis and 3D-SSP display. Ann Nucl Med 18: 13–21
19. Nakagawara J (2007) Cerebral ischemia and single photon emission computed tomography. Jpn J Neurosurg (Tokyo) 16: 753–761
20. JET Study Group (2002) Japanese EC-IC Bypass Trial (JET study): study design and interim analysis. Surg Cereb Stroke (Jpn) 30: 97–100
21. Rosen BR, Belliveau JW, Vevea JM, et al (1990) Perfusion imaging with NMR contrast agents. Magn Reson Med 14: 249–265
22. Warach S, Gaa J, Siewert B, et al (1995) Acute human stroke studied by whole brain echo planar diffusion-weighted magnetic resonance imaging. Ann Neurol 37: 231–241
23. Wu O, Koroshetz WJ, Ostergaard L, et al (2001) Predicting tissue outcome in acute human cerebral ischemia using combined diffusion- and perfusion-weighted MR imaging. Stroke 32: 933–942
24. Kudo K, Sasaki M, Ogasawara K, et al (2009) Difference in tracer delay-induced effect among deconvolution algorithms in CT perfusion analysis: quantitative evaluation with digital phantoms. Radiology 251: 241–249

Brain Perfusion SPECT in Moyamoya Disease

Jin Chul Paeng and Dong Soo Lee

Imaging Techniques

Equipments and Radiopharmaceuticals

For brain single photon emission computed tomography (SPECT), gamma cameras with multiple detectors (multihead cameras) are recommended. Although a single-head camera may be used for image acquisition, multihead cameras have two- or three-times higher sensitivity than those of single-head cameras, which can reduce scan time and enhance image quality. However, as only a few multihead gamma cameras that have more than three detectors are commercially available, dual-head cameras are at present used for brain SPECT in many institutes.

Three radiopharmaceuticals are currently in clinical use for brain perfusion SPECT, including ^{123}I-iodoamphetamine (IMP), ^{99m}Tc-hexamethyl propylene amine oxime (HMPAO), and ^{99m}Tc-ethyl cysteinate dimer (ECD). ^{123}I-IMP has excellent characteristics for brain perfusion SPECT, such as high lipophilicity, high first-pass extraction ratio, and linear correlation with blood flow over wide range of cerebral flow. Furthermore, absolute quantification of cerebral blood flow (CBF) is possible with ^{123}I-IMP SPECT. However, ^{123}I-IMP is almost exclusively used in Japan because the supply of ^{123}I is limited in other countries. In contrast, ^{99m}Tc is easily accessible worldwide and both ^{99m}Tc-HMPAO and ^{99m}Tc-ECD are currently used for most brain perfusion SPECT. The mechanisms of brain uptake are considered to be reduction by glutathione for ^{99m}Tc-HMPAO and hydrolysis by esterase for ^{99m}Tc-ECD.

Both the ^{99m}Tc-labeled radiopharmaceuticals can provide high-quality images of perfusion SPECT, while each has its own specific characteristics. For example, hyperperfusion in a reperfused area after subacute infarct is usually not observed in ^{99m}Tc-ECD SPECT [1], probably due to loss of esterase activity in nonviable ischemic brain. In cerebrovascular diseases, ^{99m}Tc-ECD is usually expected to represent perfusion and viability and thus is more sensitive

J.C. Paeng
Department of Nuclear Medicine, Seoul National University Hospital, Seoul National University College of Medicine, 101 Daehang-ro Jongno-gu Seoul, 110-744, Seoul, Republic of Korea

D.S. Lee (✉)
Department of Nuclear Medicine, and Department of Molecular Medicine and Biopharmaceutical Sciences, Seoul National University, 101 Daehang-ro Jongno-gu, Seoul 110-744, Republic of Korea
e-mail: dsl@snu.ac.kr

B.-K. Cho and T. Tominaga (eds.), *Moyamoya Disease Update*,
DOI 10.1007/978-4-431-99703-0_26, © Springer 2010

in detecting injured ischemic areas than ^{99m}Tc-HMPAO. Though the uptake of ^{99m}Tc-HMPAO in the brain is also partly dependent upon glutathione activity of the ischemic brain tissues, ^{99m}Tc-HMPAO represents rather the perfusion status alone of ischemic regions of the brain. In addition, ^{99m}Tc-ECD shows less soft tissue uptake which is washed out 30 min after injection, while ^{99m}Tc-HMPAO is better for single-day consecutive acquisition acetazolamide SPECT studies. However, both the radiopharmaceuticals have been effective for clinical use [2], although the perfusion patterns are somewhat different between the two radiopharmaceuticals. Generally, ^{99m}Tc-ECD shows more uptake in the parietal and occipital cortex, while ^{99m}Tc-HMPAO shows more uptake in the thalamus, medial temporal cortex, and midbrain [3].

Acetazolamide-Stress Study

In moyamoya disease (MMD) or other chronic obstructive cerebrovascular diseases, cerebrovascular reserve (CVR) is a more sensitive and specific parameter for vascular insufficiency than CBF itself. CVR is assessed by the ratio of regional cerebral blood volume (CBV) versus CBF, or by the vasoreactivity in response to CO_2 or acetazolamide in stress SPECT. In a stress test using CO_2, 5–7% of CO_2 is administered by inhalation, and cerebral vessels are induced to dilate by hypercarbia. However, a CO_2 stress study is not so commonly used because of its inconvenience and relatively high rate of adverse effects such as nausea, tachycardia, and hypertension.

Acetazolamide is a more convenient and safer stress agent. Acetazolamide is a carbonic anhydrase inhibitor, which inhibits conversion between CO_2 and H_2CO_3. As a result, local concentration of CO_2 is increased in cerebral tissue, and reactive cerebral vasodilation occurs. Intravenous administration of acetazolamide (1 g in an adult, and 20 mg/kg in a child) can induce a significant increase in CBF, with its peak at 20 min after injection. The effect of acetazolamide on cerebral perfusion persists for about 1 h, and CBF is increased with acetazolamide stress by about 30% in a normal adult [4]. Although some adverse effects such as mild dizziness, paresthesia, and short-term diuresis have been reported with the use of acetazolamide, they are usually ignorable.

Imaging Protocols and Analysis Methods

In brain perfusion SPECT using ^{99m}Tc-HMPAO or ^{99m}Tc-ECD, 555–1,110 MBq (15–30 mCi) of radioactivity is injected in an adult and the injected dose is adjusted in a pediatric patient according to the body weight. The radiation exposure in this protocol is estimated to be about 7–8 mSv [5].

According to the condition of each institute, a 1-day or 2-day protocol is used for stress SPECT. In a 1-day protocol, basal and acetazolamide-challenged SPECT images are acquired consecutively with the same position, and the stress image is reconstructed by subtraction of images. In this case, two times more radioactivity is injected for the second scan to achieve equivalent signal-to-noise ratio of the subtracted acetazolamide study [6]. In a 2-day protocol, basal and stress images are acquired on separate days. Although the 1-day protocol requires close cooperation of a patient or even sedation of a pediatric patient because of longer imaging time for consecutive scans, it is more convenient for patients and easier to register and match the specific location of a lesion between basal and stress images than the coregistered images from 2-day studies.

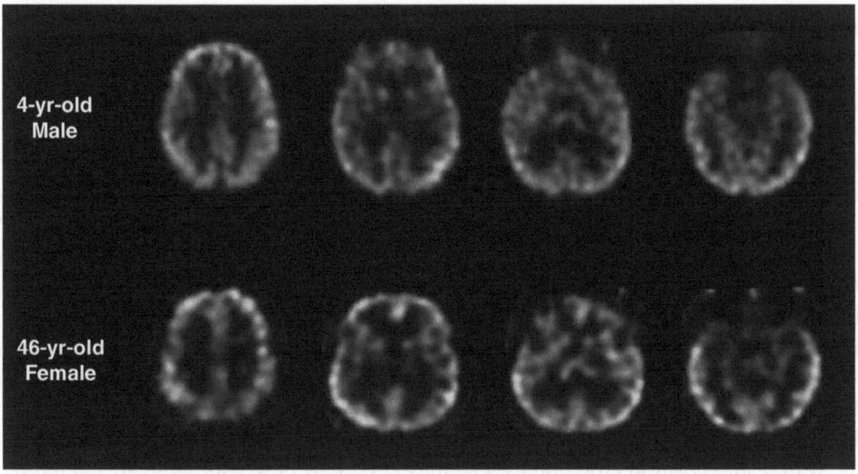

Fig. 1 Normal brain perfusion SPECT images of a 4-year-old male and a 46-year-old female MMD patients

In the analysis of SPECT images, semiquantitative analysis using region of interest (ROI) is commonly adopted in addition to conventional visual analysis and laborious quantitative analysis [7]. For example, in MMD, ROIs may be drawn for a specific cerebral artery territory and the radioactivity in the ROI is measured. The measurement of radioactivity is used as a surrogate parameter for CBF in each ROI, and this is in good correlation with quantitative measurements [8]. Furthermore, recently developed algorithms for image normalization and registration have markedly enhanced the quality of semiquantitative analyses. For example, different brain images can be normalized into a standard template and analyzed automatically pixel-by-pixel, adopting the algorithm of statistical parametric mapping [9]. Also, specific anatomical localization such as a vascular territory can be determined automatically using a statistical probabilistic anatomical mapping algorithm [10–12].

The SPECT/CT fusion scanner, which was recently introduced to the clinical field, is expected to upgrade the quality of image analysis by simultaneous acquisition of solid anatomical coordinate images.

Clinical Applications

Normal Brain Perfusion SPECT

Normal brain perfusion changes according to age. Brain perfusion of a neonate is globally lower, but gradually increases to be even higher than that of an adult until the age of 7 years. Afterwards, global brain perfusion gradually decreases to be similar to that of an adult at adolescence. Although there are some age-related variations of regional cerebral perfusion, the perfusion patterns are similar between different ages more than 10 years old [13]. In a normal brain perfusion SPECT, high perfusion is observed in the gray matter including basal ganglia and thalami, and especially in the primary visual cortex. Normal brain perfusion SPECT images are demonstrated in Fig. 1.

Hemodynamic Changes in MMD

In a normal adult, cerebral perfusion is 70–90 mL/min/100 g in the gray matter, 20–30 mL/min/100 g in the white matter, and around 50 mL/min/100 g on average. In chronic progressive vascular obstruction, perfusion is preserved until a critical point by the autoregulation of cerebral vascular resistance. In the early phase of vascular obstruction, the autoregulation induces lowering of vascular resistance in response to decreasing cerebral perfusion pressure (CPP). This compensatory mechanism results in increased CBV, decreased CVR, and preservation of CBF. A further fall in CPP is accompanied with decrease in CBF. However, cerebral metabolic rate of O_2 ($CMRO_2$) and metabolic rate of glucose (CMR_{glu}) are still preserved by an increase in oxygen extraction fraction (OEF) of brain tissue. A fall of average CBF under 20–25 mL/min/100 g may cause neurologic deficit, which would become irreversible under 10 mL/min/100 g of average CBF.

Most of the above-mentioned hemodynamic parameters can be evaluated noninvasively using SPECT and positron emission tomography (PET). SPECT with radiolabeled red blood cells is used for measurement of CBV. OEF or $CMRO_2$ can be measured by $^{15}O–H_2O$ and ^{15}O PET, and CMR_{glu} by ^{8}F-FDG PET. CBF and CVR are evaluated by brain perfusion SPECT, as described above.

Preoperative Assessment

In MMD, the characteristic hemodynamic change is 'decreased CVR' in the brain region subtending the affected cerebral artery, which is demonstrated as aggravated perfusion on acetazolamide-stress SPECT (Fig. 2). A basal perfusion study may also show various degrees of decreased radioactivity reflecting hypoperfusion probably coupled with hypometabolism in the region. Ischemic infarct is demonstrated as a defect area in perfusion SPECT (Fig. 3), and common in watershed zones. In some cases, brain regions that are functionally connected with

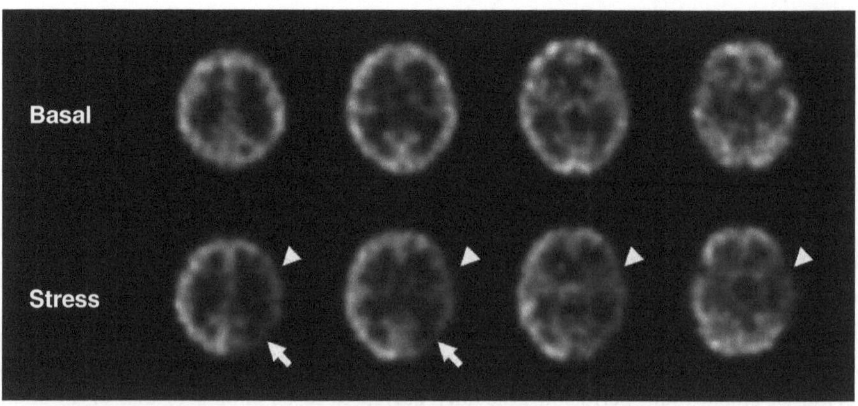

Fig. 2 Brain perfusion SPECT images of a typical MMD case (5-year-old male). While basal SPECT shows just subtle perfusion abnormality, stress SPECT demonstrates definite abnormality of CVR in the whole left internal carotid artery territory (*arrow* and *arrowhead*), with its most severity in the left posterior watershed zone (*arrow*)

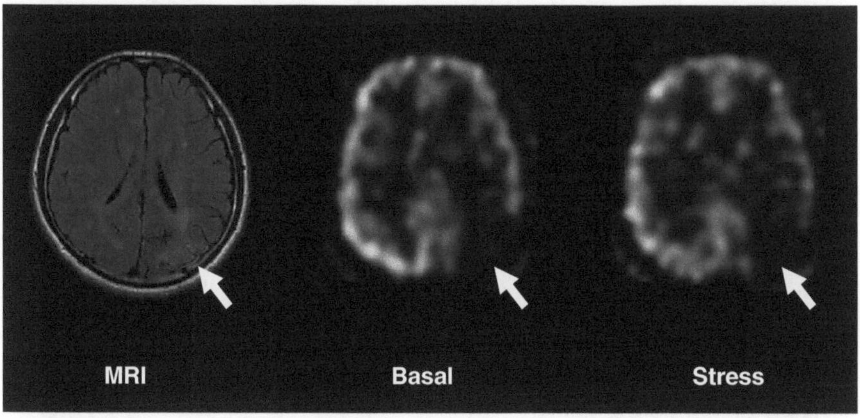

Fig. 3 Cerebral infarct of a 22-year-old patient with MMD. In the left posterior border zone, large perfusion defect that does not change between stress and rest is observed (*arrow*)

the primarily affected area may show hypoperfusion without hemodynamic impairment, which is known as "diaschisis." This phenomenon results from functional inhibition by neuronal deafferentation from the affected lesion. The region of diaschisis shows preserved vasoreactivity to acetazolamide stress in spite of decreased basal perfusion [14]. Abnormal basal perfusion usually recovers after successful revascularization surgery in the noninfarct area.

Hemodynamic status assessed on acetazolamide-stress SPECT is closely correlated with the manifestations of patients. Decrease in CBF and CVR is more severe in symptomatic MMD patients, and specific symptoms from MMD are related to the specific regions of hemodynamic impairment. Movement disorders such as chorea and dystonia are presented in cases where CBF and CVR are decreased in the striatum [15]. Visual symptoms such as visual field defects are observed in cases where the occipital lobe is involved in hemodynamic impairment [16]. However, the most commonly involved areas are the parietal and frontal areas subtending the middle cerebral artery. The caudate nucleus is often spared by the supply from posterior circulation. In cases where the anterior cerebral artery is affected, the medial frontal area shows deteriorated hemodynamics. As can be expected, however, the occipital lobes subtending posterior circulation are usually spared in MMD, because MMD predominantly affects the internal carotid arteries. However, in cases where the posterior circulation is impaired, more severe ischemia is presented due to loss of the source for collateral supply [17].

In cerebrovascular diseases, medical treatment is inappropriate in patients with decreased CBF and CVR, and revascularization surgery is recommended [18]. Patients with decreased CVR but with preserved basal CBF may demonstrate marked improvement of ischemic symptoms after revascularization surgery [19], while postoperative improvement of symptoms is not so marked in patients with preexisting infarct.

Postoperative Assessment

Acetazolamide-stress SPECT is a very useful modality for postoperative assessment of patients, because it is noninvasive, quantitative or semiquantitative, and easy to perform, compared with conventional cerebral angiography. Hemodynamic improvement after revascularization

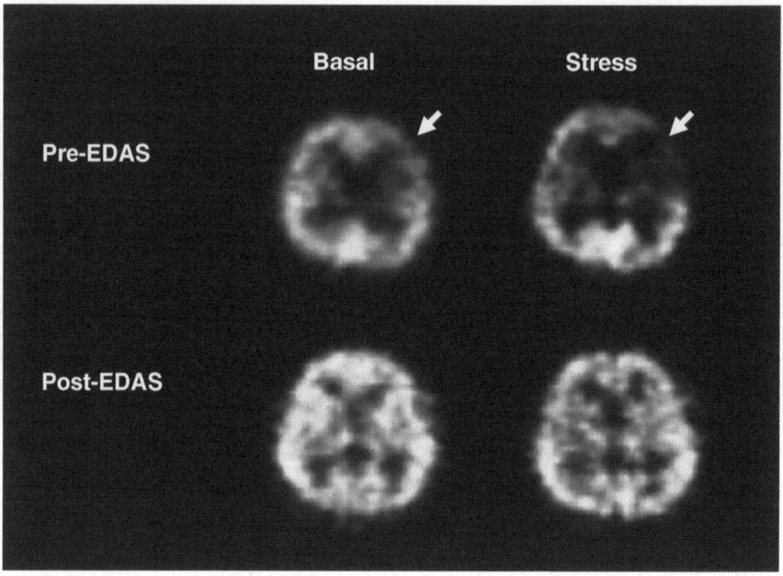

Fig. 4 Postoperative improvement of hemodynamic status. Decreased CBF and CBV are improved after indirect revascularization surgery of encephalo-duro-arterio-synangiosis (EDAS)

surgery is well demonstrated on acetazolamide-stress SPECT (Fig. 4). Infrequently, basal CBF has shown temporary increase within several days or a week after surgery reflecting some hyperperfusion, which returns to normal after a while. After successful surgery, CVR usually shows gradual improvement up to several months after surgery.

Postoperative hemodynamic status measured on acetazolamide-stress SPECT after the completion of the surgery on both hemispheres is closely related to further prognosis. In a study on clinical outcome of MMD patients after revascularization surgery, regional CVR status on postoperative SPECT was the most significant predictor for the symptomatic outcome of patients [20]. If a patient's CVR was still poor after revascularization surgery, prognosis on symptoms or neurologic deficits was also poor. Therefore, additional surgical intervention is recommended if a patient's hemodynamic status after initial revascularization surgery still shows abnormality [21].

Acetazolamide-stress SPECT has also been used to evaluate the efficacy of newly introduced surgical techniques. In addition to direct revascularization such as the external to internal carotid bypass surgery, the efficacy of indirect revascularization surgery such as encephalo-duro-arterio-synangiosis and encephalo-galeo-synangiosis (EGS) were verified by comparison of pre- and postoperative acetazolamide-stress SPECT [22, 23].

Other Issues with Spect

Postoperative Hyperperfusion Syndrome

Hyperperfusion syndrome (HPS) is one of the major complications after revascularization surgery in chronic obstructive cerebrovascular diseases. The pathophysiology of HPS is restoration of CPP in the regions of impaired vasoreactivity. It may occur in indirect revascularization, although it is more common in high-flow direct revascularization surgery. The symptoms of HPS include headache, transient neurological deficit, seizure, cerebral edema, and hemorrhage, and so on. Therefore, in cases where acute neurological deficit after revascularization surgery is presented, HPS is considered in addition to sustained or even aggravated hemodynamic impairment. Brain perfusion SPECT has been used in postoperative HPS, and has shown the hyperperfusion status with quantitative or semiquantitative measurements. In some studies, severe hyperperfusion such as about 100% more perfusion than the contralateral side was reported [24]. However, even mild to moderate hyperperfusion by about 10–40% may cause HPS, because vascular reactivity and permeability are impaired in the affected regions [25]. Brain perfusion SPECT is an excellent tool to assess HPS.

Future Perspectives

One of recent trends of development in medial imaging is the fusion of multimodal images between computed tomography (CT), magnetic resonance image (MRI), SPECT, and PET. Among these, fusion images between structural images (CT or MRI) and functional images (SPECT or PET) are of most interest. Many software fusion methods have been used for more than a decade, and, recently, hardware fusion became available with commercial products of PET/CT and SPECT/CT. Also, PET/MRI is under development and expected to be available within a couple of years. Fusion with optical imaging will be more helpful for surgery because it can visualize perfusion or other specific imaging targets directly in the surgical field. Neurological disorders including MMD will benefit from these new modalities, and a recent study showed a potential of fusion images in which the recipient for cerebral artery anastomosis surgery was selected by fusion images between MRI and perfusion SPECT [26].

Another trend in medical imaging is the adoption of molecular imaging, which means imaging for the molecular level affairs. In MMD, very few functional imaging over perfusion imaging have been tried. For example, ^{123}I-iomazenil SPECT has been tried for the assessment of neuronal loss, in which iomazenil binds to a ubiquitous neuronal receptor of the central benzodiazepine receptor [27]. In the future, such molecular imaging as hypoxia, apoptosis, and angiogenesis imaging are expected to be introduced to clinical fields. At present, several molecular imaging probes have already been developed and tried in preclinical or clinical studies, including ^{99m}Tc-labeled nitroimidazole for hypoxia imaging, ^{99m}Tc-annexin V for apoptosis imaging, and RGD derivatives for angiogenesis imaging. These molecular imaging methods are expected to be helpful in the diagnosis and treatment of MMD patients, as well as in other diseases.

References

1. Nakagawara J, Nakamura J, Takeda R (1994) Assessment of postischemic reperfusion and diamox activation test in stroke using 99mTc-ECD SPECT. J Cereb Blood Flow Metab 14:S49–S57
2. Dormehl IC, Oliver DW, Langen KJ et al (1997) Technetium-99 m-HMPAO, technetium-99 m-ECD and iodine-123-IMP cerebral blood flow measurements with pharmacological interventions in primates. J Nucl Med 38:1897–1901
3. Hyun Y, Lee JS, Rha JH et al (2003) Different uptake of 99mTc-ECD and 99mTc-HMPAO in the same brains: analysis by statistical parametric mapping. Eur J Nucl Med Mol Imaging 28:191–197
4. Okazawa H, Yamauchi H, Sugimoto K et al (2001) Effects of acetazolamide on cerebral blood flow, blood volume, and oxygen metabolism: a positron emission tomography study with healthy volunteers. J Cereb Blood Flow Metab 21:1472–1479

5. Bushberg JT, Stabin MG (2003) Radiopharmaceutical dosimetry. In: Sandler MP, Coleman RE, Patton JA et al (ed) Diagnostic nuclear medicine, 4th edn. Lippincott Willams & Wilkins, Philadelphia
6. Lee DS, Lee TH, Kim KM et al (1997) Optimization of subtraction brain perfusion SPECT with basal/acetazolamide consecutive acquisition. Korean J Nucl Med 31:330–338
7. Kim KM, Lee DS, Kim SK et al. (2000) Quantification of cerebrovascular reserve using Tc-99 m HMPAO brain SPECT and Lassen's algorithm. Korean J Nucl Med 34:322–335
8. Saito N, Nakagawara J, Nakamura H, et al (2004) Assessment of cerebral hemodynamics in childhood moyamoya disease using a quantitative and a semiquantitative IMP-SPECT study. Ann Nucl Med 18:323–331
9. Lee HY, Paeng JC, Lee DS et al (2004) Efficacy assessment of cerebral arterial bypass surgery using statistical parametric mapping and probabilistic brain atlas on basal/acetazolamide brain perfusion SPECT. J Nucl Med 45:202–206
10. Lee JS, Lee DS, Kim YK et al (2004) Probabilistic map of blood flow distribution in the brain from the internal carotid artery. Neuroimage 23:1422–1431
11. Kim SJ, Kim IJ, Kim YK et al (2008) Probabilistic anatomic mapping of cerebral blood flow distribution of the middle cerebral artery. J Nucl Med 49:39–43
12. Lee JS, Lee DS (2005) Analysis of functional brain images using population-based probabilistic atlas. Curr Med Imaging Rev 1:81–87
13. Ogawa A, Sakurai Y, Kayama T et al (1989) Regional cerebral blood flow with age: changes in rCBF in childhood. Neurol Res 11:173–176
14. Kuwabara Y, Ichiya Y, Sasaki M et al (1996) Cerebellar vascular response to acetazolamide in crossed cerebellar diaschisis: a comparison of 99mTc-HMPAO single-photon emission tomography with 15O-H2O positron emission tomography. Eur J Nucl Med 23:683–689
15. Hong YH, Ahn TB, Oh CW et al (2002) Hemichorea as an initial manifestation of moyamoya disease: reversible striatal hypoperfusion demonstrated on single photon emission computed tomography. Mov Disord 17:1380–1383
16. Chu MK, Lee IH, Kim DI (2001) Moyamoya disease initially presenting visual field defect. Yonsei Med J 42:566–570
17. Yamada I, Murata Y, Umehara I et al (1996) SPECT and MRI evaluations of the posterior circulation in moyamoya disease. J Nucl Med 37:1613–1617
18. Jeffree RL, Stoodley MA (2009) STA-MCA bypass for symptomatic carotid occlusion and haemodynamic impairment. J Clin Neurosci 16:226–235
19. Lee DS, Hyun IY, Wang KC et al (1998) Evaluation of surgical outcome with pre- and post-operative rest/acetazolamide Tc-99 m HMPAO SPECT in children with moyamoya disease. Kor J Nucl Med 32:314–324
20. So Y, Lee HY, Kim SK et al (2005) Prediction of the clinical outcome of pediatric moyamoya disease with postoperative basal/acetazolamide stress brain perfusion SPECT after revascularization surgery. Stroke 36:1485–1489
21. Hayashi T, Shirane R, Tominaga T (2009) Additional surgery for postoperative ischemic symptoms in patients with moyamoya disease: the effectiveness of occipital artery-posterior cerebral artery bypass with an indirect procedure: technical case report. Neurosurgery 64:E195–E196
22. Kim SK, Wang KC, Kim IO et al (2002) Combined encephaloduroarteriosynangiosis and bifrontal encephalogaleo (periosteal) synangiosis in pediatric moyamoya disease. Neurosurgery 62:1456–1464.
23. Park JH, Yang SY, Chung YN et al (2007) Modified encephaloduroarteriosynangiosis with bifrontal encephalogaleoperiosteal synangiosis for the treatment of pediatric moyamoya disease. Technical note. J Neurosurg 106:237–242
24. Hosoda K, Kawaguchi T, Ishii K et al (2003) Prediction of hyperperfusion after carotid endarterectomy by brain SPECT analysis with semiquantitative statistical mapping method. Stroke 34:1187–1193
25. Lee JW, Kim YK, Lee SM et al (2008) Assessment of hyperperfusion by brain perfusion SPECT in transient neurological deterioration after superficial temporal artery-middle cerebral artery anastomosis surgery. Nucl Med Mol Imaging 42:267–274
26. Kikuta K, Takagi Y, Fushimi Y et al (2008) "Target bypass": a method for preoperative targeting of a recipient artery in superficial temporal artery-to-middle cerebral artery anastomoses. Neurosurgery 62:1434–1441
27. Sato S, Shirane R, Maruoka S et al (1999) Evaluation of neuronal loss in adult moyamoya disease by 123I-iomazenil SPECT. Surg Neurol 51:158–163

Iomazenil SPECT (BZP-Receptor)

Jyoji Nakagawara

Introduction

^{123}I-Iomazenil (IMZ) [1] is a specific radioligand for the central benzodiazepine (BZ) receptor that may be useful as an indicator of cortical neuron loss after focal cerebral ischemia using SPECT [2, 3]. The reduction of BZ receptor density in reperfused cortex that remained structurally intact is likely to be the result of injury to only a limited number of neurons (i.e., incomplete brain infarction) [3]. The study of permanent or transient ischemia (lasting 3–6 h) in baboons by Sette et al. [4], who used ^{18}F-flumazenil as a BZ receptor ligand and PET, has a more direct relevance to the study of the incomplete brain infarction in reperfused cortex using IMZ-SPECT. They observed a decrease of BZ receptor binding not only in the infracted area but also, albeit to a lesser degree, in the CT-intact opercular cortex overlying the hypodense area. Selective neuronal necrosis with sparing of glia and microvessels is seen after transient occlusion of the MCA in macaque monkey and rats [5, 6]. The extent of ischemic neuronal damage depends on both the magnitude and duration of cerebral ischemia. In the study by Garcia et al. [7], up to 60 min of MCA occlusion followed by 7 days of survival in rats resulted in neuronal necrosis that involved isolated groups of cortical neurons (i.e., incomplete brain infarction), while no cases of cortical infarction were found. A close correlation existed between the number of necrotic neurons and the severity of the neurological deficits.

Incomplete brain infarction defined by the reduction of central BZ receptor density using IMZ-SPECT had been observed within ischemic penumbra salvaged by restored CBF in the acute stroke [3] and could be occurred within long-term hemodynamic cerebral ischemia such as misery perfusion in the chronic stroke [8]. More recently, the relationship between long-term hemodynamic ischemia and the occurrence of incomplete brain infarction in patients with moyamoya disease was estimated to establish functional neuroimagings of the higher brain dysfunction by IMZ-SPECT.

J. Nakagawara (✉)
Department of Neurosurgery, Nakamura Memorial Hospital,
South-1, West-14, Chuo-ku, Sapporo 060-8570, Japan
e-mail: george@med.nmh.or.jp

B.-K. Cho and T. Tominaga (eds.), *Moyamoya Disease Update*,
DOI 10.1007/978-4-431-99703-0_27, © Springer 2010

Kinetics of Iomazenil and the Indicator of the Intactness of the Cortical Neurons

IMZ has a high affinity for the central BZ receptors. This receptor, part of the GABA-ergic complex [9], is widely distributed in high concentration in the cerebral cortex as a reflection of the numerous GABA-ergic inhibitory synapses that exist there. Therefore, measuring the binding potential of central BZ receptor radioligand could correspond to an approximate measure of the number of synapses and hence be taken as an indicator of the intactness of the cortical neurons.

To estimate the binding potential of IMZ to central BZ receptor, three-compartment, four-parameter (K1–k4) model can be mathematically solved using serial image dataset (Fig. 1) [10–12]. However, the non-specific binding fraction involving free ligand of this tracer is approximately 1–2% of the specific binding fraction in normal cortex, the distribution volume (V_d=K1/k2) of IMZ in relative units using a two-compartment, two-parameter model is practically proportional to the binding potential, which in turn is proportional to central BZ receptor concentration [13]. Furthermore, V_d distribution in relative units (IMZ-V_d image) is remarkably proportional to the tracer distribution in relative units under pseudo-equilibrium state 3 h after tracer injection (IMZ-3 h image) (Fig. 2). Therefore, a IMZ-3 h image can practically provide the indicator of the intactness of the cortical neurons.

IMZ-3 h image can be estimated by semiquantitative ROI analysis [3], and statistical imaging analysis such as 3-dimensional stereotactic surface projections (3D-SPP) [14]. In semiquantitative ROI analysis, the cortical neuron loss could be calculated by the side-to-side asymmetry (i.e., SPECT value of an ROI divided by that of the opposite symmetrical region). In statistical imaging analysis such as 3D-SSP, axial images of IMZ-SPECT from subjects are transformed to the frame of Talairach's standard brain reference pixel by pixel, then relative tracer distribution of the cortex is compared with the database from normal volunteers in which all pixels have both mean value and standard deviation (S.D.) normalized by specific brain territories. Differences between the subject's data and the normal database in each pixel are converted to

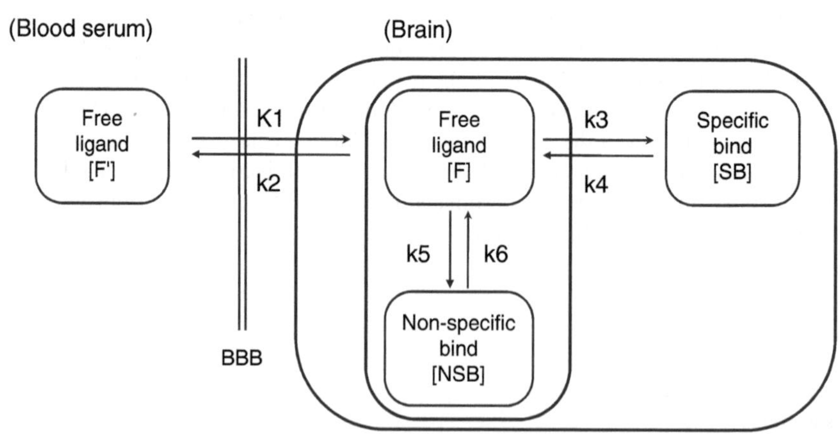

Fig. 1 To estimate the binding potential (BP) of IMZ to central BZ receptor, three-compartment, four-parameter (K1–k4) model and two-compartment, two-parameter (K1, k2) model could be mathematically solved using serial image data set. Three-compartment model: BP=B_{max}/K_d=BP=K1/k2*k3/k4, two-compartment model: BP=$B_{max}/K_d = 1/f\,(V_d - \lambda)$ [11, 12]. *Bmax* The tissue concentration of the BZ receptor, K_d the equilibrium dissociation constant, *f* the ratio of free to total plasma ligand, V_d the distribution volume: the equilibrium ratio of the brain and plasma concentration (V_d=K1/k2), λ the non-specific V_d in the brain

Z-score as a multiple of SD, then the cluster of pixels which have significant differences (Z-score > 2) can be identified as the specific area with the cortical neuron loss on the stereotactic surface projections (total eight directions).

Diagnosis of Incomplete Brain Infarction in Moyamoya Disease

In patients with moyamoya disease, long-standing hemodynamic ischemia can lasted in their anterior circulation. Atrophic changes of frontal lobe were occasionally observed in CT or MRI. However, frontal cortical neuron damages involving incomplete brain infarction have not been estimated until IMZ-SPECT became available for clinical use. On the other hand, hemodynamic cerebral ischemia can be stratified by both resting and acetazolamide-activated CBF-SPECT quantification. The stage of hemodynamic cerebral ischemia can be stratified as follows [15]: Stage 0: cerebrovascular reserve [(acetazolamide-activated CBF-resting CBF)/resting CBF × 100%] is preserved more than 30%; Stage I: cerebrovascular reserve is reduced from 10 to 30%, or cerebrovascular reserve is reduced less than 10% and resting CBF is preserved more than 80% of normal mean CBF; Stage II: cerebrovascular reserve is reduced less than 10% and resting CBF is reduced less than 80% of normal mean CBF.

Based on the development of these functional neuroimagings, relationship between long-standing hemodynamic ischemia and the occurrence of incomplete brain infarction in patients with moyamoya disease was studied by stratification of hemodynamic cerebral ischemia using quantified CBF-SPECT and central BZ receptor mapping using IMZ-SPECT. Ten patients with moyamoya disease (seven with TIA or infarction, three with ICH) were enrolled in this study. The stage of hemodynamic ischemia (0–II) was estimated by CBF-SPECT quantification using the ^{123}I-IMP-ARG method. The stage of hemodynamic ischemia in the cerebral cortex was estimated using stereotactic extraction estimation (SEE) analysis [16] (see "Overview" chapter). In SEE analysis, resting and acetazolamide-activated CBF-SPECT are stereotactically and quantitatively conversed to brain surface CBF. The conversions are performed pixel by pixel on the frame of Talairach's standard brain reference which has been utilized in 3D-SSP analysis. Then, stereotactic estimations of cerebrovascular reserve and stereotactic stratification of hemodynamic cerebral ischemia (Stages 0–II) [15] can be completed pixel by pixel on the same frame (Fig. 3). On the other hand, incomplete brain infarction was defined as a significant reduction of BZ receptor density by 3D-SSP analysis of IMZ-SPECT. Delayed image 3-h after tracer injection was dealt as equivalent map to BZ receptor density.

As a study result, the areas of incomplete brain infarction were displayed on 3D-SSP by the cluster of pixels which consisted of *Z*-score value more than 2 SD. Incomplete brain infarction defined by 3D-SSP analysis of IMZ-SPECT was observed not only in Stage II ischemic area but also in part of Stage I ischemic area (Figs. 4 and 5). In cases with ICH, selective loss of cortical neuron was occasionally observed by undercutting of cortex (white matter lesions).

In conclusion, long-standing hemodynamic ischemia in patients with moyamoya disease can result in selective loss of cortical neuron (incomplete brain infarction). Cortical neuron can be damaged by long-standing hemodynamic ischemia, even though the degree of hemodynamic ischemia has been mildly reduced (Fig. 6). Statistical imaging analysis of incomplete brain infarction in moyamoya disease could be valuable for assessing the prognosis of surgical revascularization and the evidence of higher brain dysfunction.

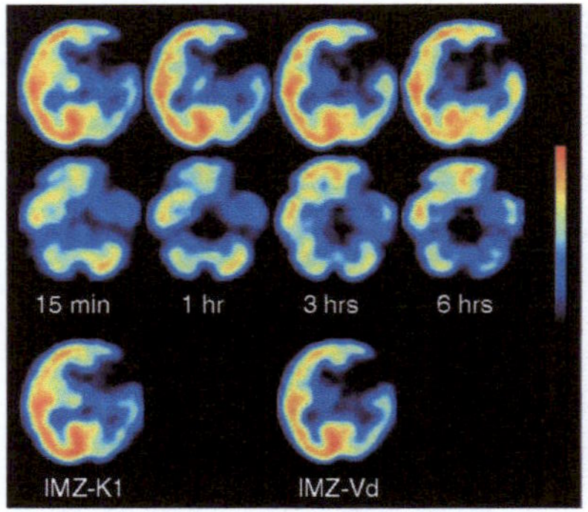

Fig. 2

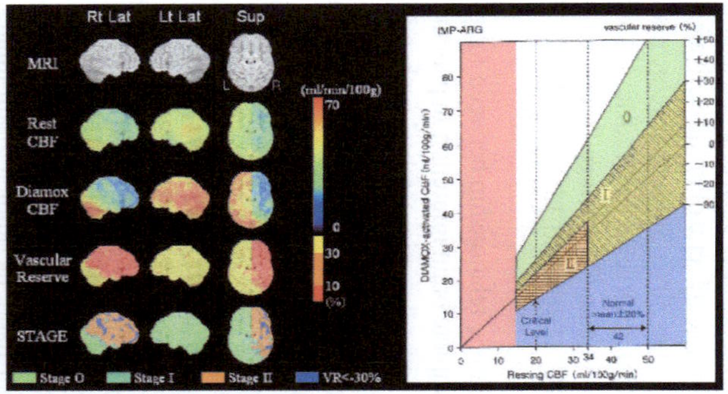

Fig. 3

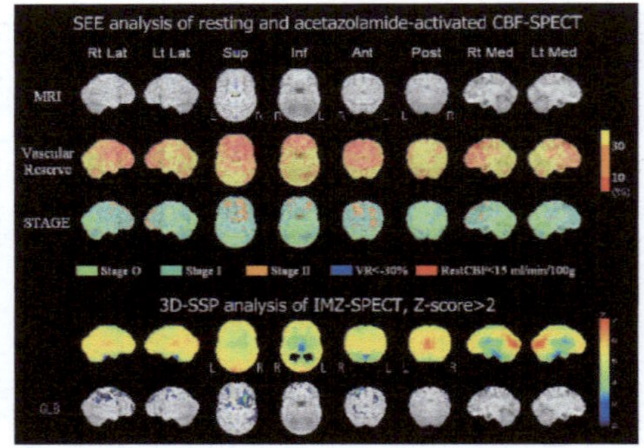

Fig. 4

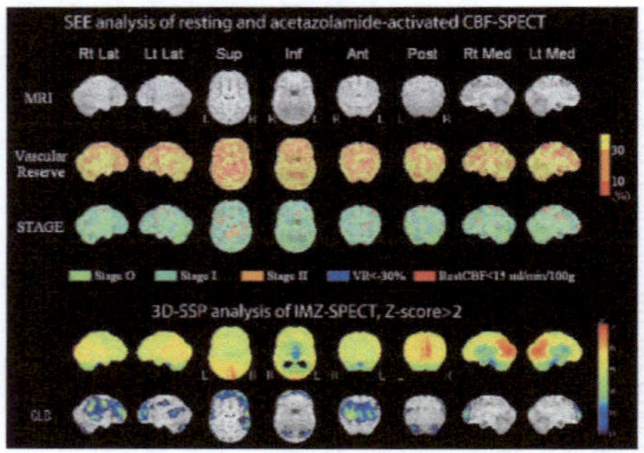

Fig. 5

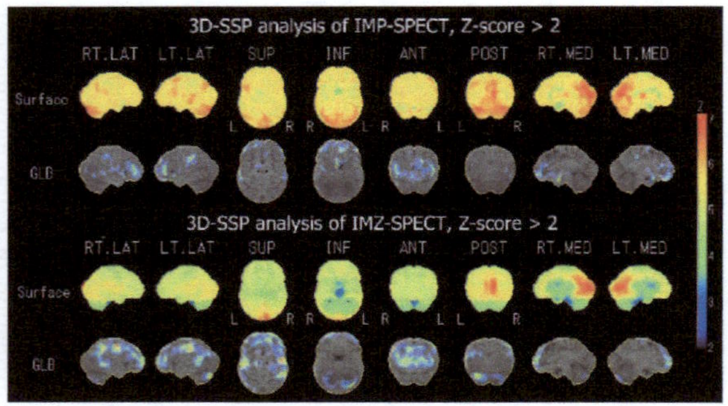

Fig. 7

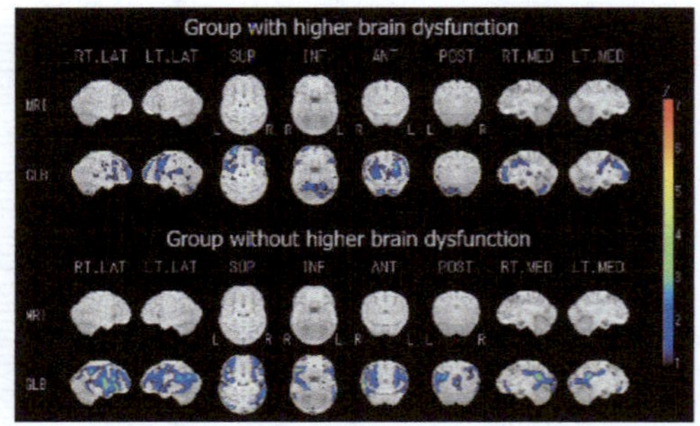

Fig. 8

Fig. 2 (*Upper 2 rows*) A serial change of IMZ distribution after intravenous tracer injection was demonstrated in a patient with the left MCA embolism. The fast-in, fast-out of the tracer distribution was observed in the left cerebellar cortex, the slow-in, slow-out of the tracer distribution was observed in the right cerebellar cortex. Three hours after tracer injection, pseudo-equilibrium state was obtained on IMZ-3 h image. (*Lower row*) IMZ-K1 and IMZ-V_d images were calculated using two-compartment model. The binding potential of IMZ in relative units corresponding to IMZ-V_d images is practically proportional to the tracer distribution in relative units on IMZ-3 h image. Correlation between asymmetry index (AI) of IMZ-V_d (Y) and AI of IMZ-3 h (X): $Y=0.971X+2.193$ ($r^2=0.995$) (AI; circle ROI on affected side/circle ROI on unaffected side (%); size of circle ROI=10 pixels)

Fig. 3 Hemodynamic cerebral ischemia could be quantitatively and stereotactically assessed using stereotactic extraction estimation (SEE) analysis. (*Left*) From the upper low, brain surface images of standardized brain MRI, resting CBF, acetazolamide-activated CBF, cerebrovascular reserve and stage of hemodynamic ischemia are indicated. (*Right*) Stratification of hemodynamic cerebral ischemia using quantified resting and acetazolamide-activated CBF-SPECT. Stages 0–II are defined in the text

Fig. 4 A 30-year-old female, suffered from TIA such as the left hemiparesis. After the bilateral EC-IC bypass surgery was performed, no TIA episode was noted. However, a wide decrease of cerebrovascular reserve and a partial Stage II ischemia was persisted in bilateral frontal lobes using SEE analysis. Incomplete brain infarction defined by 3D-SSP analysis of IMZ-SPECT (Z-score>2) was observed in the right high frontal lobe corresponding to persisted Stage II ischemia

Fig. 5 A 47-year-old female, suffered from TIA such as the right hemiparesis. After the left EC-IC bypass surgery was performed, severity of hemodynamic cerebral ischemia in the left cerebral hemisphere using SEE analysis was improved form Stage II ischemia to Stage I ischemia. However, incomplete brain infarction defined by 3D-SSP analysis of IMZ-SPECT (Z-score>2) was observed in the right MCA territory and bilateral frontal pole (estimated as Stage I ischemia) where surgical revascularization was not performed

Fig. 7 In a patient with higher brain dysfunctions defined by neuropsychological tests, a partial CBF reduction (*upper row*) and cortical neuron loss (*lower row*) were observed in bilateral medial and lateral frontal lobes. Z-score images were normalized by global hemisphere (GLB)

Fig. 8 In a group comparison between patients with higher brain dysfunction and normal database, cortical neuron loss was observed in bilateral medial frontal lobes involving the anterior cingulate cortex (*upper row*). On the other hand, in a group comparison between patients without higher brain dysfunction and normal database, there is no cortical neuron loss in bilateral medial frontal lobes involving the anterior cingulate cortex but cortical neuron loss in the bilateral posterior cingulate cortex (*lower row*)

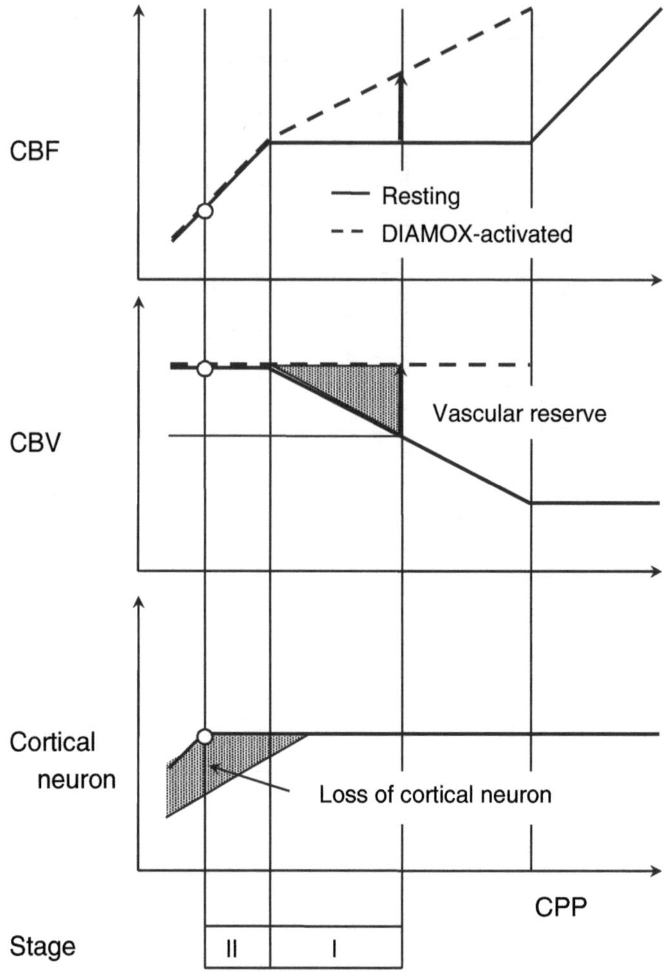

Fig. 6 In moyamoya disease, cortical neuron can be damaged by long-standing hemodynamic ischemia, even though the degree of hemodynamic ischemia has been mildly reduced within Stage I ischemia

Diagnosis of Higher Brain Dysfunction in Moyamoya Disease

In patients with adult moyamoya disease, higher brain dysfunctions which consist of cognitive impairments such as memory, attention, performance, and social behavioral disturbances are becoming increasingly apparent. These cognitive impairments can occur in patients with medial frontal lobe damage including the anterior cingulate cortex [17, 18]. These patients should be supported by social welfare as psychologically handicapped persons. In general, psychologically handicapped patients with adult moyamoya disease should be certified by both neuropsychological findings and obvious brain damage on neuroimagings such as CT or MRI. In patients with adult moyamoya disease, diagnosis of higher brain dysfunctions without obvious brain damages on morphological neuroimagings such as CT or MRI could be a social issue to be solved.

Based on these social backgrounds, relationships between cortical neuron damages in the frontal lobe and higher brain dysfunction in patients with adult moyamoya disease was studied by central BZ receptor mapping using IMZ-SPECT. Thirteen patients with moyamoya disease without obvious frontal lobe damage on morphological neuroimagings were enrolled in this study (Table 1). Statistical imaging analysis using 3D-SSP of both ^{123}I-IMZ-SPECT and ^{123}I-IMP-SPECT were performed. A normal database of 3D-SSP analysis was prepared for both ^{123}I-IMZ-SPECT and ^{123}I-IMP-SPECT, respectively. *Z*-score images were normalized by global hemisphere. The areas of incomplete brain infarction in the frontal lobe were defined as the cluster of pixels which consisted of *Z*-score value more than 2 SD in a comparison between single patients and the normal database. In group comparison between patients with higher brain dysfunction and the normal database using 3D-SSP, a statistical decrease of cortical neuron was defined as the cluster of pixels which consisted of *Z*-score value more than 1 SD.

As a study result, in four patients with higher brain dysfunctions defined by neuropsychological tests (upper four patients in Table 1), both cortical neuron loss and significant CBF reduction were observed in bilateral medial frontal lobes without obvious brain damage on morphological neuroimagings (Fig. 7). In the group comparison between patients with higher brain dysfunction and the normal database, cortical neuron loss was observed in bilateral medial frontal lobes involving the anterior cingulate cortex (Fig. 8). On the other hand, in nine patients without higher brain dysfunctions (lower nine patients in Table 1), there is no case with both cortical neuron loss and significant CBF reduction in bilateral medial frontal lobes. In the group comparison between patients without higher brain dysfunction and normal database, there is no cortical neuron loss in bilateral medial frontal lobes involving the anterior cingulate cortex (Fig. 8).

In conclusion, long-standing hemodynamic ischemia in the anterior circulation of adult moyamoya disease can lead to incomplete brain infarction (selective loss of cortical neuron) defined by a reduction of central BZ receptor density within the frontal brain cortex. Statistical imaging analysis using 3D-SSP of IMZ-SPECT can demonstrate cortical neuron loss in bilateral medial frontal lobes involving the anterior cingulate cortex in adult moyamoya patients with higher brain dysfunctions without obvious brain damage on morphological neuroimagings.

Table 1 Cortical neuron loss and significant CBF reduction in the frontal lobe on *Z*-score map of 3D-SSP for IMZ-SPECT and IMP-SPECT in 13 patients with moyamoya disease (upper 4 patients with higher brain dysfunction, and lower 9 patients without higher brain dysfunction)

Case	Type	Neuron loss in FL (IMZ)	CBF reduction in FL (IMP)
M.F. 55F	TIA	Bil. med. frontal	Bil. med. frontal
E.F. 26F	TIA	Bil. med. frontal	Bil. med. frontal
S.K. 46F	TIA	Bil. med. & lat. frontal	Bil. med. & lat. frontal
K.H. 26M	TIA	Bil. med. & lat. frontal	Bil. med. & lat. frontal
M.F. 38F	TIA	Rt. Lat. frontal	(–)
Y.K. 18F	TIA	(–)	Bil. med. frontal pole
M.M. 30F	TIA	Rt. med. high frontal	Bil. Lat. frontal
A.N. 51F	TIA	Lt. lat. frontal	Lt. lat. frontal
A.T. 40F	IVH	(–)	(–)
M.T. 31F	IVH	(–)	Bil. med. frontal base
S.M. 32F	TIA	(–)	Bil. med. frontal
M.M. 36F	TIA	(–)	(–)
Y.T. 55F	ICH	(–)	(–)

FL: frontal lobe

References

1. Beer HF, Blauenstein PA, Hasler PH, et al (1990) In vitro and in vivo evaluation of iodine-123 Ro 16-0154: a new imaging agent for SPECT investigations of benzodiazepine receptors. J Nucl Med 31: 1007–1014
2. Hatazawa J, Satoh T, Shimosegawa E, et al (1995) Evaluation of cerebral infarction with iodine-123-iomazenil SPECT. J Nucl Med 36: 2154–2161
3. Nakagawara J, Sperling B, Lassen NA (1997) Incomplete brain infarction of reperfused cortex may be quantitated with iomazenil. Stroke 28: 124–132
4. Sette G, Baron JC, Young AR, et al (1993) In vivo mapping of brain benzodiazepine receptor changes by positron emission tomography after focal ischemia in the anesthetized baboon. Stroke 24: 2046–2058
5. DeGirolami U, Crowell RM, Marcoux FW (1984) Selective necrosis and total necrosis in focal cerebral ischemia: neuropathologic observations on experimental middle cerebral artery occlusion in the macaque monkey. J Neuropathol Exp Neurol 43: 57–71
6. Garcia JH, Liu KF, Ho KL (1995) Neuronal necrosis after middle cerebral artery occlusion in Wistar rats progresses at different time intervals in the caudoputamen and the cortex. Stroke 26: 636–643
7. Garcia JH, Wagner S, Liu K-F, et al (1995) Neurological deficit and extent of neuronal necrosis attributable to middle cerebral artery occlusion in rats: statistical validation. Stroke 26: 627–635
8. Nakagawara J (2006) Assessment of brain function by neuron maker on SPECT imaging. Cereb Blood Flow Metab (Jpn) 18: 149–151
9. Abadie P, Baron JC (1991) In vivo studies of the central benzodiazepine receptors in the human brain with positron emission tomography. In: Diksic M, Reba RC, eds. Radiopharmaceuticals and Brain Pathology Studies with PET and SPECT. CRC Press, Boca Raton
10. Videbaek C, Friberg L, Holm S, et al (1993) Benzodiazepine receptor equilibrium constants for flumazenil and midazolam determined in humans with the single photon emission computer tomography tracer [^{123}I]iomazenil. Eur J Pharmacol 249: 43–51
11. Koeppe RA, Holthoff VA, Frey KA, et al (1991) Compartmental analysis of [^{11}C] flumazenil kinetics for the estimation of ligand transport rate and receptor distribution using positron emission tomography. J Cereb Blood Flow Metab 11: 735–744
12. Lassen NA (1992) Neuroreceptor quantitation in vivo by the steady-state principle using constant infusion or bolus injection of radioactive tracers. J Cereb Blood Flow Metab 12: 709–716
13. Holthoff VA, Koeppe RA, Frey KA, et al (1991) Differentiation of radioligand delivery and binding in the brain: validation of a two-compartment model for [^{11}C] flumazenil. J Cereb Blood Flow Metab 11: 745–752
14. Minoshima S, Frey KA, Koeppe RA, et al (1995) A diagnostic approach in Alzheimer's disease using three-dimensional stereotactic surface projections of fluorine-18-FDG PET. J Nucl Med 36: 1238–1248
15. Nakagawara J (2007) Cerebral ischemia and single photon emission computed tomography. Jpn J Neurosurg (Tokyo) 16: 753–761
16. Mizumura S, Nakagawara J, Takahashi M, et al (2004) Three-dimensional display in staging hemodynamic brain ischemia for JET study: objective evaluation using SEE analysis and 3D-SSP display. Ann Nucl Med 18: 13–21
17. Baird A, Dewar BK, Critchley H, et al (2006) Cognitive functioning after medial frontal lobe damage including the anterior cingulate cortex: a preliminary investigation. Brain Cogn 60: 166–175
18. Rudebeck PH, Bannerman DM, Rushworth MF (2008) The contribution of distinct subregions of the ventromedial frontal cortex to emotion, social behavior, and decision making. Cogn Affect Behav Neurosci 8: 485–497

Perfusion Imaging in Moyamoya Disease

Jung-Eun Cheon and In-One Kim

Introduction

Moyamoya disease is a chronic, occlusive cerebrovascular disorder involving the distal internal carotid artery and/or the proximal portion of the anterior and middle cerebral arteries (ACAs and MCAs, respectively). Moyamoya disease is characterized by the extensive development of collateral pathways. The first pathway is known as the "basal moyamoya," and includes an abnormal dilation of the perforating arteries and a true neoangiogenesis around the circle of Willis. Other collateral pathways may occur via pial-to-pial anastomoses from other less compromised territories, particularly the posterior circulation, or in more advanced cases, via a dural-to-pial collateral pathway, which is known as the "vault moyamoya." These collateral networks seemingly provide an alternative route of cerebral perfusion in moyamoya disease [1–3].

Magnetic resonance imaging (MRI) and MR angiography are useful imaging tools for the diagnosis of moyamoya disease. MRI can localize the parenchymal lesions and MR angiography can delineate the status of the major intracranial arteries noninvasively [4–6]. In children with moyamoya disease, transient ischemic attacks (TIAs) or cerebral infarctions are the most common clinical manifestations, and hemodynamically-mediated perfusion failure has been implicated in ischemic manifestations of childhood moyamoya disease [7, 8]. Therefore, identification of abnormal tissue perfusion is an important aspect of the evaluation in these patients. However, conventional MRI and MR angiography are not sufficient to provide adequate hemodynamic information.

Recent advances in imaging techniques allow non-invasive investigation of tissue perfusion. Currently, MR perfusion imaging has been performed using fast T2*-weighted imaging to detect signal changes that occur during the first-pass of contrast material [9–14]. Computed tomography (CT) perfusion using dynamic contrast enhancement techniques can demonstrate cerebral hemodynamic status by direct visualization of contrast material [15–17].

J.-E. Cheon and I.-O. Kim (✉)
Department of Radiology, Seoul National University Hospital, Seoul National University College of Medicine, 101 Daehang-ro, Jongro-gu, Seoul 110-744, Republic of Korea
e-mail: kimio@radcom.shu.ac.kr

B.-K. Cho and T. Tominaga (eds.), *Moyamoya Disease Update*,
DOI 10.1007/978-4-431-99703-0_28, © Springer 2010

MR Perfusion Imaging

MR perfusion imaging is an advanced MR technique to evaluate cerebral perfusion dynamics. Currently, there are two commonly available MR techniques for assessing cerebral perfusion: dynamic susceptibility contrast-enhanced (DSC) MRI and arterial spin labeling (ASL) techniques. These techniques use exogenous tracer agents, such as paramagnetic contrast material, or endogenous tracer agents, such as magnetically-labeled blood.

DSC-perfusion MRI relies on first-pass tracer methodology. By using T2*-weighted imaging that is sensitive to magnetic susceptibility, MR perfusion shows signal changes that occur in the brain during the first pass of an exogenous contrast agent [10–12]. Gadolinium-based contrast material is injected intravenously, passing through capillary beds and inducing spin dephasing through susceptibility effects. The result is a T2 or T2* signal intensity drop that is related to the perfusion of the tissue in question (Fig. 1). It is assumed that the tracer is restricted to the intravascular compartment and does not diffuse into the extracellular space. Imaging is performed dynamically (rapid imaging over time during a bolus injection) using echo planar imaging (EPI)-based spin echo or gradient echo sequences, as both allow whole-brain imaging in the short temporal resolution needed. It is thought that the spin echo sequences are more sensitive to capillary level blood vessels, whereas gradient echo techniques are more sensitive to the larger vessels [18]. Gradient-echo EPI allows for greater contrast-to-noise ratio, but more magnetic susceptibility artifact than spin-echo EPI [18–20]. After conversion to concentration-time curves, hemodynamic parameters, such as relative cerebral blood volume (CBV), regional cerebral blood flow (rCBF), time to peak (TTP), and mean transit time (MTT), characterize tissue perfusion status (Fig. 2). CBV has been defined as the volume of blood in a region of brain tissue, commonly measured in milliliters per 100 g of brain tissue. Cerebral blood flow (CBF) refers to the volume of blood per unit time passing through a given region of brain tissue, measured in milliliters per minute per 100 g of brain tissue. TTP refers to the arrival time of the contrast material to the maximum concentration after contrast injection and MTT refers to the average time it takes blood to pass through a

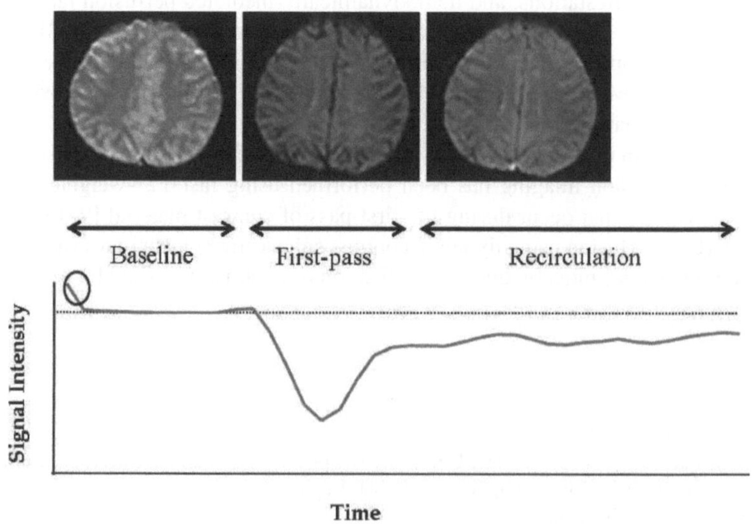

Fig. 1 The figure demonstrates changes in signal intensity in the cerebral hemisphere as bolus paramagnetic contrast material traverses the brain parenchyma (*top*). The time signal intensity curve demonstrates the transient decrease in signal intensity with first-pass of contrast media (*bottom*)

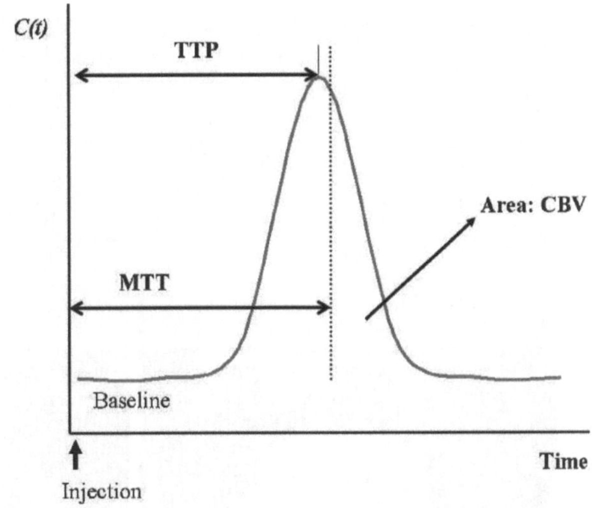

Fig. 2 Schematic concentration-time curve illustrating parameters often used to characterize the hemodynamics of tissue. $C(t)$ indicates the concentration of contrast material over time

given region of brain tissue, commonly measured in seconds [11, 12]. For young children and infants, there are challenges to intravenous access, small intravenous catheters, and limitations in the dose of contrast. Other limitations of the T2* technique include the relative quantification of CBV. However, DSC-perfusion MR remains the primary MRI method to assess cerebral hemodynamics in moyamoya disease [10–14].

ASL perfusion MRI is an alternative and emerging noninvasive method to measure CBF directly by using magnetically-labeled arterial blood water as an endogenous contrast agent (tracer). The ASL technique requires no contrast materials because it uses an endogenous contrast agent (the patient's own magnetically-labeled blood) [21, 22]. Arterial blood water is magnetically-labeled through inversion or saturation proximal to the tissue of interest, and image acquisition is usually performed after a delay time that allows the labeled blood to flow into the imaging slices. Images with and without the spin label are acquired and then subtracted. Repeated measurements of interleaved label and control acquisitions are performed to improve the signal-to-nose ratio of perfusion images, which often require a few minutes of scan time. The advantages of the ASL technique include the lack of intravenous contrast, the ability to repeat the study, and comparison of CBF values within and between patient examinations. However, the signal to-noise ratio, anatomic coverage, and shorter imaging time are currently better for the DSC perfusion techniques compared with the ASL.

MR perfusion has been used as a valuable tool for characterizing and monitoring ischemia in moyamoya disease. MR perfusion provides additional functional information not available from conventional MRI and has a potential role comparable to single photon emission computed tomography (SPECT) in the evaluation of cerebral hemodynamics [23, 24]. Kim et al. [14] described four patterns of MR perfusion abnormalities: (1) normal rCBV and TTP; (2) normal rCBV and delayed TTP; (3) increased rCBV and delayed TTP; and (4) decreased rCBV and delayed TTP. Patients who present with TIAs, no focal parenchymal lesions on MRI, early angiographic stages, and decreased vascular reserve on SPECT usually show delayed TTP without significant rCBV abnormalities. In patients with abundant collateral channels, perfusion MR showed increase of rCBV with delayed TTP (Fig. 3). The presence of collateral vessels introduces large delays and is likely to disperse contrast agent, therefore maps generated by deconvolution may result in significantly increased TTP and rCBV values. In patients with large areas of cerebral infarction, a decrease in the rCBV with delayed TTP and a perfusion defect on SPECT at the corresponding area was shown (Fig. 4).

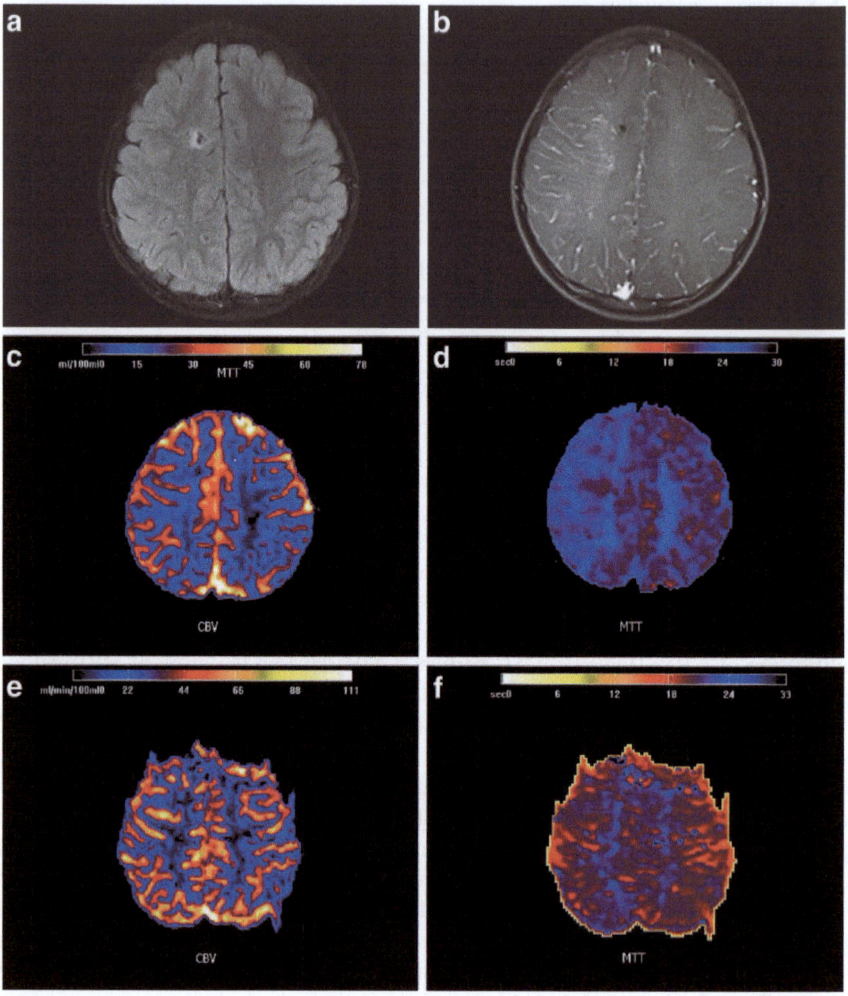

Fig. 3 An 11-year-old girl with left-sided weakness shows a focal infarct in the right centrum semiovale (**a**, **b**) and increased leptomeningeal enhancement on post-contrast T1-weighted image (**b**). Pre-operative MR perfusion images show that slightly increased CBV (**c**) and delayed MTT (**d**) in the right frontal lobe. Follow-up MR perfusion images after right EDAS and frontal EGS obtained 3 months later demonstrate improvement of the cerebral perfusion in the right frontal area and bilateral symmetric cerebral perfusion (**e**, **f**)

MR perfusion provides information regarding cerebral hemodynamic changes after revascularization surgery in moyamoya disease [25, 26]. Surgical revascularization is aimed at augmenting blood flow to the affected hemisphere, either directly with extracranial–intracranial bypass surgery, or indirectly via different techniques, including encephalo-duro-arterio-synangiosis (EDAS), encephalo-duro-arterio-myo-synangiosis, encephalo-myo-synangiosis, and placement of multiple burr holes. Most studies have documented clinical benefits and hemodynamic improvements after revascularization surgery [2, 3, 8, 26]. These studies have demonstrated an improvement in the cerebral vascular reserve and lowering of the CBV and O_2 extraction fraction. Benefits may be seen as early as 3 months after the post-revascularization procedure [3]. Lee et al. [25] reported that all 13 of their patients showed delayed TTP in the

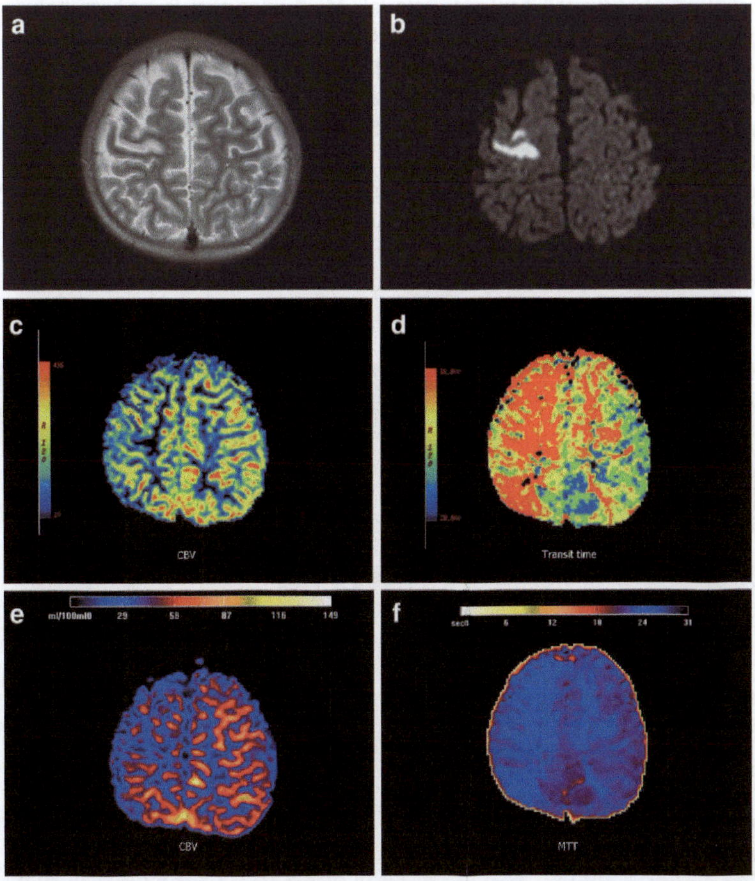

Fig. 4 An 8-year-old girl with recent aggravation of left-sided weakness. Brain MR images, including diffusion-weighted images, demonstrate acute focal infarction in the right frontal lobe (**a**, **b**). MR perfusion using an arterial spin labeling technique show a decrease of cerebral perfusion in the right hemisphere, especially the right frontal lobe (**c**, **d**). MR perfusion images obtained DSC technique demonstrate a decrease of CBV and delayed TTP and MTT in the corresponding right fontal area (**e**, **f**)

MCA territory before EDAS, as compared with normal controls, and that TTP values were significantly reduced after EDAS. In our retrospective analysis of 67 patients with moyamoya disease [26], regional TTP and rCBV values were significantly reduced after revascularization surgery (Fig. 3e, f). Furthermore, the results of the present study concerning reductions in TTP and rCBV agree well with those of earlier studies [12, 13, 25]. It appears that these phenomena are probably due to rapid parenchymal perfusion after revascularization surgery.

CT Perfusion Imaging

The main principle of the CT perfusion method is based on the analysis of noncontrast and contrast-enhanced CT scans obtained at different times. CT perfusion data involve only the sequential acquisition of cerebral CT sections achieved in an axial mode during intravenous administration of iodinated contrast material. Most important is a sharp bolus of contrast medium resulting from rapid injection [15]. CT perfusion relies on direct visualization of the contrast material. The linear relationship between contrast concentration and attenuation in CT more readily lends itself to evaluate the CBV, CBF, and MTT. Wintermark et al. [16] reported a good correlation between CT perfusion imaging of rCBF and xenon CT.

The clinical application of CT perfusion in moyamoya disease has been limited to a few clinical studies [27, 28]. In clinical application of CT perfusion in pediatric moyamoya disease, there are several limitations. First, there are challenges of intravenous access for young children and infants, small intravenous catheters, and limitations in the dose of contrast, which also exist for DSC-MR perfusion imaging. Second, in the CBF calculations with CT perfusion

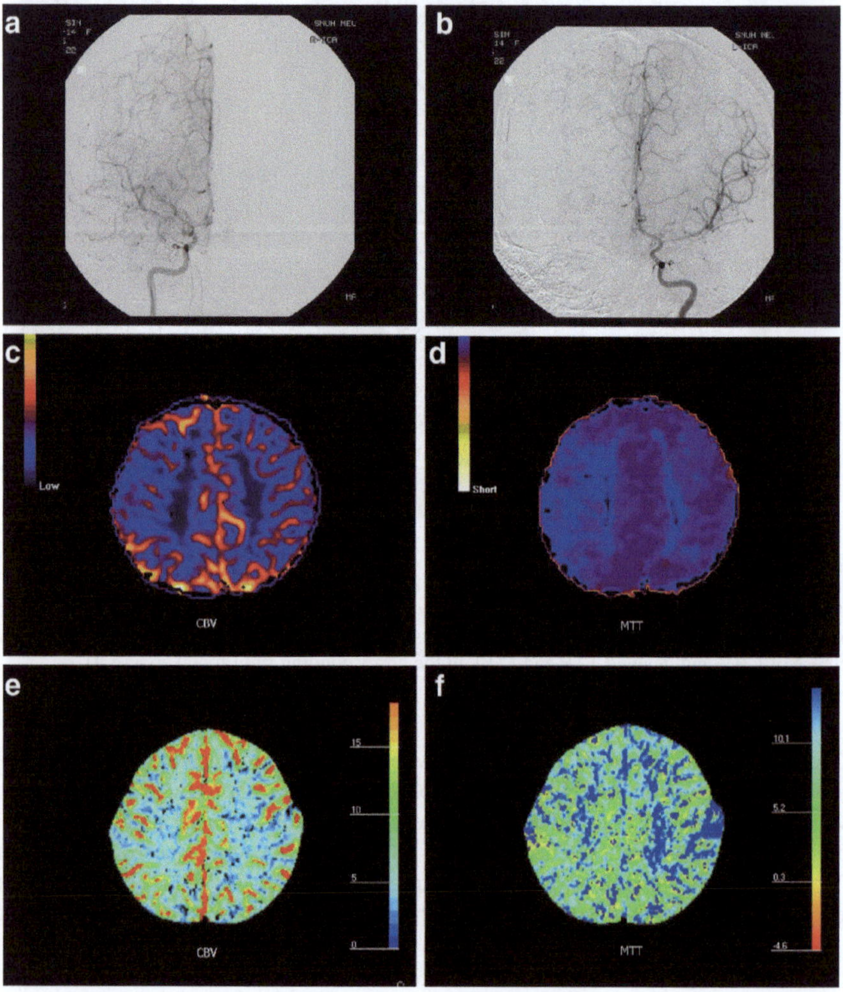

Fig. 5 A 16-year-old girl with left-sided weakness demonstrates bilateral distal ICA narrowing and prominent basal collateral formation in the right hemisphere (**a**, **b**). There is no focal parenchymal lesion in the conventional MR image (not shown here). Perfusion MR images depict a decrease of CBV (**c**) and delayed MTT (**d**) in the right frontoparietal area. Follow-up perfusion imaging using CT perfusion after bilateral EDAS and frontal EGS demonstrate symmetric perfusion in the cerebral hemisphere (**e**, **f**)

imaging, the choice of a reference artery is critical for the arterial input function. In a patient with moyamoya disease, occlusion of the ACAs and/or MCA and multiple collateral vessels always leads to a delay and dispersion of the bolus of the contrast materials. Third, the above limitations may result in a wide range of absolute measurements. The use of the hemispheric ratio or normalization of the hemodynamic parameters can improve the quantification problems [15, 27]. Finally, there is radiation issue for CT perfusion if the patients need follow-up evaluation. In spite of these limitations, a preliminary CT perfusion study for the evaluation of the cerebral vascular reserve has provided promising results [29, 30]. In our limited experience, CT perfusion demonstrates pre- and postoperative hemodynamic status of moyamoya disease well (Fig. 5). CT perfusion has an advantage over a postoperative cerebral perfusion evaluation because distortion of perfusion data due to metallic artifact is less than that of DCS-MR perfusion (Fig. 3e, f). Kang et al. [28] reported that CT perfusion is suitable for quantitative evaluation of the cerebral vascular reserve after acetazolamide challenge.

Conclusion

Perfusion imaging for moyamoya disease supports the diagnosis of the disease as early as possible, and provides accurate information about intracranial vasculature and brain perfusion. The information of cerebral perfusion obtained by combining various imaging techniques may help with guidance in selecting the appropriate therapy and monitoring the postoperative hemodynamic state.

References

1. Suzuki J, Takaku A (1969) Cerebrovascular “moyamoya” disease. Disease showing abnormal net-like vessels in base of brain. Arch Neurol 20:288–299
2. Scott RM, Smith ER (2009) Moyamoya disease and moyamoya syndrome. N Engl J Med 360:1226–1237
3. Kuroda S, Houkin K (2008) Moyamoya disease: current concepts and future perspectives. Lancet Neurol 7:1056–1066
4. Yoon HK, Shin HJ, Chang YW (2002) “Ivy sign” in childhood moyamoya disease: depiction on FLAIR and contrast-enhanced T1-weighted MR images. Radiology 223:384–389
5. Yamada I, Nakagawa T, Matsushima Y et al (2001) High-resolution turbo magnetic resonance angiography for diagnosis of Moyamoya disease. Stroke 32:1825–1831
6. Hasuo K, Mihara F, Matsushima T (1998) MRI and MR angiography in moyamoya disease. J Magn Reson Imaging 8:762–726
7. Kuroda S, Houkin K, Kamiyama H et al (1995) Regional cerebral hemodynamics in childhood moyamoya disease. Childs Nerv Syst 11:584–590
8. Touho H, Karasawa J, Ohnishi H (1996) Preoperative and postoperative evaluation of cerebral perfusion and vasodilatory capacity with 99mTc-HMPAO SPECT and acetazolamide in childhood Moyamoya disease. Stroke 27:282–289
9. Tsuchiya K, Inaoka S, Mizutani Y et al (1998) Echo-planar perfusion MR of moyamoya disease. Am J Neuroradiol 19:211–216
10. Yamada I, Himeno Y, Nagaoka T et al (1999) Moyamoya disease: evaluation with diffusion-weighted and perfusion echo-planar MR imaging. Radiology 212:340–347
11. Petrella JR, Provenzale JM (2000) MR perfusion imaging of the brain: techniques and applications. Am J Roentgenol 175:207–219

12. Calamante F, Ganesan V, Kirkham FJ et al (2001) MR perfusion imaging in Moyamoya Syndrome: potential implications for clinical evaluation of occlusive cerebrovascular disease. Stroke 32:2810–2816
13. Togao O, Mihara F, Yoshiura T et al (2006) Cerebral hemodynamics in Moyamoya disease: correlation between perfusion-weighted MR imaging and cerebral angiography. Am J Neuroradiol 27:391–397
14. Kim SK, Wang KC, Oh CW et al (2003) Evaluation of cerebral hemodynamics with perfusion MRI in childhood moyamoya disease. Pediatr Neurosurg 38:68–75
15. Srinivasan A, Goyal M, Azri FA et al (2006) State of the art imaging of stroke. Radiographics 26:S75–S95
16. Wintermark M, Thiran JP, Maeder P et al (2001) Simultaneous measurement of regional cerebral blood flow by perfusion CT and stable xenon CT: a validation study. Am J Neuroradiol 22: 905–914
17. Koenig M, Klotz E, Luka B et al (1998) Perfusion CT of the brain: diagnostic approach for early detection of ischemic stroke. Radiology 209:85–93 20
18. Rowley HA, Roberts TP (2004) Clinical perspectives in perfusion: neuroradiologic applications. Top Magn Reson Imaging 15:28–40
19. Luypaert R, Boujraf S, Sourbron S et al (2001) Diffusion and perfusion MRI: basic physics. Eur J Radiol 38:19–27
20. Speck O, Chang L, DeSilva NM et al (2000) Perfusion MRI of the human brain with dynamic susceptibility contrast: gradient-echo versus spin-echo techniques. J Magn Reson Imaging 12:381–387
21. Detre JA, Alsop DC (1999) Perfusion magnetic resonance imaging with continuous arterial spin labeling: methods and clinical applications in the central nervous system. Eur J Radiol 30:115–124
22. Lee M, Zaharchuk G, Guzman R et al (2009) Quantitative hemodynamic studies in moyamoya disease: a review. Neurosurg Focus 26:E5
23. Kim JH, Lee EJ, Lee SJ et al (2002) Comparative evaluation of cerebral blood volume and cerebral blood flow in acute ischemic stroke by using perfusion-weighted MR imaging and SPECT. Acta Radiol 43:365–370
24. Hatazawa J, Shimosegawa E, Toyoshima H et al (1999) Cerebral blood volume in acute brain infarction: a combined study with dynamic susceptibility contrast MRI and 99mTc-HMPAO-SPECT. Stroke 30:800–806
25. Lee SK, Kim DI, Jeong EK et al (2003) Postoperative evaluation of moyamoya disease with perfusion-weighted MR imaging: initial experience. Am J Neuroradiol 24:741–747
26. Yun TJ, Cheon JE, Kim IO et al (2009) Childhood moyamoya disease: quantitative evaluation of perfusion MR imaging: correlation with clinical outcome after revascularization surgery. Radiology 251:216–223
27. Rim NJ, Kim HS, Shin YS et al (2008) CT perfusion parameter best reflects cerebrovascular reserve?: correlation of acetazolamide-challenged CT perfusion with single-photon emission CT in Moyamoya patients. Am J Neuroradiol 9:1658–1663
28. Kang KH, Kim HS, Kim SY (2008) Quantitative cerebrovascular reserve measured by acetazolamide-challenged dynamic CT perfusion in ischemic adult Moyamoya disease: initial experience with angiographic correlation. Am J Neuroradiol 29:1487–1493
29. Sakamoto S, Ohba S, Shibukawa M et al (2006) CT perfusion imaging for childhood moyamoya disease before and after surgical revascularization. Acta Neurochir (Wien) 148:77–81
30. Chen A, Shyr MH, Chen TY et al (2006) Dynamic CT perfusion imaging with acetazolamide challenge for evaluation of patients with unilateral cerebrovascular steno-occlusive disease. Am J Neuroradiol 27:1876–1881

Positron Emission Tomography in Moyamoya Disease

Tadashi Nariai

Abbreviations

CBF	cerebral blood flow
CBV	cerebral blood volume
$CMRO_2$	cerebral metabolic rate for oxygen
CPP	cerebral perfusion pressure
CVD	cerebrovascular disease
MTT	mean vascular transit time
OEF	oxygen extraction fraction
PET	positron emission tomography

Introduction

The hallmark features of moyamoya disease are a progressive occlusion of bilateral internal carotid arteries and the development of collateral networks to compensate for the reduced cerebral perfusion [1,2]. Besides these very specific changes, several other conditions can also lead to the chronic cerebral ischemia encountered mainly in younger patients. It thus becomes necessary to evaluate the hemodynamic condition of patients with moyamoya disease in order to understand the pathophysiology of the syndrome and select appropriate treatments for patients individually.

The author and colleagues have long been using positron emission tomography (PET) for the clinical evaluation of this syndrome. Earlier, we reported that PET measurements of moyamoya disease, like those of other occlusive cerebrovascular diseases (CVDs), reflect the hemodynamic condition with only weak uniformity [3]. In that report, we proposed that PET information is important for both the practical management of moyamoya patients and for clinical research on the disease. This chapter will explain the rationale for using PET in moyamoya disease. The features of the measurement, present limitations, and future perspectives will be described.

T. Nariai
Department of Neurosurgery, Tokyo Medical and Dental University, 1-5-45 Yushima, Bunkyo-ku, Tokyo 113-8519, Japan
e-mail: nariai.nsrg@tmd.ac.jp

B.-K. Cho and T. Tominaga (eds.), *Moyamoya Disease Update*,
DOI 10.1007/978-4-431-99703-0_29, © Springer 2010

Strength of PET in Cerebrovascular Diseases

PET is a useful medical imaging modality for monitoring biological events inside the human body. PET can quantify the distribution of positron-labeled molecules in living tissue by coincidence detection of gamma rays and attenuation correction with an external positron-emitting source [4]. Thus, the images obtained by PET serve well as in vivo analogs of autoradiographs [5,6].

For application in CVD, the strength of PET lies in the use of $C^{15}O_2$ and $H_2{}^{15}O$, two inert diffusible tracers which enable the quantification of cerebral blood flow (CBF) based on the Fick principle and the Kety–Schmidt equation, the gold standard technique for organ blood flow measurement [7]. Another, maybe the biggest, advantage of PET is its ability to quantify the cerebral metabolism using $^{15}O_2$ (cerebral metabolic rate for oxygen, $CMRO_2$) or ^{18}F-fluorodeoxyglucose (glucose metabolism). The oxygen extraction fraction (OEF) can be obtained by taking serial measurements of CBF and $CMRO_2$. An abnormally elevated OEF is now recognized as the best parameter for detecting viable brain tissue at high risk of a future stroke, tissue which may benefit from bypass surgery [8,9].

Cerebral blood volume (CBV), a parameter quantified by inhalation of $C^{15}O$, is also important for understanding the pathophysiology of CVDs. Cerebral perfusion pressure (CPP) is defined as CBF/CBV. The inverse of CBF/CBV, from a theoretical standpoint, is the mean vascular transit time (MTT) of red blood cells through the cerebral vessels. Powers et al. used these PET parameters to propose a famous theoretical model of the compensatory mechanism in the process of occlusive cerebral vascular diseases [10,11]. Within this model, the phase of compensation by vascular reserve is categorized as Stage I, and that by metabolic reserve, as Stage II (Fig. 1) [10,11]. The latter condition is also described as "misery perfusion" [12]. We note, with interest, that this theoretical model accurately describes the hemodynamic condition of moyamoya disease.

Hemodynamics of Moyamoya Disease as Examined by PET

As described in the last paragraph, multiple hemodynamic parameters obtained by PET can serve well in the analysis of moyamoya disease. These can include $^{15}O_2$ gas studies, serial measurements of CBF, $CMRO_2$, OEF, and CBV, and calculations of CPP or MTT with inhalation of $C^{15}O_2$, $^{15}O_2$, and $C^{15}O$. Variations of these factors based on the hemodynamic model are more clearly seen in moyamoya disease than in atherosclerotic diseases, presumably due to the slowly progressive nature of the former. Nariai et al. [3] observed elevated CBV without accompanying reductions of CBF in nonsymptomatic cases. When the compensation by vascular reserve reaches maximum, transient ischemic attack (TIA) is observed. When infarction begins to appear and TIA remains, an elevated OEF can be detected in the viable cerebral cortex (Fig. 2). This indicates that the model from Powers et al. [10,11] accurately depicts the hemodynamic condition of moyamoya disease and can be used to interpret the pathophysiology and determine the treatment strategy.

Repeated measurement of CBF with $H_2{}^{15}O$ has proven to be another important source of information on the hemodynamics of moyamoya disease [13]. To take advantage of the short duration required for image acquisition and the short half-life of tracer radioactivity (2 min), $H_2{}^{15}O$ PET has been used in activation studies for the mapping of brain function [14]. Our group and several others have investigated the vascular responses of moyamoya patients against various tolerance tests such as CO_2 inhalation, hyperventilation, and acetazolamide

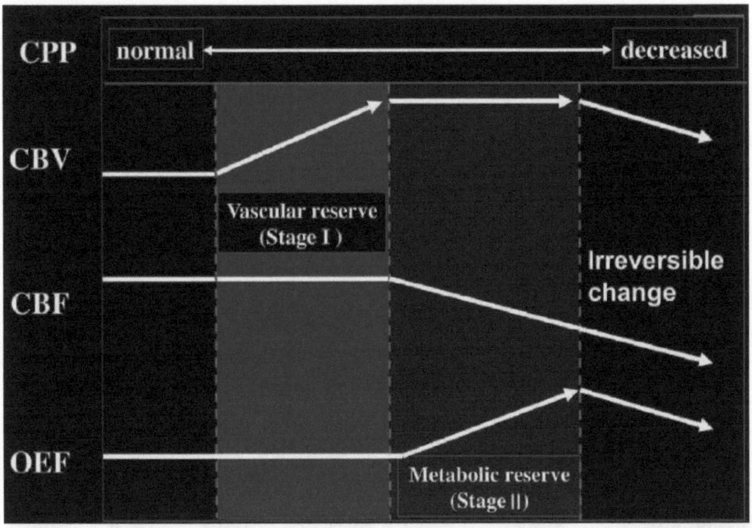

Fig. 1 Theoretical model of a compensatory mechanism against chronic decrease in CPP. The stage of hemodynamic compensation by elevated CBV was termed Stage I, and that of metabolic compensation by elevated OEF was termed Stage II [10,11]

loading [15,16]. According to these examinations, vascular responses against various stimuli are often badly disturbed in the areas affected by moyamoya disease. Thus, the CBF is influenced by the normal vascular response of the surrounding area, and a paradoxical decrease by vasodilatory stimuli and paradoxical increase by vasoconstrictive stimuli are often observed (Fig. 3). This abnormal response in moyamoya disease may be one of causes of the frequent TIAs or prolonged hypoperfusion induced by hyperventilation. It may also be one of the reasons behind the limited effectiveness of medical treatments in controlling ischemia in this syndrome.

Clinical Use of PET for Moyamoya Disease: Limitation and Resolution

As described earlier, hemodynamic parameters measured by PET offer definite benefits for the precise treatment of this syndrome. Yet in clinical practice, PET studies are not feasible for routine use. The public health insurance system in Japan covers the cost of ^{15}O-gas studies, and the number of institutions equipped with PET systems has been rapidly increasing, yet PET is still used chiefly for ^{18}F-FDG studies for cancer patients, and the number of ^{15}O-gas examinations has actually been declining. It may be that the arterial blood sampling and other complicated procedures required to obtain reliable data for decision-making, such as the OEF, discourage clinicians from performing the examinations. In cases with unilateral internal carotid disease, there are methods to obtain the ratio of OEF to the contralateral side without arterial blood sampling [17]. Yet the bilateral involvement in moyamoya disease renders these unsuitable for moyamoya patients. To promote the use of PET for moyamoya disease, it will

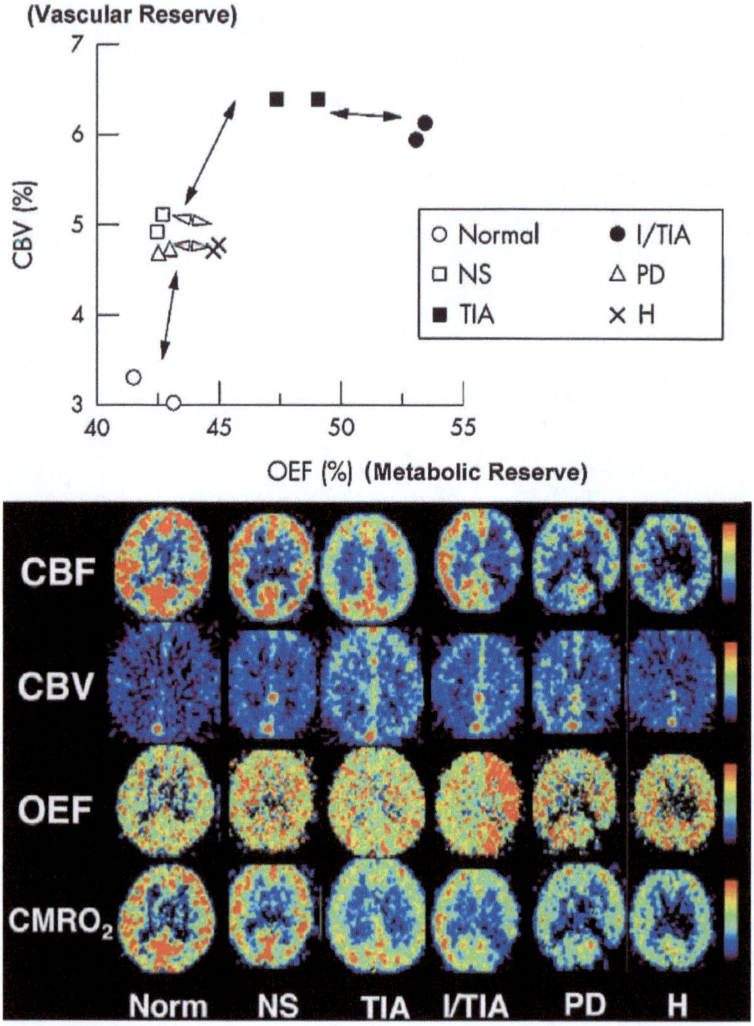

Fig. 2 Two-dimensional plotting of the couplings between the OEF (*x*-axis) and CBV (*y*-axis) among various clinical subtypes of patients with moyamoya disease (modified from a figure in [3]). The NS, H, and PD groups all manifested elevated CBV in the range of normal OEF (Stage I). In the TIA group, the CBV peaked and the OEF began to rise (border between Stages I and II). The I/TIA group had maximally increased CBV and OEF (Stage II). PET images of representative patients from the respective groups also represented the changes quite clearly. *Norm* normal control, *NS* nonsymptomatic patients, *TIA* patients presenting TIA without infarction, *I/TIA* patients presenting TIA with infarction, *PD* patients with infarction and permanent neurological deficit, *H* patients with hemorrhagic onset

be important to provide more clinical evidence on the utility of hemodynamic measurements by PET. We are currently interpreting PET data on moyamoya disease based on theories focused on atherosclerosis of the major cerebral arteries. The significance of CBF, OEF, and CBV on the natural course of moyamoya disease remains uncertain. Clinical data on long-term follow-ups of many more patients will be required. A prospective observational study of

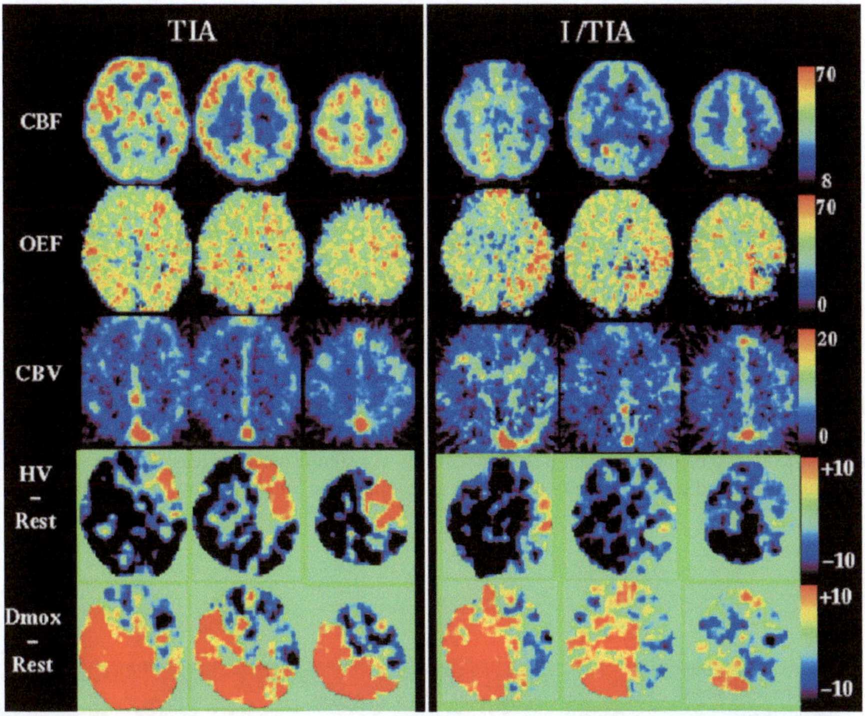

Fig. 3 Vascular response of two patients with moyamoya disease. The area with maximally elevated CBV and increased OEF showed a paradoxical CBF response. Vasoconstrictive stimuli by hyperventilation induced an increase in CBF in the affected area. Vasodilatory stimulation by acetazolamide (DMOX) loading induced a decrease in CBF

moyamoya patients based on PET measurement, a study now underway in the USA, may help to significantly clarify the clinical features of this syndrome [18]. It will also be important to accumulate data on the hemodynamic changes accompanying surgical revascularization. The work by Ikezaki et al. in the early 1990s [19] is the only report on changes of PET hemodynamic parameters induced by operative treatment. Yet, according to their results, the interventions failed to bring about significant increases in CBF. We presume that the variable preoperative hemodynamics of this syndrome were not considered in their analysis. We showed that the area with elevated OEF is benefited by angiogenesis induced by indirect bypass surgery [20]. Our preliminary statistical analysis of CBF and OEF also clearly indicated that CBF was significantly increased in bilateral frontal lobes, and that the elevated OEF was significantly ameliorated in exactly the same regions (Fig. 4). Further subgroup analyses on the contributions of factors such as age, surgical procedures, and preoperative clinical subtypes to the surgical effects may help lead the way to the establishment of proper guidelines for the application of surgery.

The complicated procedures of ^{15}O-gas studies also make PET difficult to use it for pediatric cases. To help solve this problem, we performed a comparative study between PET and dynamic susceptible contrast enhancement-magnetic resonance perfusion study (DSC-MRI) [21]. In that study, we demonstrated that a prolonged mean transit time exceeding a certain threshold examined by DSC-MRI corresponded well with an area with abnormally elevated OEF (Fig. 5). The success of this study led the way to the routine use of a noninvasive

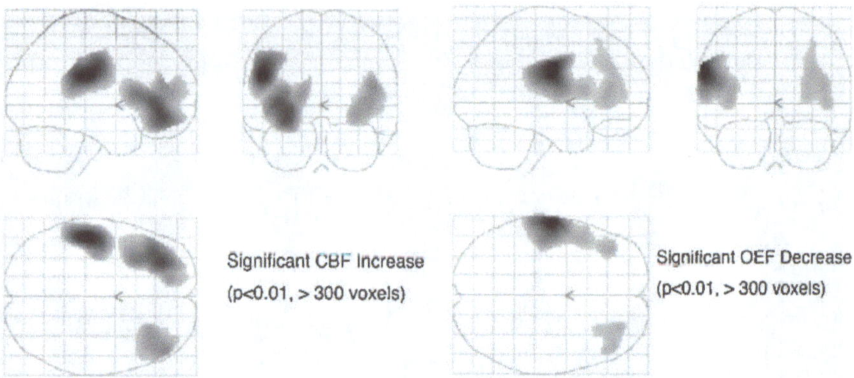

Fig. 4 Statistical image analysis of 48 patients who underwent bilateral indirect bypass surgery. Glass brain expression using SPM2 demonstrated a significant elevation of CBF in bilateral frontal lobes and in the parietal lobe of the dominant hemisphere. OEF was significantly decreased in the same territory. The results indicated that the surgery effectively ameliorated the Stage II hemodynamic stress

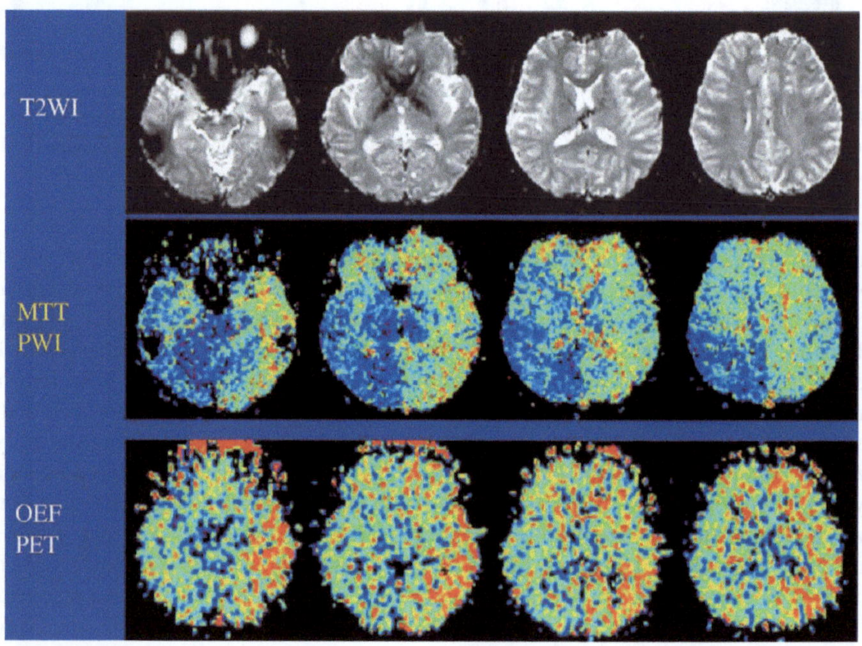

Fig. 5 Comparison between PET-measured OEF and MTT obtained by dynamic susceptible contrast enhancement-magnetic resonance perfusion study (DSC-MRI) (modified from a figure in [21]). By setting a certain threshold in prolongation of MTT, the area with abnormally elevated OEF could be detected with high specificity and sensitivity

hemodynamic evaluation of moyamoya disease and contributed much to the establishment of tailor-made management for patients individually.

Conclusion

The measurement of multiple hemodynamic parameters in moyamoya disease with PET is likely to contribute significantly to the establishment of an appropriate clinical management protocol for this syndrome. To benefit moyamoya patients in a meaningful way, it will be necessary to prospectively accumulate more PET data on this disease.

References

1. Suzuki J, Takaku A (1969) Cerebrovascular "moyamoya"" disease. Disease showing abnormal net-like vessels in base of brain. Arch Neurol 20:288–299
2. Matsushima Y (1999) Moyamoya disease. In: Albright A, Pollack I, Adelson P (eds) Principle and practice of pediatric neurosurgery. Thieme, New York, pp 1053–1069
3. Nariai T, Matsushima Y, Imae S, et al. (2005) Severe haemodynamic stress in selected subtypes of patients with moyamoya disease: a positron emission tomography study. J Neurol Neurosurg Psychiatry 76:663–669
4. Phelps ME, Hoffman EJ, Mullani NA, et al. (1975) Application of annihilation coincidence detection to transaxial reconstruction tomography. J Nucl Med 16:210–224
5. Phelps ME, Mazziotta JC (1985) Positron emission tomography: human brain function and biochemistry. Science 228:799–809
6. Herscovitch P, Markham J, Raichle ME (1983) Brain blood flow measured with intravenous $H_2{}^{15}O$. I. Theory and error analysis. J Nucl Med 24:782–789
7. Kety SS, Schmidt CF (1948) The nitrous oxide method for the quantitative determination of cerebral blood flow in man: theory, procedure and normal values. J Clin Invest 27:476–483
8. Grubb RL, Jr., Derdeyn CP, Fritsch SM, et al. (1998) Importance of hemodynamic factors in the prognosis of symptomatic carotid occlusion. JAMA 280:1055–1060
9. Yamauchi H, Fukuyama H, Nagahama Y, et al. (1999) Significance of increased oxygen extraction fraction in five-year prognosis of major cerebral arterial occlusive diseases. J Nucl Med 40:1992–1998
10. Powers WJ (1991) Cerebral hemodynamics in ischemic cerebrovascular disease. Ann Neurol 29:231–240
11. Powers WJ, Grubb RL, Jr., Raichle ME (1984) Physiological responses to focal cerebral ischemia in humans. Ann Neurol 16:546–552
12. Baron JC, Bousser MG, Rey A, et al. (1981) Reversal of focal "Misery-perfusion syndrome" by extra-intracranial arterial bypass in hemodynamic cerebral ischemia. A case study with ^{15}O positron emission tomography. Stroke 12:454–459
13. Raichle ME, Martin WRW, Herscovitch P, et al. (1983) Brain blood flow measured with intravenous $H_2{}^{15}O$. II. Implementation and validation. J Nucl Med 24:790–798
14. Cherry S, Phelps M (1996) Imaging brain function with positron emission tomography. In: Toga A, Mazziotta J (eds) Brain mapping: the methods. Academic, San Diego, pp 191–221
15. Kuwabara Y, Ichiya Y, Sasaki M, et al. (1997) Response to hypercapnia in moyamoya disease. Cerebrovascular response to hypercapnia in pediatric and adult patients with moyamoya disease. Stroke 28:701–707
16. Nariai T, Senda M, Ishii K, et al. (1998) Posthyperventilatory steal response in chronic cerebral hemodynamic stress: a positron emission tomography study. Stroke 29:1281–1292
17. Derdeyn CP, Videen TO, Simmons NR, et al. (1999) Count-based PET method for predicting ischemic stroke in patients with symptomatic carotid arterial occlusion. Radiology 212:499–506

18. Zipfel GJ, Sagar J, Miller JP, et al. (2009) Cerebral hemodynamics as a predictor of stroke in adult patients with moyamoya disease: a prospective observational study. Neurosurg Focus 26:E6
19. Ikezaki K, Matsushima T, Kuwabara Y, et al. (1994) Cerebral circulation and oxygen metabolism in childhood moyamoya disease: a perioperative positron emission tomography study. J Neurosurg 81:843–850
20. Nariai T, Suzuki R, Matsushima Y, et al. (1994) Surgically induced angiogenesis to compensate for hemodynamic cerebral ischemia. Stroke 25:1014–1021
21. Tanaka Y, Nariai T, Nagaoka T, et al. (2006) Quantitative evaluation of cerebral hemodynamics in patients with moyamoya disease by dynamic susceptibility contrast magnetic resonance imaging-comparison with positron emission tomography. J Cereb Blood Flow Metab 26:291–300

Part IX
Diagnostic Evaluation III: Electrophysiology

Electroencephalography (EEG) in Moyamoya Disease

Jong-Hee Chae and Ki Joong Kim

Introduction

Moyamoya disease (MMD) is one of the most common causes of cerebrovascular disease in East Asian populations, especially of Japan, China and Republic of Korea. This condition is characterized by progressive stenosis of both terminal internal carotid arteries in the supraclinoid portion with the development of a network of cerebral collaterals, referred to as the moyamoya vessels. Interestingly, clinical symptoms are different between children and adults. Children present most frequently with the symptoms of episodic cerebral ischemia like transient reversible hemiplegia, which are often precipitated by hyperventilation situation such as when crying, playing the harmonica, eating hot and spicy food, and taking a deep breath when emotionally upset, while in adults, they are intracranial hemorrhages. We can diagnose the patients by brain magnetic resonance (MR) imaging, an MR angiography, an electroencephalography (EEG), and a cerebral angiography without any difficulties [1–3].

EEG changes in MMD have been described in many reports [4–7]. Here, we review the electroencephalographic features in MMD as a diagnostic implication and suggest the pathophysiology of abnormal EEG generation, especially the "re-build-up phenomenon."

Electroencephalographic Changes in Moyamoya Disease

Although EEG is not a specific diagnostic tool for MMD, EEG can play an important role as a means of screening, especially in children.

J.H. Chae (✉) and K.J. Kim
Department of Pediatrics, Pediatric Clinical Neuroscience Center,
Seoul National University Children's Hospital, Seoul National University College of Medicine,
101 Daehangno, Jongno-gu, Seoul 110-744, Republic of Korea
e-mail: chaeped1@snu.ac.kr

J.H. Chae
Research Center for Rare Disease, Seoul, Republic of Korea

B.-K. Cho and T. Tominaga (eds.), *Moyamoya Disease Update*,
DOI 10.1007/978-4-431-99703-0_30, © Springer 2010

The commonly associated abnormal EEG findings in MMD are high amplitude slow waves on the posterior or centrotemporal area and sleep spindle depression, which are often associated with other nonspecific brain injuries or cerebral ischemia. Interestingly, theses abnormal high amplitude monorhythmic posterior slow waves on the posterior head region (P slow activities) and high amplitude, polyrhythmic centrotemporal waves (CT slow activities) tend to be observed in the more involved side, which correspond to the side of the more prominent neurologic symptoms in MMD patients. In addition, Kodama et al. pointed out that P slow activities appear within a relatively short time after the onset of the disease. The CT slows activities at mid-stage, and the diffuse low voltage background pattern at a later time, in which the EEG changes with time may reflect the degree of progressive circulatory disturbance [4].

The characteristic EEG features in MMD have been reported to be: a "build-up" phenomenon, the appearance of monorhythmic high voltage generalized slow activities during hyperventilation (Fig. 1a); and "re-build-up", the reappearance of polymorphic high amplitude slow waves several minutes after the cessation of hyperventilation, followed by the build-up phenomenon (Fig. 1b).

The clinical difference between children and adults have been described previously. The appearance of abnormal EEG changes after hyperventilation, so-called re-build-up is almost exclusively in children with MMD. Interestingly these re-build-up phenomena disappear with increasing age and are not seen in adults, independent of the clinical stages. One possible explanation could be that a hyperventilation response is hardly detectable even in healthy adults [7–9].

Pathophysiology of the Re-Build Up Phenomenon

The mechanism of build-up during hyperventilation and re-build-up after hyperventilation has not yet been clarified. However, several studies have suggested possible mechanisms. The build-up during hyperventilation is known to originate from the deep regions of the brain and to be induced by a decrease in partial pressure of carbon dioxide ($PaCO_2$) caused by vasoconstriction of small arterioles during hyperventilation, and to disappear after the termination of hyperventilation in about 80% of normal children [6, 10–12]. In contrast, the re-build-up phenomenon is suggested to have a different origin from that of the build up phenomenon [13]. Kemeyama et al. measured the regional cerebral blood flow (rCBF) and the regional cerebral metabolite for oxygen ($rCMRO_2$) before and after hyperventilation. They observed a decrease in rCBF and a greater decrease in $rCMRO_2$ after hyperventilation and suggested that the re-build-up phenomenon results not only from ischemic hypoxia but also from hypoxic hypoxia [14]. The concentration of oxygenated hemoglobin increased during hyperventilation and gradually decreased further after hyperventilation for 5–7 min. During this period, the re-build-up occurs with an increase of deoxygenated hemoglobin [15, 16]. In a region where cerebrovascular reactivity is disturbed, regional cerebral perfusion reserve after hyperventilation decreases more with the reduction of oxygenated hemoglobin and regional cerebral hypoxia [13, 17]. Therefore, the regional cerebral hypoxia resulting from the impairment of cerebrovascular reactivity and disturbance of oxygen metabolism could contribute to the occurrence of the re-build-up phenomenon after hyperventilation.

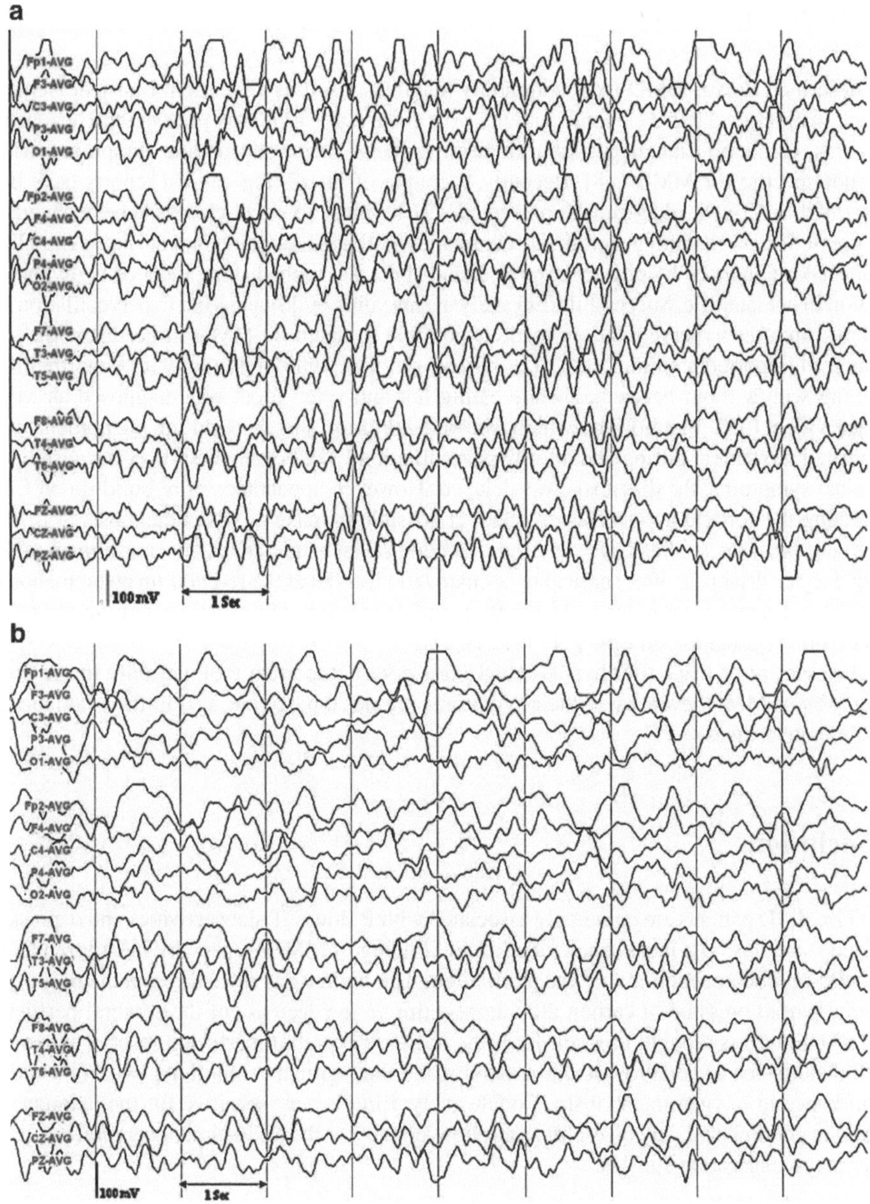

Fig. 1 High voltage delta wave activities in the 120-s hyperventilation (**a**) and re-build-up phenomenon, showing high A polymorphic delta waves 6 min after cessation of hyperventilation (**b**)

Clinical Implications

As described above, MMD most commonly manifests itself as a recurrent transient ischemic attack in children. However, some patients with the juvenile type may present with headaches, seizures, incoherent languages, abnormal movements, or psychosomatic symptoms, which are not specific for MMD [18]. Recently, a couple of interesting clinical reports have been described. A 13-year-old girl, who presented with atypical absence seizures in her early years, progressed to partial and generalized seizures, unmotivated laughing and crying, generalized limb shaking induced by physical exercise, and abnormal limb shaking induced by hyperventilation in her later life. Successful EEG analysis, revealing build-up during hyperventilation and re-buil- up after hyperventilation, made it possible to diagnose MMD in her later life [19]. Kim et al. reported a similar case of a 39-year-old man, who presented with abnormal limb shaking with/without headaches while eating hot and spicy food, was diagnosed as MMD under video EEG monitoring, which showed build-up and re-build-up phenomena with abnormal movement during and after hyperventilation [20]. For the first time, because of the atypical symptoms, the diagnosis was delayed. However, appearance of re-build-up on EEG, reflecting the cortical hypoperfusion, made it possible to make a correct diagnosis of MMD.

Many previous studies have reported that cerebral ischemic attacks decrease markedly in frequency or disappear after surgical revascularization, and that the re-build-up phenomenon on EEG also disappears or reduces the duration and distribution after surgery with improvement of cerebral regional blood flow [11, 13, 21].

Assessment of EEG after hyperventilation is a very important tool, not only in the initial diagnosis of MMD, even when their symptoms are not typical, but also in the evaluation of postoperative cases.

Conclusion

EEG in MMD patients are commonly associated with P slow, CT slow activities and depression of sleep spindles. The most characteristic EEG finding of MMD, especially in children, is the re-build-up phenomenon after hyperventilation. The build-up is related to a reduction of the arterial partial pressure of carbon dioxide resulting in the decrease of the cerebral perfusion, and re-build-up is thought to result from the decreased cerebral perfusion reserve associated with disturbance of cerebrovascular reactivity and the regional cerebral hypoxia followed by disturbance in oxygen metabolism. Conclusively, EEG is very sensitive for the diagnosis of MMD in children and may be useful as a follow-up tool for the evaluation of cerebral perfusion after revascularization surgery.

References

1. Suzuki J, Kodama N (1986) Moyamoya disease – review. Stroke 14:104–109
2. Fukui M, Kono S, Sueishi K et al (2000) Moyamoya disease. Neuropathology 20(Suppl):61–64
3. Manceau E, Giroud M, Dumas R (1997) Moyamoya disease in children: a review of the clinical and radiological features and current treatment. Childs Nerv Syst 13:595–600
4. Kodama N, Aoki Y, Hiraga H et al (1979) Electroencephalographic findings in children with moyamoya disease. Arch Neurol 36:16–19

5. Sunder TR, Erwin CW, Duboid PJ (1980) Hyperventilation induced abnormalities in the electroencephalogram of children with moyamoya disease. Electroencephalogr Clin Neurophysiol 49:414–420
6. Konish T (1987) The standardization of hyperventilation on EEG recording in childhood II. The quantitative analysis of build-up. Brain Dev 9:21–25
7. Kurlemann G, Fahrendorf G, Wolfgang K et al (1992) Characteristic EEG findings in childhood moyamoya syndrome. Neurosurg Rev 15:57–60
8. Aoki Y, Hiraga H, Ichijo S (1977) EEG or the moyamoya disease. Electroencephalogr Clin Neurophysiol 43:490
9. Tagawa T, Naritomi H, Mimaki T et al (1984) Mechanism of EEG abnormality caused by hyerventilation in children with moyamoya disease-hemodynamic study be Xe^{133} inhalation method. Brain Dev 6:217
10. Prestwick G, Reivich M, Hill ID (1965) The EEG effects of combined hyperventilation and hypoxia in normal subjects. Electroencephalogr Clin Neurophysiol 18:56–65
11. Kim DS, Ko TS, Ra YS et al (2006) Postoperative electroencephalogram for follow up of pediatric moyamoya disease. J Korean Med Sci 21:495–499
12. Achenbach-NG, Mavroudakis N, Chippa KH et al (1990) Effects of routine hyperventilation on PCO2 and PO2 in normal subjects: implication form EEG interpretations. J Clin Neurophysiol 11(2):220–225
13. Kuroda S, Kamiyama H, Isobe M et al (1995) Cerebral hemodynamics and "re-build up" phenomenon on electroencephalogram in children with moyamoya disease. Childs Nerv Syst 11:214–219
14. Kameyama M, Shirane R, Tsurumi Y et al (1986). Evaluation of cerebral blood flow and metabolism in childhood moyamoya disease: an investigation into "re-build up" on EEG by positron CT. Childs Nerv Syst 2:130–133
15. Touho H, Karasawa J, Shishido H et al (1990) Mechanism of the re-build up phenomenon in moyamoya disease. Neurol Med Chir (Tokyo) 30:721–726
16. Lin Y, Yoshiko K, Negoro T et al (2000) Cerebral oxygenation state in childhood moyamoya disease: a near-infrared spectroscopy study. Pediatr Neurol 22:365–369
17. Kuroda S, Houkin K, Hoshi Y et al (1996) Cerebral hypoxia after hyperventilation causes "re-build up" phenomenon and TIA in childhood moyamoya disease: a near-infrared spectroscopy study. Childs Nerv Syst 12:448–453
18. Fernandez-Fernandez S, Vazquez-Lopez M, Carrasco-Marina LL et al (2003) An association between moyamoya disease and morning glory anomaly. Rev Neurol 37:541–544
19. Kacinski M, Kubik A, Kroczka S et al (2007) Clinical and video-EEG findings in a girl with juvenile moyamoya disease. Brain Dev 29:603–606
20. Kim HY, Chung CS, Lee J et al (2003) Hyperventilation-induced limb shaking TIA in moyamoya disease. Neurology 60:137–139
21. Karasawa J, Touho H, Ohnishi H et al (1992) Long-term follow up study after extracranial intracranial bypass surgery for anterior circulation ischemia in childhood moyamoya disease. J Neurosurg 77:84–89

Magnetoencephalography (MEG): Its Application to Moyamoya Disease

Nobukazu Nakasato, Akitake Kanno, and Teiji Tominaga

Introduction

The re-build-up phenomenon in electroencephalography (EEG) was first described as a pathognomonic phenomenon of moyamoya disease in 1977 (in Japanese) [1] and in 1979 (in English) [2]. Slow wave discharges are known to "build-up" during hyperventilation used as a routine provocation method in clinical EEG. Moreover, slow wave discharges also appear a few minutes after the termination of hyperventilation exclusively in patients with moyamoya disease. This "re-build-up" phenomenon was once thought to occur only in pediatric patients [1, 2], but was later also found in adult patients. Interestingly, the re-build-up phenomenon is often accompanied by ischemic symptoms. However, the cortical or deep structural origin of the generator mechanism remains controversial.

In this review chapter, we summarize recent advances in magnetoencephalography (MEG) as a diagnostic tool of cerebral ischemia. Previous, and our own, experience of MEG indicates that the re-build-up phenomenon can be considered to represent cortical dysfunction caused by transient ischemia. Our present study in healthy young subjects also suggests that marked respiratory depression after hyperventilation causing transient hypoxia must be intense enough to provoke ischemic symptoms in patients with moyamoya disease.

N. Nakasato (✉) and A. Kanno
MEG Laboratory, Kohnan Hospital, 4-20-1 Nagamachi-minami, Taihaku-ku, Sendai 982-8523, Japan

N. Nakasato
Department of Neurosurgery, Kohnan Hospital, 4-20-1 Nagamachi-minami, Taihaku-ku, Sendai 982-8523, Japan
e-mail: nobukazun@mac.com

T. Tominaga
Department of Neurosurgery, Tohoku University Graduate School of Medicine, 1-1 Seiryo-cho, Aoba-ku, Sendai 980-8574, Japan

B.-K. Cho and T. Tominaga (eds.), *Moyamoya Disease Update*,
DOI 10.1007/978-4-431-99703-0_31, © Springer 2010

MEG Localization of Re-Build-Up Phenomenon

EEG often demonstrates slow waves such as delta (below 4 Hz) and theta (4–8 Hz) activity in patients with cerebral infarction [3–7]. Previous MEG studies have indicated that the slow waves are generated from the adjacent cortical areas, rather than from the centre of the infarct lesions [8, 9]. MEG may be more suitable than EEG to detect focal or local ischemic abnormality because the spatial resolution is both theoretically [10] and practically higher [11, 12].

The re-build-up phenomenon in MEG and haemodynamic studies using single-photon emission computed tomography (SPECT) were first reported in 2003 [13]. Re-build-up slow waves were measured in four children using a whole-head MEG system. Equivalent current dipoles of the re-build-up phenomenon were predominantly located in the deep cortical sulci in the area with impaired reactivity to acetazolamide revealed by SPECT [13].

We treated a patient in whom re-build-up discharges were localized near the cortex that could explain the transient ischemic attacks in his right arm and hand (Fig. 1). The re-build-up phenomenon in MEG was exactly congruent with the ischemic symptoms in time and space, so that further studies are needed to evaluate the possible clinical applications of MEG as a presurgical diagnostic indicator of revascularization surgery for moyamoya disease. However, there are ethical concerns whether hyperventilation can be allowed and to what intensity in patients with moyamoya disease. The following experiment was conducted to design a non-invasive method to monitor the length and intensity of hyperventilation during MEG measurement.

Hypoxic State Caused by Post-Hyperventilation Respiratory Depression

EEG, MEG, respiration rate, end-tidal CO_2, oxygen saturation, pH, pO_2, and pCO_2 were measured in eight normal subjects (seven males), aged 18–21 years. Arterial blood samples were obtained sequentially from a catheter in a radial artery. Subjects were instructed to perform maximum voluntary ventilation for 2 and 3 min separated by an interval of more than 2 h.

During the measurements, no subject suffered ischemic symptoms such as motor weakness or sensory disturbance except for mild numbness of the hands and lips. Some subjects showed build-up discharges in EEG and MEG but not re-build-up discharges. Figure 2 shows the time courses of end-tidal CO_2, oxygen saturation, pH, pO_2, and pCO_2.

During hyperventilation, arterial pCO_2 decreased rapidly, which can also be monitored by end-tidal CO_2. Arterial pH and pO_2 rapidly increased, but oxygen saturation remained stable at around 99–100%. Immediately after the termination of hyperventilation, breath frequency spontaneously decreased to as low as 2 or 3 per min. Consequently, arterial pCO_2 and end-tidal pCO_2 gradually increased and recovered to normal levels within 4–6 min after the termination of hyperventilation. The most striking results were the decreases in arterial pO_2 and oxygen saturation. Two to five minutes after the termination of hyperventilation, arterial pO_2 decreased to as low as 60 mm Hg and oxygen saturation to around 93%. Although EEG or MEG detected no abnormal slow waves in the normal subjects, such hypoxia is sufficiently intense to provoke transient ischemic attacks in patients with moyamoya disease. Therefore, the well-known timing of the re-build-up phenomenon corresponded to the hypoxic time in the present study.

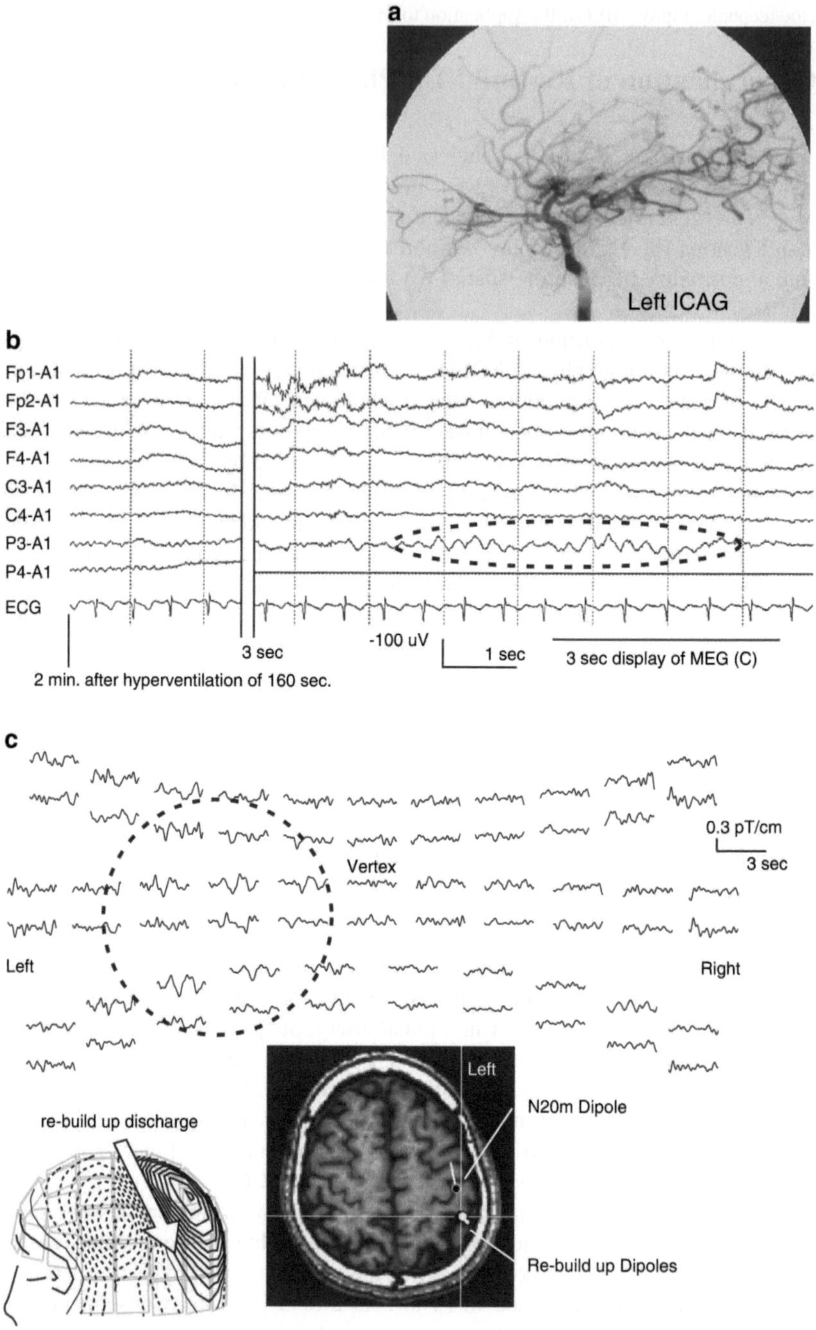

Fig. 1 Re-build-up phenomenon in a 35-year-old male patient who suffered transient right hemiparesis and aphasia 7 days before the study. (**a**) Angiogram revealing moyamoya disease more prominent in the left internal carotid artery. (**b**) Electroencephalogram indicating abnormal slow waves (*broken line*) in the left parietal area 127 s after the end of hyperventilation for 160 s. Immediately afterwards, the patient complained of numbness of his right arm and hand. The symptoms resolved soon after administration of oxygen. (**c**) Simultaneous magnetoencephalogram revealing abnormal slow waves (*broken line*) in the left parietal area. Equivalent current dipoles of the slow waves were localized in the left parietal sulcus near the hand sensory cortex indicated by the N20m dipole of the somatosensory evoked fields for right median nerve stimulus

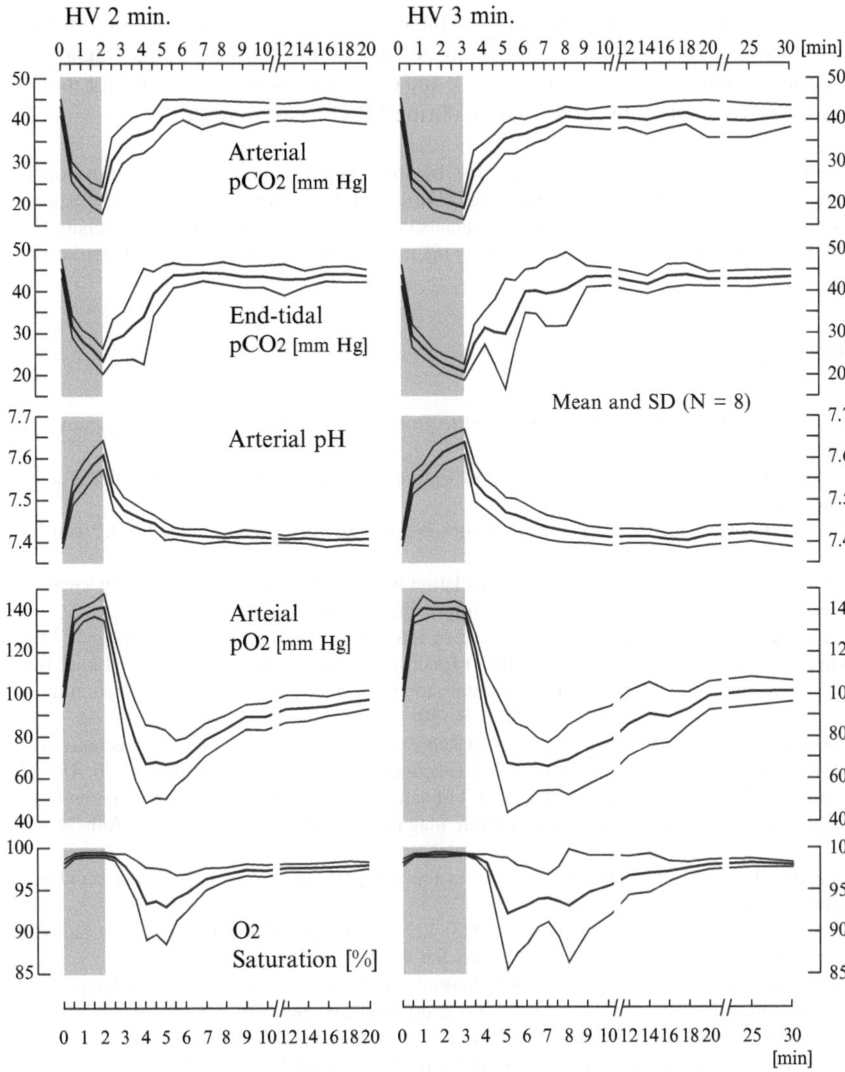

Fig. 2 Hyperventilation (HV)-induced hypoxia in young healthy subjects. Arterial pCO_2, pH, pO_2, and O_2 saturation were monitored via a catheter in a radial artery. After HV for either 2 or 3 min, spontaneous respiratory depression, as low as 2 or 3 times per min, induced marked decrease of arterial pO_2 and O_2 saturation, most severely between 2 and 4 min after the end of HV

MEG as a Possible Diagnostic Indicator of Ischemia in Moyamoya Disease

MEG has higher spatial resolution than EEG, so can be used to monitor and evaluate transient ischemic conditions. Three minutes of hyperventilation is recommended for provocation in routine clinical EEG. However, a shorter hyperventilation time should be used for patients with moyamoya disease, since 2 min of hyperventilation caused hypoxic conditions of similar intensity but shorter duration in comparison to 3 min of hyperventilation in normal subjects. Although arterial gas is difficult to monitor noninvasively and nonmagnetically in a magnetically-shielded room, end-tidal CO_2 and oxygen saturation are useful for monitoring the intensity of voluntary hyperventilation during MEG measurement.

Acknowledgements This work was supported by the Open Competition for the Development of Innovative Technology (No. 12208) from the Ministry of Education, Culture, Sports, Science and Technology, Japan. We thank Drs. Ken-ichi Nagamatsu and Masaki Iwasaki (Tohoku University Graduate School of Medicine) for the technical help during the measurement of EEG, MEG, and arterial gas.

References

1. Aoki Y, Kodama N, Hiraga H, et al (1977) Electroencephalographic findings in moyamoya disease. No To Shinkei 29: 551–559
2. Kodama N, Aoki Y, Hiraga H, et al (1979) Electroencephalographic findings in children with moyamoya disease. Arch Neurol 36: 16–19
3. Gloor P, Ball G, Schaul N (1977) Brain lesions that produce delta waves in the EEG. Neurology 27: 326–333
4. Ingvar DH, Sjölund B, Ardo A (1976) Correlation between dominant EEG frequency, cerebral oxygen uptake and blood flow. Electroencephalogr Clin Neurophysiol 41: 268–276
5. Nagata K (1989) Topographic EEG mapping in cerebrovascular disease. Brain Topogr 2: 119–128
6. Nagata K, Tagawa K, Hiroi S, et al (1989) Electroencephalographic correlates of blood flow and oxygen metabolism provided by positron emission tomography in patients with cerebral infarction. Electroencephalogr Clin Neurophysiol 72: 16–30
7. Steriade M, Gloor P, Llinas RR, et al (1990) Report of IFCN committee on basic mechanisms. Basic mechanisms of cerebral rhythmic activities. Electroencephalogr Clin Neurophysiol 76: 481–508
8. Kamada K, Saguer M, Möller M, et al (1997) Functional and metabolic analysis of cerebral ischemia using magnetoencephalography and proton magnetic resonance spectroscopy. Ann Neurol 42: 554–563
9. Vieth JB (1990) Magnetoencephalography in the study of stroke (cerebrovascular accident). Adv Neurol 54: 261–269
10. Ahonen A, Hamalainen M, Kajora MA (1993) 122-channel SQUID instrument for investigating the magnetic signals from the human brain. Phys Scr 49: 198–205
11. Seki S, Nakasato N, Ohtomo S, et al (2005) Neuromagnetic measurement of unilateral temporo-parietal theta rhythm in patients with internal carotid artery occlusive disease. Neuroimage 25: 502–510
12. Ohtomo S, Nakasato N, Shimizu H, et al (2009) Temporo-parietal theta activity correlates with misery perfusion in arterial occlusive disease. Clin Neurophysiol 120: 1227–1234
13. Qiao F, Kuroda S, Kamada K, et al (2003) Source localization of the re-build up phenomenon in pediatric moyamoya disease-a dipole distribution analysis using MEG and SPECT. Childs Nerv Syst 19: 760–764

Part X
Surgical Technique

Overview

Toshio Matsushima, Masatou Kawashima, and Jun Masuoka

Introduction

The aim of surgical treatment for ischemic type moyamoya disease is to establish an adequate and sufficient collateral circulation for the ischemic brain to prevent cerebral infarction. Many kinds of surgical procedures have been utilized [1–11], and, therefore, we explain those procedures and their advantages and disadvantages. Surgeons who perform surgical treatment for Moyamoya disease have to select a surgical procedure after understanding the advantages and disadvantages of each type.

Development of Surgical Procedures (Direct, Single Indirect, and Combined Bypass Procedures)

Surgical treatment for moyamoya disease started in the 1970s, when the superficial temporal artery to middle cerebral artery anastomosis (STA-MCA anastomosis) was first applied [2, 12]. This direct bypass procedure is a reliable method of collateral formation, but also involves some technical difficulties especially for young pediatric patients [3, 13, 14]. Young pediatric patients often do not have a large enough recipient cerebral artery to perform anastomosis [3]. If the direct anastomosis is not successful, the patient will have a postoperative infarction.

As a unique characteristic of moyamoya disease, it was revealed that spontaneous leptomeningeal anastomoses develop after placing donor materials supplied by the external carotid arteries (ECAs) directly onto the surface of the ischemic brain [15–17]. Therefore, various kinds of indirect nonanastomotic bypass procedures have been developed (Table 1). However, single indirect bypass procedures have a few drawbacks. Some of the patients who received the procedures failed to produce sufficient collateral vessels [14, 18, 19]. Therefore, combined indirect surgical procedures have been developed [5–8, 20–22]. When the collateral circulation is sufficiently developed, indirect bypass procedures tare also useful [23–26]. Furthermore, they

T. Matsushima (✉), M. Kawashima, and J. Masuoka
Department of Neurosurgery, Faculty of Medicine, Saga University,
5-1-1, Nabeshima, Saga 849-8501, Japan
e-mail: matsuto@cc.saga-u.ac.jp

B.-K. Cho and T. Tominaga (eds.), *Moyamoya Disease Update*,
DOI 10.1007/978-4-431-99703-0_32, © Springer 2010

Table 1 Various kinds of bypass procedures for moyamoya disease

A	Direct anastomosis	
		STA-MCA anastomosis
B	Indirect anastomosis	
	B-1	Single indirect anastomosis
		EMS (encephalo-myo synangiosis)
		EDAS (encephalo-duro-arterio synangiosis)
		EMAS (encephalo-myo-arterio synangiosis)
		EAS (encephalo-arterio synangiosis)
		Transplantation of the omentum
	B-2	Multiple combined indirect anastomoses
		Fronto-temporo-parietal combined indirect bypass procedure (Frontal EMAS, fronto-temporo EDAS and temporoparieto EMS)
		EDAMS (encephalo-duro-arterio-myo-synangiosis)
		Dual EDASs using the anterior and posterior branches of the STA
		Multiple (three) EDASs
	B-3	Additional indirect anastomosis
		Frontal EMAS
		Ribbon EDAMS
		Use of a split dura
C	Direct and indirect combined anastomoses	
		STA-MCA anastomosis with EMS
		STA-MCA anastomosis and EDAMS

are safe and easy even for young pediatric patients, and can be done in any areas including the frontal or parieto-occipital region [26, 27].

Direct Bypass Procedure: STA-MCA Anastomosis with Encephalo-Myo-Synangiosis (Fig. 1)

The STA-MCA anastomosis, double anastomoses if possible, is performed as a direct anastomosis in the regions around the Sylvian fissure. We usually utilize a flap method and then obtain a wide craniotomy in the parietotemporal region. The angular artery is usually the biggest cortical branch. Young pediatric patients often do not have a large enough recipient cerebral artery for anastomosis. The diameter of the recipient artery is sometimes smaller than 1 mm. In addition, the arteries of moyamoya patients are also fragile. We perform the anastomosis using the interrupted suture method with 10-0 or 11-0 mono-filament nylon sutures. Just before starting the anastomosis, we always use piokutanin to clearly visualize the cutting edges of the donor and recipient arteries. After the anastomosis, the exposed cortices are covered with the temporal muscle as encephalo-myo-synangiosis (EMS) [13].

Various Kinds of Indirect Bypass Procedure

Karasawa first reported EMS as an indirect nonbypass procedure [3]. He performed it in some cases in which he could not find a MCA cortical branch that was large enough to be the recipient artery for the direct anastomosis. After his report, several indirect procedures were developed, including encephalo-duro-arterio-synangiosis (EDAS) [9, 10], encephalo-arterio-synangiosis (EAS) [28], encephalo-myo-arterio-synangiosis (EMAS) [27], omental transplantation [4], and utilization of the split dura mater [29]. EDAS was very popular in the 1990s. The extent of collateral formation even after the same bypass procedure varies considerably from patient to patient and/or from area to area. Thus, it seems wiser to design surgical fields after mapping the misery perfusive area when possible [18, 24, 30, 31]. Most indirect bypass procedures are effective, but some single indirect procedures sometimes fail to produce collateral formation. Our experience revealed that about 20% of sites treated surgically by EDAS or EMS failed to produce sufficient collateral vessels [18, 19]. In some cases, a reoperation was required [14, 30, 32, 33]. To overcome these problems, we have gradually changed our indirect method to the combined indirect procedure, and now always select the fronto-temporo-parietal combined indirect bypass procedure as an indirect procedure [6–8, 25] (Fig. 2). In this procedure, three indirect bypass procedures are used in combination, i.e., EMAS in the frontal region and EDAS and EMS in the temporo-parietal region, while using the anterior and the posterior branches of the STA and the frontal and the temporal muscles. With this combined procedure, a collateral formation through at least one of the three indirect bypasses is achieved and the postoperative collaterals cover a wider area [8, 34] (Fig. 3).

Management of Cases of Treatment Failure with Indirect Bypass Procedures

We first give anticoagulants to patients with persistent ischemic symptoms after surgery. During the next few months, we examine changes of symptoms and collateral formation on the MRA and conditions of the cerebral circulation and metabolism on the SPECT or PET [32]. We have to consider a reoperation for patients with the following conditions: (1) symptoms do not improve or become worse postoperatively, (2) postoperative collaterals are only found slightly or are not sufficient on cerebral angiograms, and (3) studies on the cerebral circulation and metabolism still show misery perfusion.

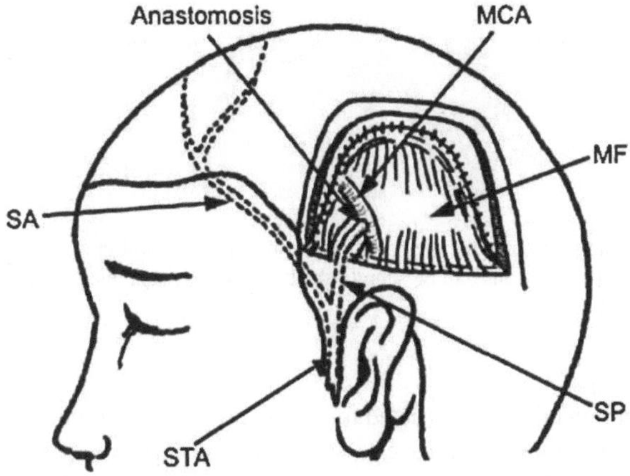

Fig. 1 The operative procedure of the STA-MCA anastomosis with encephalo-myo-synangiosis as a direct anastomosis. *MF* Temporal muscle flap, *SA* anterior branch of the STA, *SP* posterior branch of the STA

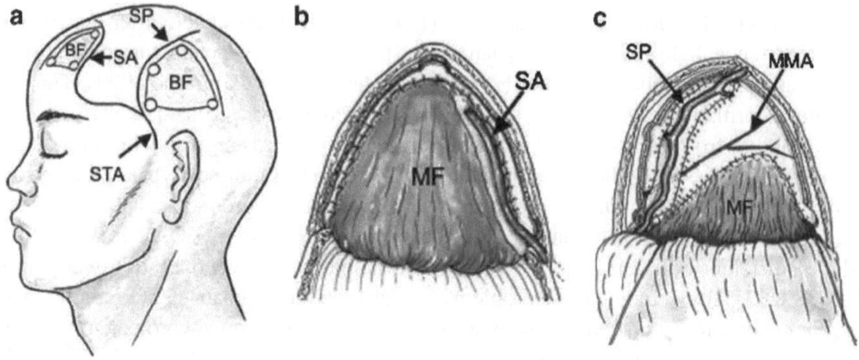

Fig. 2 The operative procedures of the fronto-temporo-parietal combined procedure as a indirect combined anastomosis. (**a**) Skin incisions and bony openings. (**b**) Frontal encephalo-myo-arterio synangiosis (EMAS). (**c**) Encephalo-duro-arterio synangiosis (EDAS) and encephalo-myo synangiosis (EMS) in the temporo-parietal region. *BF* Bone flap

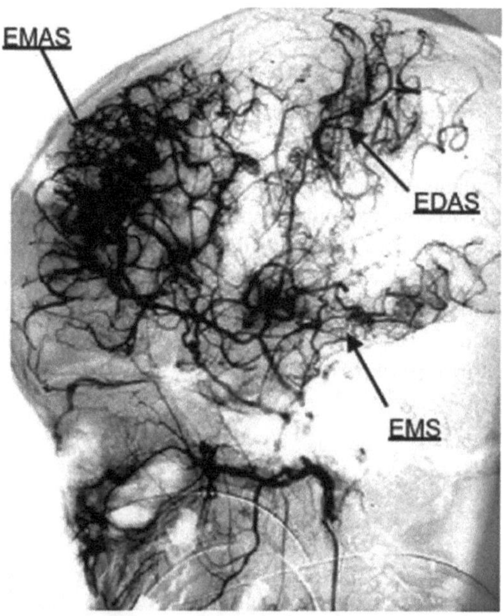

Fig. 3 Postoperative angiogram after the fronto-temporo-parietal combined indirect bypass procedure, Lateral view. Collateral formations can be seen in the three bypass regions: frontal EMAS and temporo-parietal EDAS and EMS

The reoperation procedure is restricted to bypass procedures previously utilized. The area for the reoperation is limited. We have to select an appropriate procedure for each patient from among the following procedures: STA-MCA anastomosis, additional EMS or EDAS, and omentum transplantation etc. [4, 14, 22, 30, 32]. When the posterior branch of the STA can be used, the STA-MCA anastomosis is the first choice for the MCA territory.

In cases completely refractory to EDAS, the posterior branch of the STA used for EDAS can be stripped and used as a donor artery for the anastomosis [14, 32, 33]. In cases in which the branches of the STA cannot be used, EMS or transplantation of the omentum should be selected [3, 4]. To improve symptoms, the surgical field for the second bypass surgery is also very important. Collaterals should be formed in an appropriate distribution of the anterior cerebral artery (ACA), MCA, and/or posterior cerebral artery (PCA) territories responsible for the patient's symptoms [5, 21, 26, 27].

Selection of the Initial Surgical Procedure

Selection of the initial procedure depends on the size of the recipient artery, which cannot be known preoperatively. They are anticipated from the patient's age and the Suzuki's stage of the patient. Therefore, we recommend the direct bypass procedure for an adult patient and the indirect procedure for a young pediatric patient. When treating pediatric patients under the age of 5 years, a combination of indirect bypass procedures, such as the one explained above, is the first choice. In cases in which surgical procedure cannot be decided before surgery, we decide the direct or indirect procedure during surgery after exposing the cortical branches of the MCA. In such a case, we have to expose the posterior branch of the STA using the cutting method and the distal end of the branch should not be cut before making the decision. When we are able to find a recipient artery large enough for the direct anastomosis, we select it.

Conclusion

Bypass procedures for Moyamoya disease can be divided basically into 2 groups: direct and indirect non-anastomotic bypass procedures. The former is represented by the STA-MCA anastomosis, which is a reliable method but its surgical techniques are difficult. On the other hand, indirect bypass procedures are easy and safe, but have some drawbacks. Generally, the direct bypass procedure is recommended for adult patients and the multiple combined indirect procedures are recommended for young pediatric patients.

References

1. Houkin K, Kamiyama H, Takahashi A et al (1997) Combined revascularization surgery for childhood moyamoya disease. STA-MCA and encephalo-duro-arterio-myo-synangiosis. Childs Nerv Syst 13:24–29
2. Karasawa J, Kikuchi H, Furuse S et al (1978) Treatment of moyamoya disease with STA-MCA anastomosis. J Neurosurg 49:679–688
3. Karasawa J, Kikuchi H, Furuse S et al (1977) A surgical treatment of moyamoya disease – encephalo-myo-synangiosis. Neurol Med Chir 17:29–37
4. Karasawa J, Kikuchi H, Kawamura J et al (1980) Intracranial transplantation of the omentum for cerebrovascular moyamoya disease; a two-year follow-up study. Surg Neurol 14:444–449
5. Kinugasa K, Mandai S, Kamata I et al (1993) Surgical treatment of moyamoya disease: operative technique for encephalo-duro-arterio-myo-synangiosis: its follow-up, clinical results, and angiograms. Neurosurgery 32:527–531

6. Matsushima T, Inoue T, Ikezaki K et al (1995) Fronto-temporo-parietal combined indirect bypass for children with moyamoya disease, Part 1: surgical procedure and techniques (Japanese). Nerv Syst Child 20:317–321
7. Matsushima T, Inoue TK, Suzuki SO et al (1997) Surgical techniques and the results of a fronto-temporo-parietal combined indirect bypass procedure for children with moyamoya disease – a comparison with the results of encephalo-duro-arterio-synangiosis alone. Clin Neurol Neurosurg 99:S123–S127
8. Matsushima T, Inoue TK, Ikezaki K et al (1998) Multiple combined indirect procedure for the surgical treatment of children with moyamoya disease. A comparison with single indirect anastomosis with direct anastomosis. Neurosurg Focus 5(5), Article 4:1–5
9. Matsushima Y, Fukai N, Tanaka K et al (1981) A new surgical treatment of moyamoya disease in children: a preliminary report. Surg Neurol 15:313–320
10. Matsushima Y, Inaba Y (1984) Moyamoya disease in children and its surgical treatment: introduction of a new surgical procedure and its follow-up angiograms. Childs Brain 11:155–170
11. Takeuchi S, Tsuchida T, Kobayashi K et al (1983) Treatment of moyamoya disease by temporal muscle graft "encephalo-myo-synangiosis". Childs Brain 10:1–15
12. Krayenbuhl HA (1975) The moyamoya syndrome and neurosurgeon. Surg Neurol 4:353–360
13. Matsushima T, Inoue T, Suzuki SO et al (1992) Surgical treatment of moyamoya disease in pediatric patients – comparison between the results of indirect and direct revascularization procedures. Neurosurgery 31:401–405
14. Miyamoto S, Kikuchi H, Karasawa J et al (1988) Pitfalls in the surgical treatment of moyamoya disease: operative techniques for refractory cases. J Neurosurg 68:537–543
15. Spetzler RF, Roski RA, Kopaniky DR (1980) Alternative superficial temporal artery to middle cerebral artery revascularization procedure. Neurosurgery 7:484–485
16. Suzuki J, Takaku A (1969) Cerebrovascular "moyamoya" disease. Disease showing abnormal net-like vessels in base of brain. Arch Neurol 12:288–299
17. Tsubokawa T, Kikuchi M, Asano S et al (1964) Surgical treatment for intracranial thrombosis: case report of "durapexia". Neurol Med Chir 6:48–49
18. Matsushima T, Fukui M, Kitamura K et al (1990) Encephalo-duro-arterio-synangiosis in children with moyamoya disease. Acta Neurochir 104:96–102
19. Matsushima T, Fujiwara S, Nagata S et al (1989) Surgical treatment for pediatric patients with moyamoya disease by indirect revascularization procedures (EDAS, EMS, EMAS). Acta Neurochir 98:135–140
20. Matsushima Y, Aoyagi M, Suzuki R et al (1993) Dual anastomosis for pediatric moyamoya patients using the anterior and the posterior branches of the superficial temporal artery. Nerv Syst Child 18:27–32
21. Sato H (1991) Combined revascularization for moyamoya disease in children. Child Nerv Syst 7:281–282
22. Tenjin H, Ueda S (1997) Multiple EDAS (encephalo-duro-arterio-synangiosis); additional EDAS using the frontal branch of the superficial temporal artery (STA) and the occipital artery for pediatric moyamoya patients in whom EDAS using the parietal branch of STA was insufficient. Childs Nerv Syst 13:220–224
23. Houkin K, Kuroda S, Ishikawa T et al (2000) Neovascularization (angiogenesis) after revascularization in moyamoya disease. Which technique is most useful for moyamoya disease? Acta Neurochir 142:269–276
24. Kuwabara Y, Ichiya Y, Otsuka M et al (1990) Cerebral hemodynamic change in the child and the adult with moyamoya disease. Stroke 21:272–277
25. Matsushima T, Inoue T, Katsuta T et al (1998) An indirect revascularization method in the surgical treatment of moyamoya disease – various kinds of indirect procedures and a multiple combined indirect procedure. Neurol Med Chir 38(Suppl):297–302
26. Takahashi A, Kamiyama H, Houkin K et al (1995) Surgical treatment of childhood moyamoya disease-comparison of reconstructive surgery centered on the frontal region and the parietal region. Neurol Med Chir 35:231–237
27. Inoue T, Matsushima T, Nagata S et al (1992) Frontal encephalo-myo-arterio-synangiosis (EMAS) (Japanese). Surg Cereb Stroke 20:297–300
28. Nakagawa Y, Gotoh S, Shimoyama M et al (1983) Reconstructive operation for moyamoya disease. Neurol Med Chir (Tokyo) 23:464–470

29. Kashiwagi S, Kato S, Yasuhara S et al (1996) Use of a split dura for revascularization of ischemic hemispheres in moyamoya disease. J Neurosurg 85:380–383
30. Matsushima T, Fujiwara S, Nagata S et al (1990) Reoperation for moyamoya disease refractory to encephalo-duro-arterio-synangiosis. Acta Neurochir 107:129–132
31. Matsushima T, Inoue T, Kuwabara Y et al (2006) Moyamoya disease in children. In: Alexander MJ, Spetzler RF (eds) Pediatric neurovascular disease. Thieme, New York
32. Matsushima T, Natori Y, Kuwabara Y et al (2001) Management strategies for moyamoya disease. Part3: Postoperative evaluation, follow-up imaging, management of treatment failure, indication for reoperation. In: Ikezaki K, Loftus CM (eds) Moyamoya disease. American Association of Neurological Surgeons, Rolling Meadows
33. Touho H, Karasawa J, Ohnishi H et al (1993) Surgical reconstruction of failed indirect anastomosis in childhood moyamoya disease. Neurosurgery 32:935–940
34. Suzuki SO, Matsushima T, Inoue T et al (1995) Fronto-temporo-parietal combined indirect bypass procedures for children with moyamoya disease, Part 2: Surgical results (Japanese). Nerv Syst Child 20:322–326

Moyamoya Disease and Anesthesia in Children

Hee-Soo Kim

Introduction

Moyamoya disease (MMD) is an uncommon pediatric neurological disease characterized by bilateral spontaneous stenosis or obstruction of the intracranial arteries at the base of the brain and extensive collateral vessels ("moyamoya vessels"). These moyamoya vessels are dilated medullary arteries which provide collateral circulation to the brain.

The etiology of MMD is unknown. There is evidence of heredity such as HLA haplotypes and point mutation [1] but also evidence of environmental factors [2]. MMD is commonest in Japan, Republic of Korea, and China [3]. The distribution of the age of onset has two peaks: a high peak in the first decade of the life and a lower peak in the third to fourth decades [2]. The clinical presentation of MMD in children includes repeated transient ischemic attacks, [4, 5] cerebral infarction [6], and headaches [7]. Children with MMD need surgical intervention.

Diagnosis, Classifications, Treatments and Outcomes

Diagnosis and Classifications

Diagnostic guidelines differ between institutes. The Research Committee on MMD of the Japanese Ministry of Health and Welfare has identified four criteria for the diagnosis of MMD: (1) stenosis or occlusion of the terminal portion of the internal carotid artery; (2) a coexisting abnormal vascular network in the base of the brain or basal ganglia; (3) bilateral vascular involvement; and (4) no other identifiable cause for symptoms [8].

H.-S. Kim (✉)
Division of Pediatric Anesthesiology and Pain Medicine, Seoul National University Children's Hospital, Seoul National University College of Medicine, 101 Daehangno Jongnogu, Seoul 110-744, Republic of Korea
e-mail: dami0605@snu.ac.kr

B.-K. Cho and T. Tominaga (eds.), *Moyamoya Disease Update*,
DOI 10.1007/978-4-431-99703-0_33, © Springer 2010

MMD is also staged by the angiographic findings of stenosis, occlusion, and revascularization, divided into six distinct stages [9]: Stage 1, narrowing of the internal carotid arteries; Stage 2, initial appearance of moyamoya vessels; Stage 3, further definition of collateral vessels; Stage 4, minimization of collateral vessels; Stage 5, reduction of collateral vessels; and Stage 6, disappearance of collateral vessels.

Treatment

Medical treatment includes antiplatelet drugs, anticoagulants, and cerebral vasodilators. Surgery, standard for many years, is divided into direct, indirect bypass, or combined methods. Direct techniques require a specific set of preoperative conditions and are preferred by some surgeons. However, they are little used in children, in whom indirect techniques are more successful. Outcomes vary greatly; in some studies, correlation between postoperative radiological findings and relief of symptoms is poor [6, 10–17].

Our institute has recently started to use indirect revascularization techniques such as encephalo-duro-arterio-synangiosis (EDAS). Most children underwent bilateral EDAS with a superficial temporal artery, encephalo-myo-synangiosis (EMS) and encephalo-galeo-synangiosis (EGS) in two stages.

Outcomes

Overall clinical outcomes were divided into four categories [18]: (1) excellent, where preoperative symptoms (such as TIAs or seizures) had totally disappeared without any neurological deficits; (2) good, with relief of symptoms but remaining neurological deficit; (3) fair, where symptoms persisted, albeit less frequently; and (4) poor, where the symptoms remained either unchanged or increased. From a clinical viewpoint, excellent or good clinical outcomes were designated as favorable.

Preoperative Management

Preoperative Assessment

MMD has unusual characteristics and clinical findings. The most important point is to avoid aggravation of symptoms and leave the patients physically and psychologically stable. Venipuncture may cause crying, which reduces cerebral bloodflow. We use eutectic mixture of lidocaine and prilocaine (EMLA) cream before venipuncture, although this does not prevent crying from fear rather than pain.

Diazepam or midazolam have little effect on cerebral blood flow. Midazolam can be given orally, but it may be more acceptable given nasally, even though it causes an unpleasant burning sensation [19]. The antegrade amnesia is thought to be beneficial. The dose of oral midazolam is 0.5–0.75 mg/kg (maximum 20 mg); nasally, it is 0.2–0.5 mg/kg; and intravenously, it is 0.05–0.1 mg/kg (under 5 years old) or 0.025–0.5 mg/kg (over 5 years old).

Intravenous flumazenil (10 μg/kg, maximum 1 mg) can be used to reverse overdosage. Oral ketamine (3–8 mg/kg) reduces emergence agitation without affecting recovery time [20]. Thiopental and propofol reduce cerebral blood flow. Blood pressure, heart rate, and ventilation should be monitored during injection of these drugs.

For preoperative assessment, anesthesiologists should pay attention to history and image findings. If ischemic attacks are frequent, the child should be sedated to avoid crying before anesthesia.

Previous reports have inferred that preoperative TIAs are a significant risk factor for perioperative ischemic complications [21]. Adequate hydration is therefore important. Most MMD surgery is elective and normal fasting routines should be observed. Before and during fasting period, the patients should be fully hydrated. We give synthetic colloids during the fasting period, changing to normal saline once anesthesia is commenced.

Intraoperative Management

Premedication

Calming and stabilizing the patients before anesthesia or during induction is important; we premedicate with oral or intravenous midazolam [22]. Midazolam is contraindicated in impulsive patients but beneficial in anxious children [23]. Intravenous midazolam 0.1 mg/kg allows the child to be easily separated from its parents.

Monitoring and Anesthesia

On arriving at the operating room, a calm atmosphere is important during establishment of baseline values. Anesthesia is induced with thiopental (5–6 mg/kg) or propofol (2–3 mg/kg) and fentanyl (2 μg/kg). Propofol should be preceded by lidocaine or remifentanil, to avoid crying and aggravation of the ischemic symptoms. After loss of consciousness, invasive arterial blood pressure monitoring is established; this is important for maintaining stable cerebral blood flow. Blood loss should be monitored closely and blood loss replaced appropriately. Hypercapnia has been recommended during MMD surgery [24], although it may lead to hyperemia and intracerebral steal. To stabilize regional cerebral blood flow, normocapnia should be observed.

Nondepolarizing muscle relaxants (rocuronium or vecuronium) are given for tracheal intubation; they have few direct effects on the cerebral circulation. Histamine-releasing muscle relaxants should be avoided because of the risk of changes in intracranial cerebral pressure and blood pressure.

MMD surgery can be prolonged, and airway access can be difficult. The endotracheal tube should be secured tightly. Patients normally are positioned supine with a slightly rotated head and neck; the position of the endotracheal tube should be checked again before surgical draping commences, particularly in small children.

We use the esophageal stethoscope for auscultation of heart and breathing sounds. Capnography and temperature monitoring are essential, but central venous catheterization and pressure monitoring are controversial in MMD, especially in children. There is little blood loss in simple EDAS and a large bore peripheral cannula is sufficient; however, blood loss can be greater. Central venous catheterization is not without risks in infants and children, and may be avoidable if the surgery is standardized. The subclavian route is preferred.

Urine output should be monitored; it is a significant index of the state of hydration, and good output is the only intraoperative factor associated with a low incidence of complications [25]. In our study, urinary output was maintained at all times, but there were some complications after surgery. Maintaining normovolemia may be insufficient, and hypervolemia may be more important; colloids are helpful. Hemoglobin should be maintained above 10 g/dl [26], or hematocrit above 30% [25]. Appropriate padding of bony prominences and pressure areas is important in very long procedures, although padding itself is not enough to prevent pressure sores.

Hypothermia is normally regarded as neuro-protective in neurosurgery, but in MMD, it may induce vasospasm and thus ischemia; we prefer normothermia. We maintain anesthesia with isoflurane, sevoflurane, or propofol. Inhalational anesthetics increase the cerebral blood flow to cerebral metabolic rate ratio [26], but decrease regional cortical blood flow in MMD patients, possibly by provoking intracerebral steal. Total intravenous anesthesia lacks these effects [27]. Propofol may preserve regional cerebral blood flow in the frontal lobes in MMD surgery [28]. In practice, there are no differences in early complications between inhalational and intravenous anesthetics in MMD [29]. Before skin incision, local anesthetic infiltration may help to stabilize hemodynamic changes [30] and help with postoperative pain control [31].

Postoperative Management

After surgery, most MMD patients are evaluated by CT. Midazolam (0.1–0.5 mg/kg) is given for sedation during transport whether the patients are intubated or not. However, recovery in the operating room or ICU is also possible. Postoperative pain should be treated to prevent ischemic attacks or cerebral infarction. Peripheral nerve blocks can be performed just after surgery. Preoperative skull block in pediatric MMD patients is not effective [32]; usually, supraorbital nerve, supratrochlea nerve, auriculotemporal nerve, and greater or lesser occipital nerves are targeted (Fig. 1). It is not always clear whether nerve block is successful or not. It can be performed with 1–1.5 ml of 0.25% ropivacine with epinephrine (1:2,00,000), with added triamcinolone to prolong the duration of analgesia. Patient-controlled analgesia (PCA) with fentanyl (1 μg/kg, lockout time of 7 min) and a background infusion of midazolam (2 μg/kg/min) is effective [33]. There is as yet no convincing evidence for preemptive analgesia. Meperidine [34] and nerve blocks [32] have also been used for pain relief; however, fear is also a problem, and sedation should always be adequate.

Conclusions

MMD commonly presents in Asian children. For successful recovery from anesthesia and avoidance of postoperative ischemic complication, the pediatric anesthesiologist should be aware of the importance of hydration, adequate correction of anemia, and maintenance of normocapnia and normothermia.

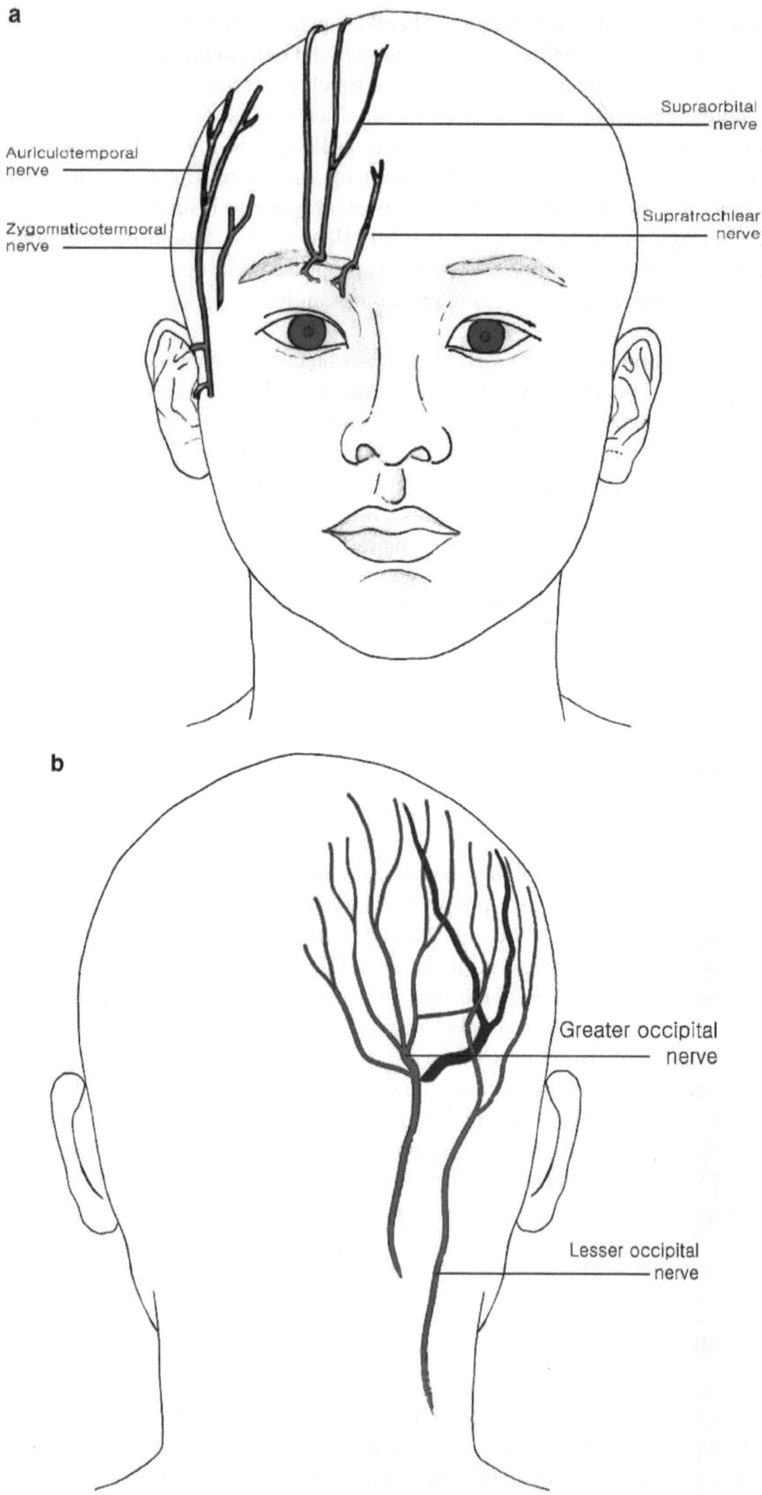

Fig. 1 Peripheral nerves which are commonly blocked in MMD patients

References

1. Pavlakis SG, Verlander PC, Gould RJ et al (1995) Fanconi anemia and moyamoya: evidence for an association. Neurology 45: 998–1000
2. Kato R, Terui K, Yokota K et al (2006) Anesthetic management for cesarean section in moyamoya disease: a report of five consecutive cases and a mini-review. Int J Obstet Anesth 15: 152–158
3. Goto Y, Yonekawa Y (1992) Worldwide distribution of moyamoya disease. Neurol Med Chir (Tokyo) 32: 883–886
4. Ikezaki K, Han DH, Kawano T et al (1997) A clinical comparison of definite moyamoya disease between South Korea and Japan. Stroke 28: 2513–2517
5. Kelly ME, Bell-Stephens TE, Marks MP et al (2006) Progression of unilateral moyamoya disease: a clinical series. Cerebrovasc Dis 22: 109–115
6. Kim SK, Wang KC, Kim IO et al (2002) Combined encephaloduroarteriosynangiosis and bifrontal encephalogaleo(periosteal)synangiosis in pediatric moyamoya disease. Neurosurgery 50: 88–96
7. Seol HJ, Wang KC, Kim SK et al (2005) Headache in pediatric moyamoya disease: review of 204 consecutive cases. J Neurosurg 103: 439–442
8. Han DH, Kwon OK, Byun BJ et al (2000) A co-operative study: clinical characteristics of 334 Korean patients with moyamoya disease treated at neurosurgical institutes (1976–1994). The Korean society for cerebrovascular disease. Acta Neurochir (Wien) 142: 1263–1273; discussion 1273–1274
9. Suzuki J, Takaku A (1969) Cerebrovascular "moyamoya" disease. Disease showing abnormal net-like vessels in base of brain. Arch Neurol 20: 288–299
10. Golby AJ, Marks MP, Thompson RC et al (1999) Direct and combined revascularization in pediatric moyamoya disease. Neurosurgery 45: 50–58; discussion 58–60
11. Mizoi K, Kayama T, Yoshimoto T et al (1996) Indirect revascularization for moyamoya disease: is there a beneficial effect for adult patients? Surg Neurol 45: 541–548; discussion 548–549
12. Matsushima T, Inoue T, Suzuki SO et al (1992) Surgical treatment of moyamoya disease in pediatric patients – comparison between the results of indirect and direct revascularization procedures. Neurosurgery 31: 401–405
13. Sakamoto S, Kiura Y, Yamasaki F et al (2008) Expression of vascular endothelial growth factor in dura mater of patients with moyamoya disease. Neurosurg Rev 31: 77–81; discussion 81
14. Kim DS, Kang SG, Yoo DS et al (2007) Surgical results in pediatric moyamoya disease: angiographic revascularization and the clinical results. Clin Neurol Neurosurg 109: 125–131
15. Houkin K, Kuroda S, Ishikawa T et al (2000) Neovascularization (angiogenesis) after revascularization in moyamoya disease. Which technique is most useful for moyamoya disease? Acta Neurochir (Wien) 142: 269–276
16. Scott RM, Smith JL, Robertson RL et al (2004) Long-term outcome in children with moyamoya syndrome after cranial revascularization by pial synangiosis. J Neurosurg 100: 142–149
17. Isono M, Ishii K, Kamida T et al (2002) Long-term outcomes of pediatric moyamoya disease treated by encephalo-duro-arterio-synangiosis. Pediatr Neurosurg 36: 14–21
18. Matsushima T, Fujiwara S, Nagata S et al (1989) Surgical treatment for paediatric patients with moyamoya disease by indirect revascularization procedures (EDAS, EMS, EMAS). Acta Neurochir (Wien) 98: 135–140
19. Yildirim SV, Guc BU, Bozdogan N et al (2006) Oral versus intranasal midazolam premedication for infants during echocardiographic study. Adv Ther 23: 719–724
20. Kararmaz A, Kaya S, Turhanoglu S et al (2004) Oral ketamine premedication can prevent emergence agitation in children after desflurane anaesthesia. Paediatr Anaesth 14: 477–482
21. Iwama T, Hashimoto N, Yonekawa Y (1996) The relevance of hemodynamic factors to perioperative ischemic complications in childhood moyamoya disease. Neurosurgery 38: 1120–1125; discussion 1125-1126
22. Kain ZN, Caldwell-Andrews AA, Krivutza DM et al (2004) Trends in the practice of parental presence during induction of anesthesia and the use of preoperative sedative premedication in the United States, 1995–2002: results of a follow-up national survey. Anesth Analg 98: 1252–1259; table of contents
23. Finley GA, Stewart SH, Buffett-Jerrott S et al (2006) High levels of impulsivity may contraindicate midazolam premedication in children. Can J Anaesth 53: 73–78

24. Yamagishi N, Hashizume K, Matsuzawa N et al (1991) Anesthetic management of revascularization for moyamoya disease. Masui 40: 1132–1137
25. Sato K, Shirane R, Yoshimoto T (1997) Perioperative factors related to the development of ischemic complications in patients with moyamoya disease. Childs Nerv Syst 13: 68–72
26. Kansha M, Irita K, Takahashi S (1997) Anesthetic management of children with moyamoya disease. Clin Neurol Neurosurg 99 (Suppl 2): S110–113
27. Sato K, Shirane R, Kato M et al (1999) Effect of inhalational anesthesia on cerebral circulation in moyamoya disease. J Neurosurg Anesthesiol 11: 25–30
28. Kikuta K, Takagi Y, Nozaki K et al (2007) Effects of intravenous anesthesia with propofol on regional cortical blood flow and intracranial pressure in surgery for moyamoya disease. Surg Neurol 68: 421–424
29. Adachi K, Yamamoto Y, Kameyama E et al (2005) Early postoperative complications in patients with moyamoya disease – a comparison of inhaled anesthesia with total intravenous anesthesia (TIVA). Masui 54: 653–657
30. Pakulski C, Nowicki R, Badowicz B et al (2001) Effect of scalp infiltration with lidocaine on the circulatory response to craniotomy. Med Sci Monit 7: 725–728
31. Saringcarinkul A, Boonsri S (2008) Effect of scalp infiltration on postoperative pain relief in elective supratentorial craniotomy with 0.5% bupivacaine with adrenaline 1:400,000. J Med Assoc Thai 91: 1518–1523
32. Ahn HJ, Kim JA, Lee JJ et al (2008) Effect of preoperative skull block on pediatric moyamoya disease. J Neurosurg Pediatr 2: 37–41
33. Chiaretti A, Genovese O, Antonelli A et al (2008) Patient-controlled analgesia with fentanil and midazolam in children with postoperative neurosurgical pain. Childs Nerv Syst 24: 119–124
34. Nomura S, Kashiwagi S, Uetsuka S et al (2001) Perioperative management protocols for children with moyamoya disease. Childs Nerv Syst 17: 270–274

ACA Territory Reinforcement

Chae-Yong Kim and Byong Cheol Kim

Introduction

Moyamoya disease (MMD) usually involves the middle cerebral artery (MCA) and the anterior cerebral artery (ACA) territories [1]. The areas of frontal lobe supplied by ACA are cardinal for lower extremity motor function, sphincter functions, and especially neurocognitive development in children. It is well known that the cerebral cortex supplied by the ACA has many important roles in neuropsychological and intellectual developments in addition to lower extremity motor function and sphincter function [2]. Consequently, ischemic brain insults in the ACA territory may lead to poor intellectual outcomes and low quality of life (QoL) status as well as motor weakness or sphincter dysfunction [2–4]. Nevertheless, many cerebral blood flow studies [4, 5] using positron emission tomography (PET) or single-photon emission computed tomography (SPECT) with acetozolamide have revealed that cerebral blood flow and metabolism in the ACA territory were significantly decreased, and were not adequately compensated by collateral flow from the external carotid arteries (ECAs), MCA, or posterior cerebral artery (PCA). The majority of previous studies have focused on the augmentation of blood flow in the MCA territory [6]. The reinforcement of the ACA territory might to be kept in mind when making the treatment plan for pediatric MMD patients.

Clinical Presentations and Importance of ACA Territory

The Ministry of Health and Welfare of Japan has defined four types of MMD with the following presentation percentages: ischemic 63.4%, hemorrhagic 21.6%, epileptic 7.6%, and others 7.5% [1]. The ischemic type of MMD predominates in childhood. Transient ischemic infarcts (TIAs)

C.-Y. Kim (✉) and B.C. Kim
Department of Neurosurgery, Seoul National University Bundang Hospital, 166 Gumi-ro, Bundang-gu, Seongnam-si, Gyeonggi-do, 463-707, Republic of Korea

Department of Neurosurgery, Seoul National University College of Medicine, Seoul, Republic of Korea
e-mail: chaeyong@snu.ac.kr

B.-K. Cho and T. Tominaga (eds.), *Moyamoya Disease Update*,
DOI 10.1007/978-4-431-99703-0_34, © Springer 2010

and infarcts result in motor weakness, and in disturbances of consciousness, speech, and sensation. Those Ischemic symptoms may present repetitively and can result in motor aphasia, cortical blindness, or even vegetative state. Cerebral ischemia in the territory of the ACA can lead to lower extremity motor weakness, and to intellectual and neuropsychological dysfunctions. Karasawa et al. [7] reported that lower extremity weakness was the second most common ischemic symptom in MMD; it was about 20% of the initial presentation. About half (48%) of MMD patients have symptoms related to ischemia in the ACA territory [6]. The course of the disease often leads to mental retardation and low intelligence quotient (IQ) with long-term follow-up, and it results in a lower level of the QoL, especially in children [1, 8]. About 10% of patients had mental retardation [7]. In rare cases, adult patients can develop cognitive dysfunction such as short-term memory disturbance, irritability, or agitation, which has been occasionally misdiagnosed as psychiatric disorders, such as schizophrenia, depression, or personality disorders [8]. Cognitive function or IQ tests may not be available in some children because they are so young and the symptoms regarding cognitive function may be indistinct; however, cognitive dysfunction would mean more undesirable conditions for the patients in the future.

Therefore, augmentation of the ACA blood flow should be taken into consideration in the ACA territory as well as the MCA in treatment of MMD patients even those who have no definite symptoms of the ACA territory.

Operations and Outcomes

Surgical treatment of MMD can be divided into three types; direct, indirect, and combined/other methods [1]. There have been a few operative techniques aimed at increasing the blood flow to the ACA territory: the transplantation of omentum [9, 10], direct anastomosis of the ACA to the STA using a vein graft or not [11, 12], multiple burr-holes, and encephalo-duro-arterio-synangiosis (EDAS) using the frontal branch of the STA, have all been suggested.

Multiple burr-hole operations for adult MMD have been reported by Kwaguchi et al. [13]; they have used one and four burr-holes in each hemisphere. The operating procedures were the same as those for burr-hole operations for external ventricular drainage. They had shown relatively good results. The multiple burr-hole technique was performed in ten patients. They reported sufficient neovascularization at 41 of the total 43 burr-holes. In the frontal lobe, improvement of reactivity to acetazolamide on brain SPECT was seen in 6 of 11 hemispheres. A modified burr-hole method was also reported by Kawamoto et al. [14, 15]. They named that method as galeo-duro-encephalo-synangiosis. The galeal flap is inserted through the burr-holes towards the interhemispheric fissure and then is fixed on the dura. This method complements the deficient neovascularization in medial frontal lobe by a multiple burr-hole operation.

Karaswa et al. [9, 16] reported good results of omental transplantation in patients having ischemic symptoms in the territory of ACA. However, some authors reported the comparatively high rates of perioperative morbidity and mortality. Omental transplantation needs more complicated procedures. Bulky mass can be the source of mass effect and needs thinning of the calvaria [10].

Direct revascularization to the ACA territory was reported by Iwama et al. [12]. They performed STA-ACA and STA-MCA anastomosis during a single procedure and reported good results. But the caliber and length of the donor artery limits the usefulness of that procedure.

In 1994, Kinugasa et al. [17] introduced a new method for increasing the CBF of the ACA territory. They inserted the galea and /or the periosteum of the frontal area into the interhemispheric space combined with encephalo-duro-arterio-myo-synangiosis (EDAMS). They called it ribbon EDAMS. They achieved excellent results and concluded that ribbon EDAMS was an effective method for MMD with symptomatic cerebral ischemia of the anterior circulation. Kim et al. [18] reported a modified ribbon EDAMS and called it the combined EDAS with bifrontal encephalo-galeo-(periosteal)-synangiosis (EGS). EDAS in combination with bifrontal EGS have shown excellent revascularization in bilateral ACA territories as well as in the MCA territories with no significant complications [6, 18]. The author (C.-Y.K.) and his colleagues [6] also reported that 88% of the 67 patients who had EDAS or EMS with bifrontal EGS have had a favorable outcome; their symptoms had disappeared totally. Thirty-one of 67 patients had symptoms related with ischemia in the ACA territory and 24 of 31 patients had experienced no ACA symptoms whatsoever postoperatively. Angiographically, 35 of the 81 hemispheres showed revascularization in more than two-thirds (good) of the ACA territory and 46 showed revascularization in between two-thirds and one-third (fair). The CBF of the ACA territory on brain SPECT improved or was maintained in the majority (58 out of 61) of patients. Kim et al. [18] presented similar results. Eighty-five percent of 92 patients had no symptoms postoperatively. Seventy-nine percent of 99 hemispheres exhibited good or fair filling in the ACA territory on cerebral angiogram. Favorable changes on brain SPECT were present in 122 of the 177 ACA territories. This method developed into expanding the coverage area by using dura flap in addition to galeoperiosteal flap with a modification of EDAS combined with bifrontal EGS [19].

The author (C.-Y.K.) [6], Kim et al. [18], and Park et al. [19] have described their bifrontal EGS or EGPS procedure as follows. The surgery is usually performed in two stages. Initially, the operation would be done in the symptomatic and hemodynamically more affected hemisphere and then later in the contralateral hemisphere. Combining of bifrontal EGS or not would depend on the patient's medical condition and symptoms. The scalp incision is incised separately for the EDAS and bifrontal EGS procedures. At the bifrontal EGS site, an S-shaped scalp incision is made anterior to the coronal suture. Epigaleal scalp dissection is performed, and the galeoperiosteal flap is incised in an H-pattern. A 4×8-cm midline bifrontal craniotomy is made crossing the superior sagittal sinus (SSS). The dura mater, the base of which is adjacent to the SSS, is incised separately in both hemispheres, and the arachnoid membrane over the cortical sulci is dissected to promote neovascular ingrowth. The incised dural flaps are inserted into each interhemispheric fissure while taking care to avoid injury of cortical veins. The prepared galeoperiosteal flap is sutured to the margin of the dura mater to cover the paramedian anterior frontal lobe (Fig. 1).

Illustrative Case

An 8-year-old girl had intermittent motor weakness of both upper and lower extremities once a month when she ate hot dishes. She was so young that she could not have the test for cognitive function or IQ. Preoperative cerebral angiography showed severe stenosis of ICA with basal moyamoya vessels and occlusion of the right MCA (Fig. 2). Basal perfusion and vascular reserve in both hemispheres was decreased on brain SPECT (Fig. 3). Vascular reserve in the right hemisphere was more decreased than in the left hemisphere. First, she had an operation of EDAS in the right hemisphere. Before she had the second operation, she had intermittent weakness of both legs. Three months later, she had the second operation of left EDAS with bifrontal ribbon EGS. Postoperative follow-up angiography (Fig. 4) and brain

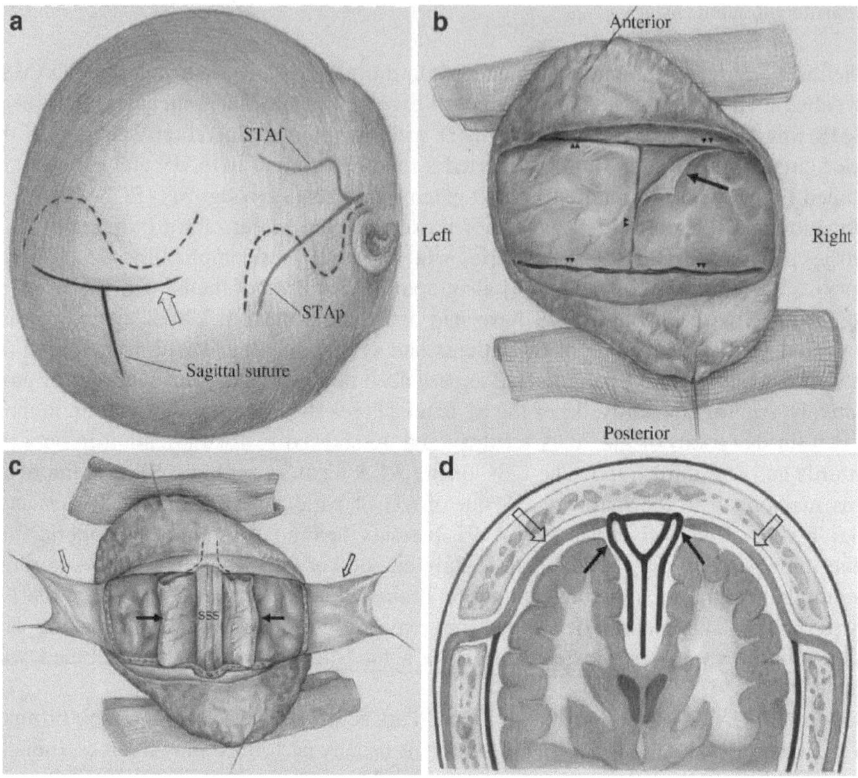

Fig. 1 Artist's drawings showing the steps of the bifrontal encephalogaleo(periosteal)synangiosis (EGPS). (**a**) At the bifrontal EGPS site, an S-shaped scalp incision (*dashed line*) is made anterior to the coronal suture. (**b**) Superior view of the EGPS site. The galeoperiosteal flap (*arrow*) is dissected and incised in an H pattern (*arrowheads*). (**c**) The incised dura (*open arrows*) is infolded into the interhemispheric fissure. The galeoperiosteal flap (*solid arrows*) is prepared to cover the paramedian anterior frontal lobe. (**d**) Coronal view illustrating the prepared galeoperiosteal flap (*solid arrows*) sutured to the margin of infolded dura (*open arrows*) to cover the paramedian frontal brain surface. STAf = frontal branch of the STA; STAp = parietal branch of the STA

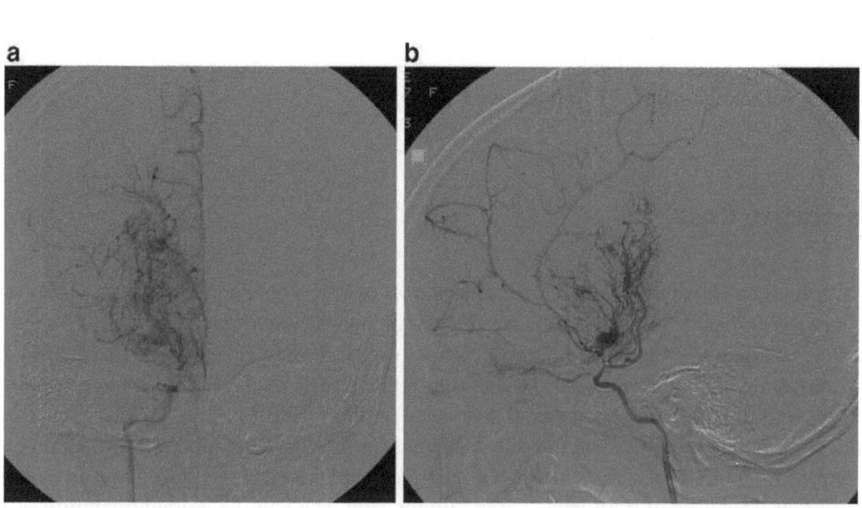

Fig. 2 Preoperative right internal cerebral artery (ICA) angiography (**a, b**) shows severe stenosis of right distal ICA with basal moyamoya vessels. Right middle cerebral artery (MCA) is occluded

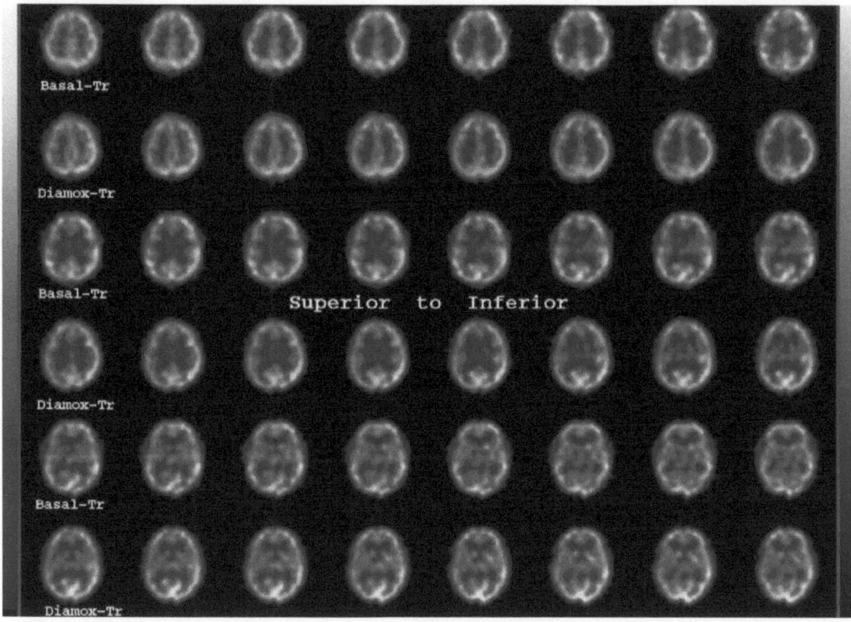

Fig. 3 Preoperative brain SPECT shows deficient basal perfusion and decreased vascular reserve in both hemisphere but more deficient in right hemisphere

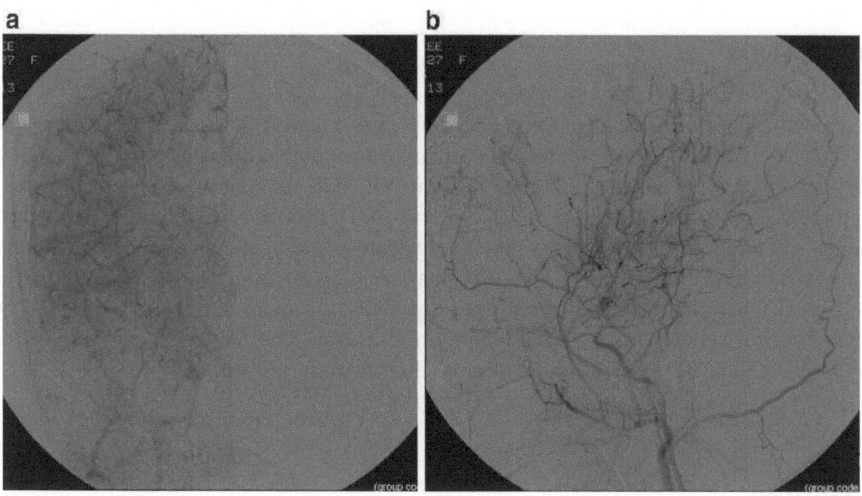

Fig. 4 Postoperative right intracranial common carotid artery angiography (**a**, **b**) shows perfusion in right frontotempoparietal area through external carotid artery. (**b**) Shows perfusion through branches of STA in galeoperiosteal flap

SPECT (Fig. 5) showed good results of revascularization and increased perfusion in MCA territory and also in ACA territory. She had a few negligible subjective symptoms and had no definite motor TIA in a more than 2-year follow-up period. Cognitive function tests will be carried out when the patient is older.

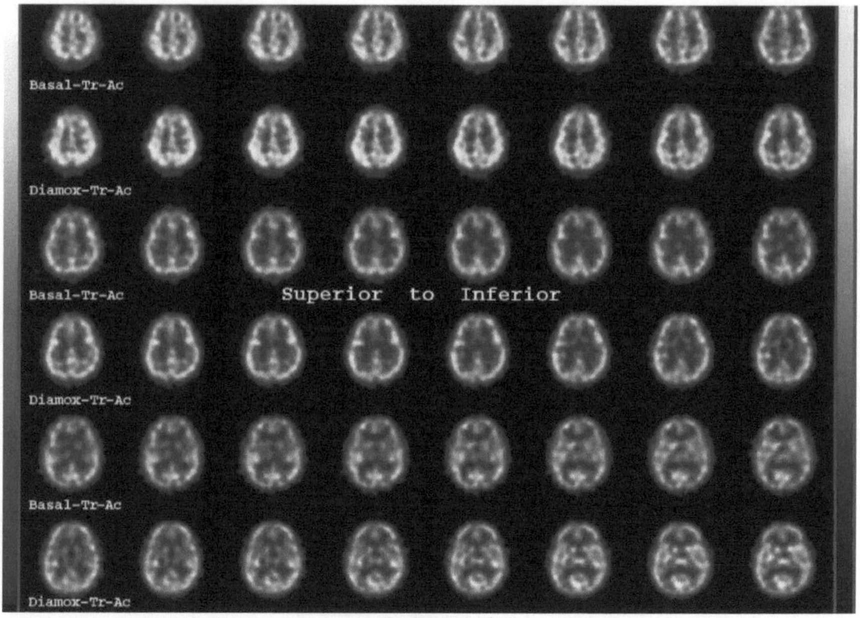

Fig. 5 Postoperative brain SPECT shows increased perfusion and vascular reserve compared with preoperative brain SPECT (Fig. 3)

Conclusions

Augmentation of the ACA territory is very important because the ACA territory has major roles related to cognition and intellectual development as well as to lower extremity motor and sphincter function. Combined EDAS with bifrontal EGS may be an excellent method for reinforcement of the ACA and the MCA territories and it may be relatively safe. Furthermore, studies of a larger number of cases may be mandatory which should show its efficacy and safety. If possible, preoperative and very long-term postoperative test for cognitive and intellectual function should be carried out, especially in young children. Finally, the QoL might also be assessed serially over a long-term follow-up. The ACA territory reinforcement may improve the QoL of MMD patients as well as their clinical symptoms.

References

1. Burke GM, Burke AM, Sherma AK et al (2009) Moyamoya disease: a summary. Neurosurg Focus 26:E11
2. Kumral E, Bayulkem G, Evyapan D et al (2002) Spectrum of anterior cerebral artery territory infarction: clinical and MRI findings. Eur J Neurol 9:615–624
3. Ishikawa T, Houkin K, Kamiyama H et al (1997) Effects of surgical revascularization on outcome of patients with pediatric moyamoya disease. Stroke 28:1170–1173
4. Ogawa A, Yoshimoto T, Suzuki J et al (1990) Cerebral blood flow in moyamoya disease. Part 1: Correlation with age and regional distribution. Acta Neurochir (Wien) 105:30–34

5. Ohtaki M, Uede T, Morimoto S et al (1998) Intellectual functions and regional cerebral haemodynamics after extensive omental transplantation spread over both frontal lobes in childhood moyamoya disease. Acta Neurochir (Wien) 140:1043–1053; discussion 1052–1043
6. Kim CY, Wang KC, Kim SK et al (2003) Encephaloduroarteriosynangiosis with bifrontal encephalogaleo(periosteal)synangiosis in the pediatric moyamoya disease: the surgical technique and its outcomes. Childs Nerv Syst 19:316–324
7. Karasawa J, Touho H, Ohnishi H et al (1992) Long-term follow-up study after extracranial-intracranial bypass surgery for anterior circulation ischemia in childhood moyamoya disease. J Neurosurg 77:84–89
8. Kuroda S, Houkin K (2008) Moyamoya disease: current concepts and future perspectives. Lancet Neurol 7:1056–1066
9. Karasawa J, Kikuchi H, Kawamura J et al (1980) Intracranial transplantation of the omentum for cerebrovascular moyamoya disease: a two-year follow-up study. Surg Neurol 14:444–449
10. Yoshioka N, Tominaga S, Suzuki Y et al (1998) Cerebral revascularization using omentum and muscle free flap for ischemic cerebrovascular disease. Surg Neurol 49:58–66
11. Ishii R, Koike T, Takeuchi S et al (1983) Anastomosis of the superficial temporal artery to the distal anterior cerebral artery with interposed cephalic vein graft. Case report. J Neurosurg 58:425–429
12. Iwama T, Hashimoto N, Miyake H et al (1998) Direct revascularization to the anterior cerebral artery territory in patients with moyamoya disease: report of five cases. Neurosurgery 42:1157–1161; discussion 1161–1152
13. Kawaguchi T, Fujita S, Hosoda K et al (1996) Multiple burr-hole operation for adult moyamoya disease. J Neurosurg 84:468–476
14. Kawamoto H, Inagawa T, Ikawa F et al (2001) A modified burr-hole method in galeoduroencephalosynangiosis for an adult patient with probable moyamoya disease – case report and review of the literature. Neurosurg Rev 24:147–150
15. Kawamoto H, Kiya K, Mizoue T et al (2000) A modified burr-hole method 'galeoduroencephalosynangiosis' in a young child with moyamoya disease. A preliminary report and surgical technique. Pediatr Neurosurg 32:272–275
16. Karasawa J, Touho H, Ohnishi H et al (1993) Cerebral revascularization using omental transplantation for childhood moyamoya disease. J Neurosurg 79:192–196
17. Kinugasa K, Mandai S, Tokunaga K et al (1994) Ribbon enchephalo-duro-arterio-myo-synangiosis for moyamoya disease. Surg Neurol 41:455–461
18. Kim SK, Wang KC, Kim IO et al (2002) Combined encephaloduroarteriosynangiosis and bifrontal encephalogaleo(periosteal)synangiosis in pediatric moyamoya disease. Neurosurgery 50:88–96
19. Park JH, Yang SY, Chung YN et al (2007) Modified encephaloduroarteriosynangiosis with bifrontal encephalogaleoperiosteal synangiosis for the treatment of pediatric moyamoya disease. Technical note. J Neurosurg 106:237–242

PCA Territory Reinforcement

Dal-Soo Kim

The PCA stenosis/occlusion in moyamoya disease (MMD) has been known to increase the risk of transient ischemic attack and/or cerebral infarction in both anterior and posterior circulation area [8]. This finding was correlated with Yamada's study in which the regional cerebral blood flow in MMD decreases proportionally with the degree of steno-occlusive lesions of the PCA because the PCA lesions decrease the number of leptomeningeal vessels to the anterior circulation in MMD [9]. However, cortical branches of the PCA territory are so small in caliber that direct anastomosis between the occipital artery and the cortical branch is very difficult to achieve and not so effective in increasing the blood flow in the PCA territory, especially in pediatric patients.

Therefore, indirect bypass surgeries such as omental transplantation [1,2] or transposition [3,4] and encephaloduroarteiorsynangiogsis [5] have been described for the revascularization of the PCA territory. However, there were also a few cases which reported the effectiveness of direct occipital artery-PCA anastmosis [6,7] for revascularization of PCA territory.

This chapter reviews surgical techniques for the PCA territory revascularization in MMD patients.

Omental Transplantation

Karasawa et al. [1, 2] reported cerebral revascularization using omental transplantation for pediatric MMD patients. Eleven (84.6%) of the 13 patients with visual symptoms showed improvement in their neurologic state following unilateral or bilateral omental transplantation to the posterior cerebral artery.

For omental transplantation, laparatomy is first performed using a midline epigastric incision to expose omentum. Perforating vessels from both the gastroepiploic artery and vein are coagulated and resected. An 8×8-cm to 13×13-cm portion of the omentum is removed with these vessels. Then a bi- or uni-occipital craniotomy is performed and the occipital artery

D.-S. Kim (✉)
Stroke Center, Department of Neurosurgery, Myong-Ji St. Mary's Hospital,
709-1, Daerim 2-dong, Yeongdeungpo-gu, Seoul 150-908, Republic of Korea
e-mail: dalskim@catholic.ac.kr

B.-K. Cho and T. Tominaga (eds.), *Moyamoya Disease Update*,
DOI 10.1007/978-4-431-99703-0_35, © Springer 2010

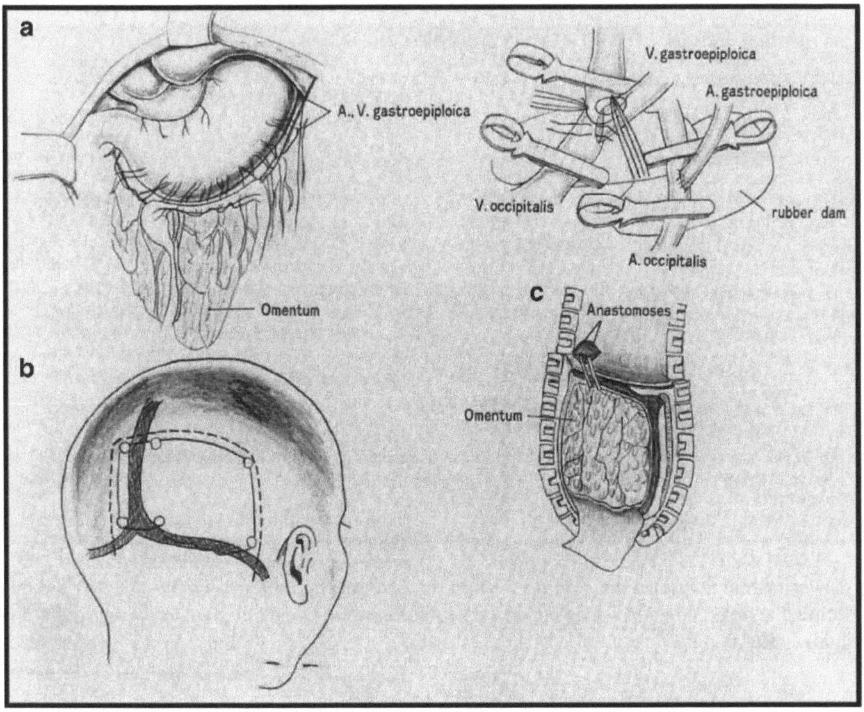

Fig. 1 Schematic representation of omental transplantation. (**a**) A portion of the omentum approximately 8×8 to 13×13 cm in area is removed complete with the gastroepiploic artery and vein. (**b**) Craniotomy is performed as indicated. In this case, the omentum is to be transplanted in the unilateral occipital lobe. (**c**) An end-to-side anastomosis between the occipital artery/vein is performed, respectively (*upper*), and the occipital lobe is covered by the omentum (*lower*). (From [2], with permission)

and vein just above the level of the transverse sinus are separated for a distance of 2 cm from the scalp. An end-to-side anastomosis between the occipital artery or superficial temporal artery and the gastroepiploic artery is performed with ten stitches of 10-0 monofilament nylon suture. Next, an end-to-side anastomosis between the occipital vein or superficial temporal vein and the gastroepiploic vein is completed with eight stitches of 10-0 monofilament nylon suture. If no adequate scalp vein is not available, the gastroepiploic vein is anastomosed to a cortical vein. The dura mater is opened bi- or uni-laterally and the omentum is spread over the cortical surface and slightly under the edges of the dura mater. The dural edges are sutured the omentum at several sites. After replacement of the bone flap, the wound is closed (Fig. 1).

Omental Transposition

Instead of anastomosing the gastroepiploic vessels to scalp vessels, the omentum can be lengthened to reach the cranium while it remains attached to the dominant gastroepiploic pedicle. The nondominant pedicle is divided. Lengthening is achieved by dividing the omentum with L-shaped incisions that pass through paralleling the greater curvature of the stomach, and a subcutaneous tunnel is made along the anterior chest wall and extending posteriorly to the ear.

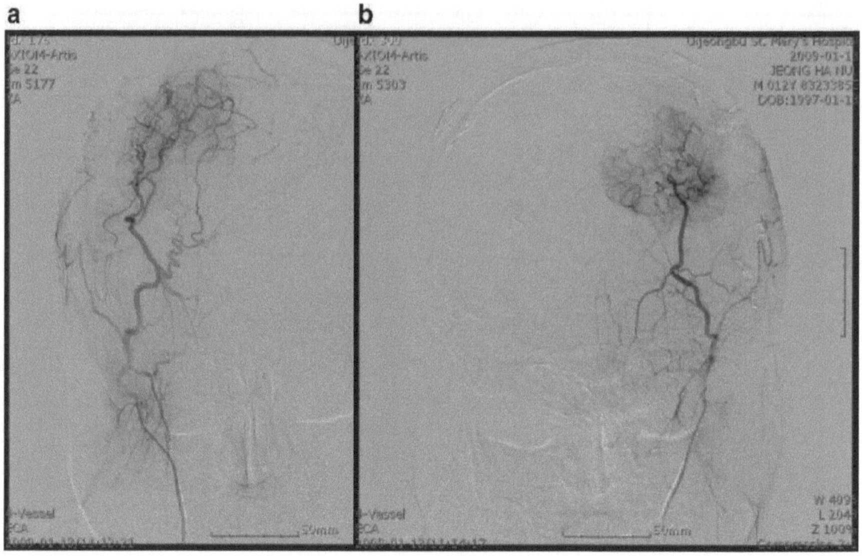

Fig. 2 Postoperative carotid angiogram showing excellent revascularization on the *right* (**a**) and the *left* (**b**) occipital regions 5 months following encephalo-duro-arterio-synangiosis in an 11-year-old boy with moyamoya disease-related recurrent visual impairment

Finally, the omental graft is spread on the exposed cortical surface and sutured along the dural edges [3, 4].

Encephaloduroarteriosynangiosis

Kim et al. [5] described encephaloduroarteriosynangiosis on the occipital cortex in his paper, combining direct and indirect reconstructive vascular surgery on the fronto-parieto-occipital region in MMD. The angiographic result demonstrated extensive and localized revascularization in each of the four sides and no evidence of revascularization in two among ten sides which underwent encephaloduroarteriosynangiosis on the occipital region.

Surgical technique was the same as Matsushimas' original description of the principle. The occipital artery was exposed from 7 to 9 cm in the length just above the transverse sinus and the galea was dissected 2–3 cm apart from the occipital artery on both its sides. The size of the bone flap was 6–8 cm in length and 4–5 cm in width (Fig. 2).

Occipital Artery-Posterior Cerebral Artery Anastomosis

Toshiaki et al. [6] made an osteoplastic craniotomy at 1 cm lateral to the sagittal sinus, anterior to the transverse sinus, and medial to the mastoid process. The periosteum was left in place on the bone, preserving the vessels that would form the future collateral networks. The occipital artery was dissected more than 5 cm in length and more than 0.5 mm in diameter from the skin flap. The cortical surface was explored via occipital craniotomy to find a suitable cortical branch of the posterior cerebral artery. The authors tried to expose the posterior cerebral artery branches in the occipital interhemispheric surface. Then end-to-side occipital artery-posterior cerebral artery anastomosis was performed with indirect bypass surgery in three patients, ranging in age from 6.0 to 35.2 years (mean age, 23.8 years) with MMD as an additional surgery for postoperative ischemic symptoms. All patients showed clinical and radiological improvement after the direct bypass surgery. Additionally, Ikeda et al. [7] performed occipital artery to calcarine artery to prevent impending cortical blindness in a 38-year-old male with MMD. The patient's neurological state was stabilized after the direct bypass surgery.

References

1. Karasawa J, Kikuchi H, Kawamura J et al (1980) Intracranial transplantation of the omentum for cerebrovascular disease: a two-year follow-up study. Surg Neurol 14:444–449
2. Karasawa J, Touho H, Ohnishi H et al (1993) Cerebral revascularization using omental transplantation for childhood moyamoya disease. J Neurosurg 79:192–196
3. Goldsmith HS (1997) Omental transposition to the brain for Alzheimer's disease. Ann NY Acad Sci 826:323–336
4. Havlik RJ, Fried I, Chyatte D et al (1992) Encephalo-omental synangiosis in the management of moyamoya disease. Surgery 111:156–162
5. Kim DS, Kye DK, Cho KS et al (1997) Combined direct and indirect reconstructive vascular surgery on the fronto-parieto-occipital region in moyamoya disease. Clin Neurol Neurosurg 99:S137–141
6. Toshiaki H, Reizo S, Teiji T (2009) Additional surgery for postoperative ischemic symptoms in patients with moyamoya disease: the effectiveness of occipital artery-posterior cerebral artery bypass with an indirect procedure: Technical case report. Neurosurgery 64:E195–196
7. Ikeda A, Yamamoto I, Sato O et al (1991) Revascularization of the calcarine artery in moyamoya disease: OA-cortical PCA anastomosis-case report. Neurol Med Chir (Tokyo) 31:658–661
8. Kuroda S, Ishikawa T, Houkin K et al (2002) Clinical significance of posterior cerebral artery atenosis/occlusion in moyamoya disease. No Shinkei Geka 30:1295–1300
9. Yamada I, Murata Y, Umehara I et al (1996) SPECT and MRI evaluations of the posterior circulation in moyamoya disease. J Nucl Med 37:1613–1617

Endovascular Treatment of Moyamoya Disease

O-Ki Kwon and Seong Hyun Kim

Endovascular Treatment of Moyamoya Disease with Hemorrhagic Presentation

Intracerebral or intraventricular hemorrhage is the second most common clinical presentation in patients with moyamoya disease (MMD). In adult patients, hemorrhage is the most common clinical manifestation and is known as the most fatal complication [1, 2]. The exact causes of bleeding from moyamoya disease have not been clarified, but saccular aneurysms formed by hemodynamic stress and fragile collateral vessels have been considered the major sources [3–6].

Although the natural history of MMD with bleeding has not been fully defined, several investigators have shown that rebleeding can occur in about 16~20% of cases and that clinical outcome after the rebleeding is poor [2, 5]. Good outcome after single episode of bleeding was 60%, but after repeated bleeding, it decreased to 40% [7].

In terms of preventing rebleeding, there has been no effective method. Several authors have proposed that surgical revascularization might play an preventive role, but its efficiency remains in question [6, 8–10].

Direct surgical intervention for saccular aneurysms could be a treatment option [4, 11]. But it carries a risk of additional brain damage because cisterns around the circle of Willis are often filled with tiny basal moyamoya vessels. In cases of peripheral aneurysms, they are usually located deeply, corresponding to the prevalent locations of hemorrhage in MMD, basal ganglia and periventricular white matter. In addition, because collateral circulation is important in patients with MMD, surgical injury of these vessels can produce additional ischemic brain damage [12]. Obviously, an endovascular approach has advantages with respect to its less invasive nature. But direct endovascular access distally through the ACA or MCA is often impossible because the supraclinoid ICA is very small.

O.-K. Kwon (✉)
Division of Cerebrovascular Surgery, Department of Neurosurgery,
Seoul National University Bundang Hospital, Seoul National University College of Medicine,
300 Gumi-dong, Bundang-gu, Seongnam-si, Gyeonggi-do 463-707, Republic of Korea
e-mail: kwonoki@korea.com

S.H. Kim
Department of Radiology, Clinical Neuroscience Center, Seoul National University Bundang Hospital,
Seoul National University College of Medicine, Gyeonggi-do, Republic of Korea

B.-K. Cho and T. Tominaga (eds.), *Moyamoya Disease Update*,
DOI 10.1007/978-4-431-99703-0_36, © Springer 2010

From the technical viewpoint, endovascular treatment of saccular aneurysms in moyamoya disease is the same as for conventional aneurysms. There's nothing special in technical aspects. Careful blood pressure monitoring and control is of importance during anesthesia. Basilar top aneurysm is the most common hemodynamically-formed saccular aneurysm in MMD. Sometimes, the basilar artery is the only artery which supplies the whole brain. In this case, preservation of bilateral P1 is critical.

Unlike conventional saccular aneurysms around the circle of Willis, peripherally located small-sized aneurysms can develop in lenticulostriate artery collaterals, so-called moyamoya vessels, and in other collateral vessels especially on the anterior or posterior choroidal arteries. These aneurysmal lesions are not commonly found in angiograms. Only occasionally, angiograms show small aneurismal lesions at collateral moyamoya vessels. They might be ruptured ones or not. If these are located at the hemorrhage site, it is reasonable to think that the aneurysms are the direct causes of the bleeding (true aneurysm) or the result of vessel rupture (pseudoaneurysm) [13, 14].

According to pathological examination, collateral vessels in moyamoya disease have weakened media with occasional segmentation of the internal elastic lamina and fibrosis. Attenuated arterial walls acquire a predisposition for microaneurysm formation or rupture under hemodynamic stress [1]. Regardless of its character, it is very difficult or often impossible to access the lesion directly without additional brain damage because of its deep location and preexisting ischemic brain condition. In this situation, an endovascular approach must be considered.

In our series of nine cases, small aneurysmal lesions were found most commonly at the distal paraventricular segment of the lateral posterior choroidal artery (LPCA), which had caused intraventricular and paraventricular hemorrhage. Eight patients underwent endovascular *N*-butyl-cyanoacrylate (NBCA) glue injection for the closure of the lesions. In one patient, Onyx (EV3; Neurovascular, Irvine, USA) was used instead of NBCA. Platinum coils were not used because of several practical problems; firstly, the artery size is very small for accepting a detachable platinum coil and forced advancement of the coil may produce dangerous straightening or rupture of the fragile vessels. Secondly, the aneurysms are also too small to allow the coil to pass. The parent artery that held the aneurysmal lesion was selected with a microcatheter (Prowler-10; Cordis Neurovascular, Miami, USA) using a micro-guidewire (Agility 10 soft; Cordis Neurovascular). The microcatheter was advanced as far as possible. Selective angiogram was performed by careful hand injection and analyzed for determining the relationship of the aneurysmal lesion and the connecting arteries. If needed, the microcatheter was repositioned to minimize the length of arterial occlusion. A 33% mixture of NBCA and lipiodol mixture was injected through the microcatheter until the glue reached and filled the aneurysm and/or if the reflux of the glue was found. After the injection, postembolization angiography was performed to verify closure of the aneurysm (Figs. 1 and 2). Neither heparin nor antiplatelet agent was given during or after the procedure. The aneurysms were successfully and completely occluded in seven patients. In one patient, microcatheter navigation into the LPCA failed because the vessel size was too small. There was neither additional neurological deficit nor newly developed ischemic lesion on the follow-up MR studies. Six patients were fully recovered at discharge and two patients with poor initial condition recovered partially and still remained with neurological deficit. Follow-up radiological studies including angiograms and MRA were performed in all patients (mean 24 months, range 11–60 months) and revealed no reappearance of the aneurysm lesion at the same site.

Theoretically, occlusion of collateral arteries with glue can affect the blood supply to brain tissue, which could then produce cerebral infarction. But it did not occur in our series, for which there may be several explanations. First, we advanced the microcatheter as far as

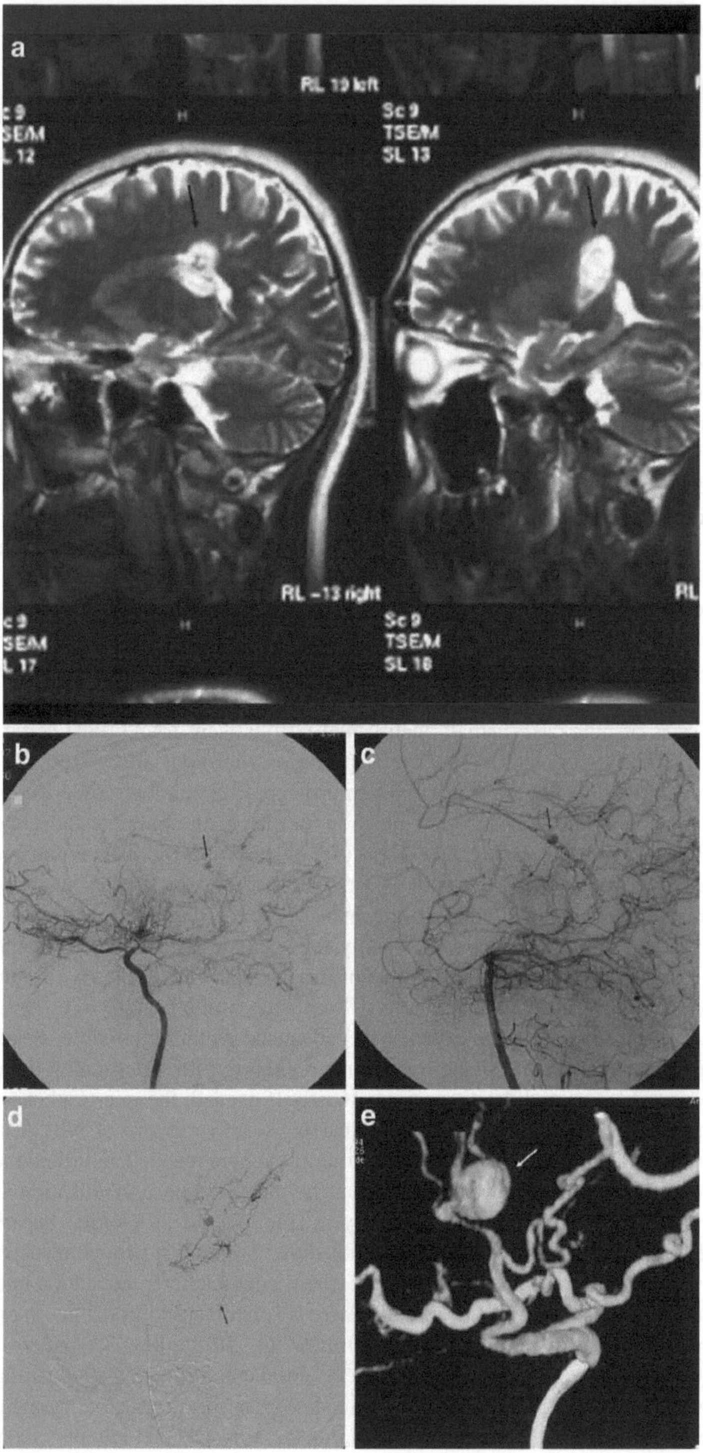

Fig. 1 This 22-year-old male patient visited emergency room with sudden severe headache and mild right hemiparesis. (**a**) MR images show paraventricular hemorrhage (*arrows*). (**b**) ICA angiogram shows an aneurysmal lesion at the site corresponding with the hemorrhage (*arrow*). (**c**) Vertebral angiogram shows the same lesion. (**d**) A microcatheter (*arrow*) is navigated distally near the aneurysm. (**e**) A three-dimensional angiographic image shows the aneurysm (*arrow*) and adjacent small collateral vessels.

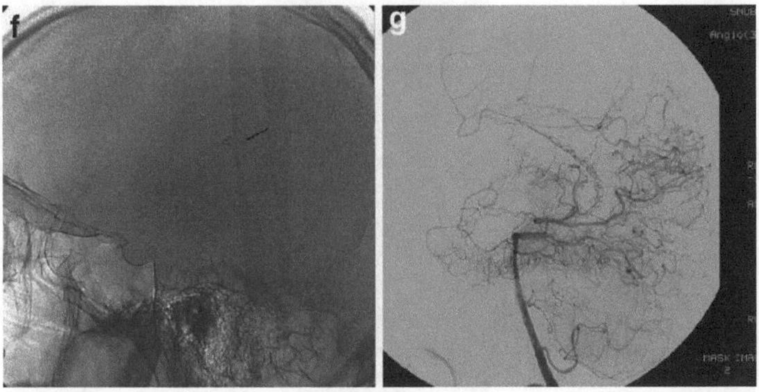

Fig. 1 (continued) (**f**) Glue (*N*-butyl cyanoacrylate, NBCA) is injected. Note that only small length of the parent artery and aneurysm is occluded (*arrow*). Glue is not injected into the collateral vessels. (**g**) Postembolization angiogram shows complete disappearance of the aneurysmal lesion

possible; branches of relatively large size were all passed. Only small collateral branches remained between the microcather tip and the aneurysm. Second, the blood flow direction was reversed in the territory of the parent vessel of the aneurysm after its selection because it was usually blocked by the catheter. We performed selective angiogram and fluoroscopic test injection several times with changing injection power and contrast volume carefully reviewing each stage. The point we tried to find was flow dominance, that is, injecting embolic agent from the microcatheter tip just to the aneurysm but not to small collateral branches of that territory. Because the parent vessel of the aneurysm was blocked, fine control of the glue was relatively easy. Thirdly, the collateral vessels are well developed in MMD. The occluded arterial part could be taken for a short segment of conduit located in ventricular wall, not in capillaries. Rich collateral networks nearby could compensate for the one conduit blockage so no infarction occurred. If any ischemia was produced it should be trivial.

Endovascular Treatment of Intracranial Arterial Stenosis of Moyamoya Disease

The introduction of endovascular techniques has allowed us to manage various cerebral vascular diseases including ischemic as well as hemorrhagic lesions with attractive minimally invasive methods. Especially in ischemic diseases, rapid development of state-of-the-art devices such as small size angioplasty balloons, flexible stents, and well-navigable delivery systems have made it possible to approach very tortuous and narrow intracranial stenosis lesions. But despite these advances, endovascular treatment has rarely been adopted for moyamoya disease which has progressive internal carotid artery stenosis as a typical feature. The reasons for this are: (1) moyamoya disease is a progressive lesion and many physicians doubt on persistent effect of angioplasty with balloons or stents; (2) brain ischemia in moymoya disease occurs mostly in pediatric patients in whom intracranial internal carotid and middle cerebral artery are frequently too small and stenotic length is relatively long for applying devices; (3) most adult patients who have larger vessels present with hemorrhage not with ischemic symptoms; and (4) in adult patients with ischemic symptoms, target vessels are often already occluded or too narrow. These explanations suggest that moyamoya disease is not a suitable indication for endovascular angioplasty. Indeed, there has been no clinical report on this issue as yet.

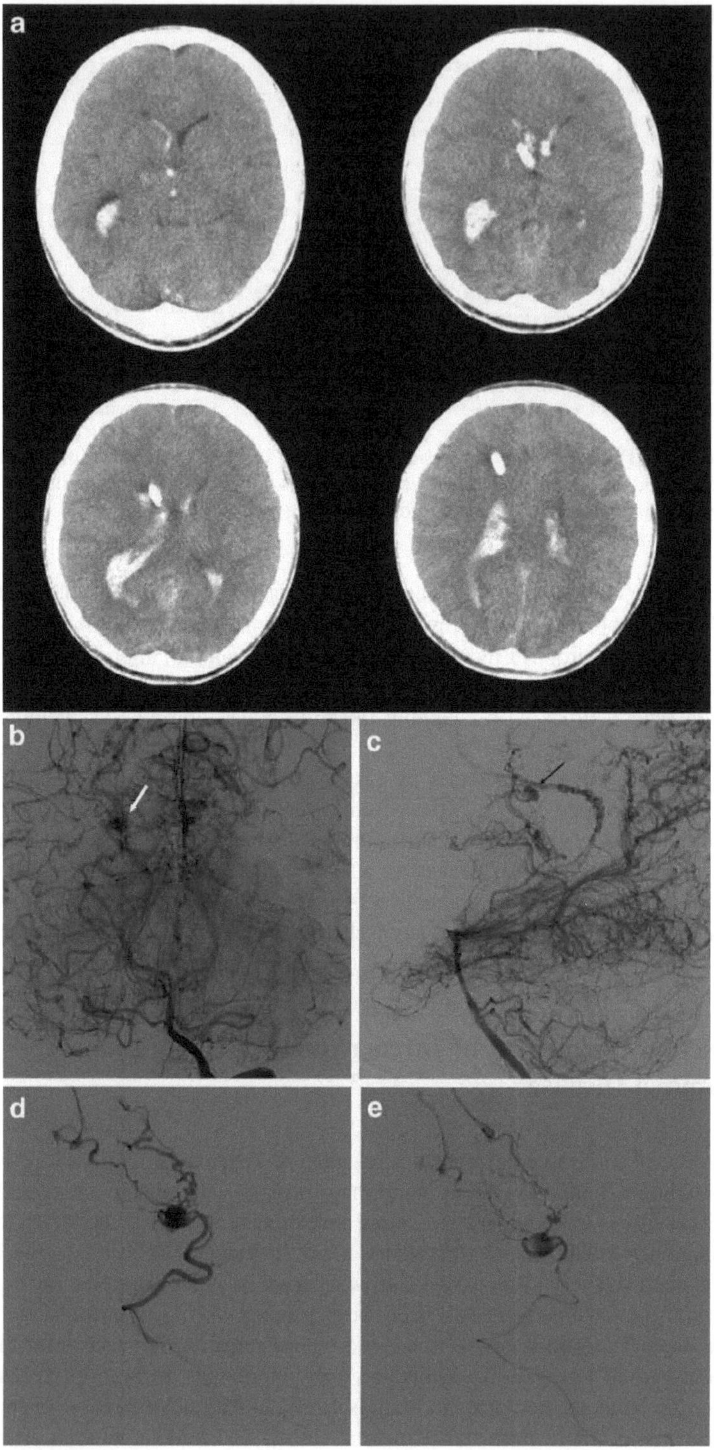

Fig. 2 This 35-year-old male patient was transferred to the emergency room with coma state. Urgent extraventricular drainage was performed. (**a**) CT images demonstrate intraventricular hemorrhage and diffuse brain swelling. (**b**) Angiogram shows an aneurysmal lesion (*white block arrow*). (**c**) A lateral view of vertebral angiogram shows the same aneurysmal lesion (*arrow*). (**d**) This lesion is selected with a microcatheter. (**e**) The microcatheter is advanced close to the aneurysm.

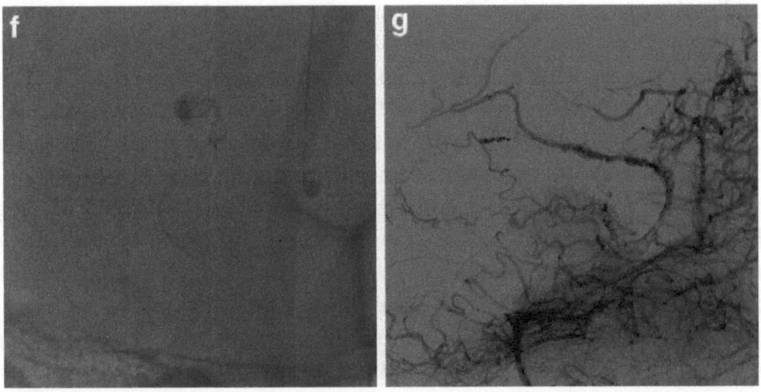

Fig. 2 (continued) (**f**) Using Onyx, the aneurysm is complete occluded with short segments of the parent artery. (**g**) Postembolization angiogram shows complete disappearance of the lesion

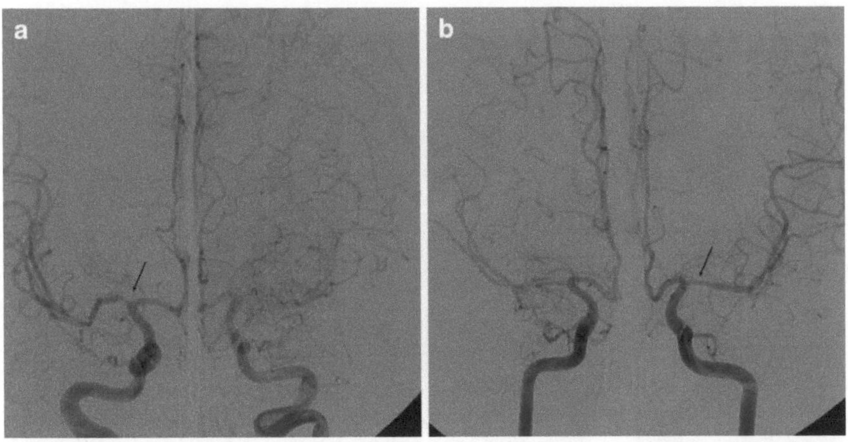

Fig. 3 (**a**) This 33-year-old female patient underwent cerebral angiography due to transient ischemic attacks. Angiograms [anterio-posterior (AP) images of right and left ICA angiogram] demonstrate complete M1 occlusion at left and stenosis at the proximal M1 at right (*arrow*). This patient did not have any evidence of other vascular diseases including atherosclerosis. (**b**) This 39-year-old male patient underwent cerebral angiography due to transient ischemic attacks, too. Angiograms (AP images of right and left ICA angiogram) demonstrate complete M1 occlusion at right and stenosis at the proximal M1 at right (*arrow*). This patient also did not have any evidence of other vascular diseases including atherosclerosis. These angiographic findings may be within a spectrum of moyamoya disease

Theoretically, moyamoya disease is a potentially good indication for angioplasty and stenting. Pathological reports of moyamoya disease have shown that intracranial artery stenosis develops by intimal hyperplasia. The intima of the diseased artery is replaced by thickened fibroelastic tissue. Inflammation does not involve in this process. These findings are same in adult and pediatric patients [15]. Fibrous intimal hyperplasia can be managed by endovascular angioplasty.

Adult and adolescent moyamoya disease patients who have intracranial stenosis and ischemic symptoms and whose target arteries are large enough to adopt angioplasty devices can be potential indications of angioplasty. Angiographically and clinically these patients could be classified as "mild." Now that angiographic features show early stage of MMD, even a definite diagnosis can be confusing. Of course, this group of patients is not common.

In the authors' experience, there is a group of patients who have common clinical and radiological features that cannot be categorized into any other cerebral vascular diseases other than MMD (Fig. 3). This patient group has intracranial stenosis at distal ICA and/or proximal M1 segments. Patients' age ranged from late teens to 70 years. Most were in their 30s and 40s. Various laboratory studies did not show evidence of atherosclerosis or any other cerebral vascular diseases. Radiological studies demonstrate tapered stenosis at distal ICA and/or proximal M1. Unlike atherosclerotic lesions, only distal ICA and M1 segments are involved. Basal moyamoya collateral vessels were scarce. In several patients, stenosis develops bilaterally but usually at a unilateral vessel. Given that angiographic and clinical features, we think that this may be a variant form of moyamoya disease.

In eight such patients, stenotic segments were dilated with angioplastic coronary balloon. The size of the balloon was mostly 2 mm in diameter. All procedures were successfully performed under general anesthesia without complication (Fig. 4). Patients did not show any symptom recurrence after treatment. Follow-up angiograms (1 year) revealed no or mild restenosis that did not require retreatment.

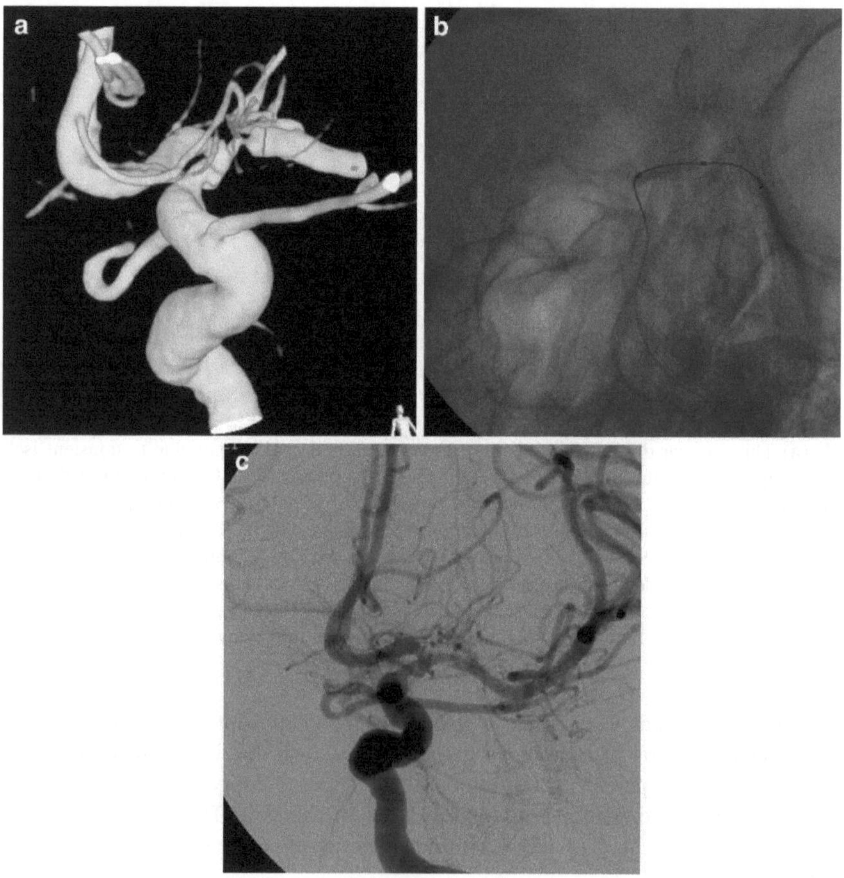

Fig. 4 This 52-year-old male patient visited our hospital due to repeated transient ischemic attacks. (**a**) A three-dimensional angiographic image reveals severe stenosis at M1 and distal ICA. (**b**) Using a 2-mm coronary balloon, angioplasty is performed. (**c**) Postangioplasty angiogram shows sufficient dilatation. The patient has been doing well for 2-year follow-up

The etiology of moyamoya disease has not been clarified and diagnosis mainly depends on radiological findings, that is, idiopathic, bilateral, progressive, distal ICA stenosis, and presence of collateral moyamoya vessels. Therefore, by definition, these patients do not have moyamoya disease. However, it cannot be classified to any other category, either. The authors believe that many characteristics represent moyamoya-like features, for example, angiographic findings, the mechanism of clinical presentation (hypoperfusion), patient ages, and ethnic background (all Korean). We think they share a common pathology with moyamoya disease. So, we believe that clinical and radiological results of angioplasty in these patients suggest that endovascular dilatation of stenotic segments in moyamoya disease might be effective at least for a short or intermediate periods.

Conclusion

Currently, endovascular approach has already become an important part in treatment of hemorrhagic moyamoya disease. The bleeding sites, especially aneurysms regardless of their location, have been treated with high success rates. Because surgical methods have obvious limitations, the role of endovascular treatment will continue for a while in treatment of moyamoya disease with hemorrhagic presentation.

In terms of intracranial arterial stenosis, endovascular angioplasty for moyamoya disease is just beginning to be used. Pathologically, intracranial stenosis of moyamoya disease is caused by fibrous intimal hyperplasia. No inflammation is involved. In many patients, the stenosis progresses to occlusion. There has been no report on angioplasty for MMD. But it could have role at least in early stage of this disease as our experiences have shown.

References

1. Yamashita M, Oka K, Tanaka K (1983) Histopathology of the brain vascular network in moyamoya disease. Stroke 14:50–58
2. Yoshida Y, Yoshimoto T, Shirane R et al (1999) Clinical course, surgical management, and long-term outcome of moyamoya patients with rebleeding after an episode of intracerebral hemorrhage: an extensive follow-up study. Stroke 30:2272–2276
3. Adams HP Jr, Kassell NF, Wisoff HS et al (1979) Intracranial saccular aneurysm and moyamoya disease. Stroke 10:174–179
4. Furuse S, Matsumoto S, Tanaka Y et al (1982) [Moyamoya disease associated with a false aneurysm – case report and review of the literature]. No Shinkei Geka 10:1005–1012
5. Ikezaki K, Fukui M, Inamura T et al (1997) The current status of the treatment for hemorrhagic type moyamoya disease based on a 1995 nationwide survey in Japan. Clin Neurol Neurosurg 99 Suppl 2:S183–186
6. Karasawa J, Kikuchi H, Furuse S et al (1978) Treatment of moyamoya disease with STA-MCA anastomosis. J Neurosurg 49:679–688
7. Saeki N, Nakazaki S, Kubota M et al (1997) Hemorrhagic type moyamoya disease. Clin Neurol Neurosurg 99 Suppl 2:S196–201
8. Karasawa J, Touho H, Ohnishi H et al (1992) Long-term follow-up study after extracranial-intracranial bypass surgery for anterior circulation ischemia in childhood moyamoya disease. J Neurosurg 77:84–89
9. Kinugasa K, Mandai S, Kamata I et al (1993) Surgical treatment of moyamoya disease: operative technique for encephalo-duro-arterio-myo-synangiosis, its follow-up, clinical results, and angiograms. Neurosurgery 32:527–531

10. Matsushima T, Inoue T, Suzuki SO et al (1992) Surgical treatment of moyamoya disease in pediatric patients – comparison between the results of indirect and direct revascularization procedures. Neurosurgery 31:401–405
11. Nakai H, Yamamoto K, Sako K et al (1992) [A ruptured aneurysm at the peripheral collateral circulation of the anterior choroidal artery in a patient with moyamoya disease: a case report]. No Shinkei Geka 20:985–990
12. Kuroda S, Houkin K, Kamiyama H et al (2001) Effects of surgical revascularization on peripheral artery aneurysms in moyamoya disease: report of three cases. Neurosurgery 49:463–467; discussion 467–468
13. Kawaguchi S, Sakaki T, Morimoto T et al (1996) Characteristics of intracranial aneurysms associated with moyamoya disease. A review of 111 cases. Acta Neurochir (Wien) 138:1287–1294
14. Yuasa H, Tokito S, Izumi K et al (1982) Cerebrovascular moyamoya disease associated with an intracranial pseudoaneurysm. Case report. J Neurosurg 56:131–134
15. Youmans J (ed) (1996) Neurological surgery. Saunders, Philadelphia

Part XI
Surgical Outcome

Overview

Byung-Kyu Cho, Seung-Ki Kim, and Kyu-Chang Wang

Introduction

Surgical revascularization (RV) methods for moyamoya disease (MMD) can be categorized into three groups: direct, indirect, and combined RV procedures. Selection of the procedure depends on the age of the patient, anatomic size of the donor/recipient vessels, preoperative extent of compromised hemodynamics (cerebral blood flow, CBF, and vascular reserve), and surgeon's preference. A report by the Japanese Ministry of Health and Welfare (1997) revealed that, of 302 patients with moyamoya disease (MMD), 162 (53.6%) patients received indirect bypass surgery, 35 (11.6%) received direct bypass surgery, 50 (16.6%) received combined indirect and direct bypass surgery, and 55 (18.2%) patients had no surgical treatment [1].

A literature review of 57 studies (1,448 patients, 2,218 hemispheres) of pediatric (<21 years of age) patients with MMD through the Ovid Medline database, most of them (74%) from Japanese institutions, revealed that 4% of patients were treated with the direct procedure, 73% with the indirect procedure (all indirect procedures were considered as a single group), and 23% with a combination of direct and indirect procedures [2].

The direct RV procedure usually involves a superficial temporal artery to middle cerebral artery (STA–MCA) cortical branch anastomosis, and rarely the occipital artery to MCA (or posterior cerebral artery) anastomosis. It is the most commonly applied method for RV of adult ischemic cerebrovascular diseases. However, the direct anastomotic RV procedure alone or in combination with the indirect RV technique is the favored procedure by many authors for most children, as well as adults with MMD [3–7]. This has the advantage of immediate high-flow RV to the ischemic brain and reduces perioperative ischemia; however, it is technically challenging, particularly in young children [8]. Reversal of flow in critical

B.-K. Cho (✉) and K.-C. Wang
Division of Pediatric Neurosurgery, Pediatric Clinical Neuroscience Center,
Seoul National University Children's Hospital, Seoul National University College of Medicine,
101 Daehangno, Jongno-gu, Seoul 110-744, Republic of Korea
e-mail: bkcho@snu.ac.kr

S.-K. Kim
Division of Pediatric Neurosurgery, Pediatric Clinical Neuroscience Center,
Seoul National University Children's Hospital, Seoul National University College of Medicine,
101 Daehangno, Jongno-gu, Seoul 110-744, Republic of Korea
Research Center for Rare Disease, Seoul, Republic of Korea

B.-K. Cho and T. Tominaga (eds.), *Moyamoya Disease Update*,
DOI 10.1007/978-4-431-99703-0_37, © Springer 2010

perforating vessel segments, blockage of the cortical blood flow of the misery perfusion state during surgery [9, 10], and immediate postoperative hyperperfusion syndrome [11, 12] are disadvantages. Furthermore, long-term efficacy of the direct technique alone in preventing ischemia has not been shown to be superior to the indirect technique in children [13]. Many authors have reported better outcomes from combined RV than from the single direct or indirect techniques in the management of MMD in children, as well as in adults [3, 13–17]. The STA–MCA anastomotic technique mainly corrects ischemia of the MCA territory; however, it does not always cover the anterior cerebral and/or posterior cerebral arterial territories.

Indirect RV is often applied to young children with MMD; however, it is also favorably applied in adults [10, 18]. Sufficient RV requires about 3–6 months to form, even though RV begins 1 or 2 weeks after surgery [19, 20]. There are some limitations to applying the direct procedure to children. The younger the child is, the smaller the diameter of the STA and/or cortical branch of the MCA, and these vessels are more fragile. Children younger than 4 years of age are usually not candidates for the direct RV procedure [7].

Children over 5–8 years of age can be considered as candidates for the direct RV procedure [4, 21]. The patency of STA–MCA anastomoses in children with MMD decreases to 53% about 3 months after the direct procedure [16].

The most basic and commonly used indirect RV procedures are encephalo-duro-arterio-synangiosis (EDAS) [19], encephalo-myo-synangiosis (EMS) [22], and encephalo-duro-arterio-myo-synangiosis (EDAMS) [20]. There are variations and combinations of indirect RV procedures, mostly toward more extensive use of donor tissues including the STA, temporal muscle (deep temporal artery), dura (middle meningeal artery), galea, and periosteum [15, 16, 23–25], or direct contact of the donor vessel to the pial surface [26].

Combined direct and indirect RV is often done by STA–MCA bypass plus one or two indirect bypasses. The most common varieties used are STA–MCA anastomosis plus EMS (or EDAS) [3, 14, 24, 27], and STA–MCA anastomosis plus EDAMS [16, 17]. This method takes advantage of direct and indirect bypass techniques at the expense of prolonged surgical time with anesthesia.

Combined multiple indirect procedures involve a wide variety of methods and modifications, and the aim is to extend coverage of the ischemic brain as much as possible, including the MCA and anterior cerebral artery (ACA) territories, which are the most commonly and simultaneously affected vessels in MMD. Multiple combined indirect procedures [24], ribbon EDAMS [28, 29], multiple EDAS [30], EDAS plus bifrontal encephalo-galeo-periosteal synangiosis (EGPS) [23], and multiple burr holes [31] are included in this category.

Indication and Timing of RV

The Committee on Moyamoya Disease from the Ministry of Health and Welfare of Japan advise surgical intervention when repeated clinical symptoms because of apparent cerebral ischemia or decreased regional cerebral blood flow (rCBF), vascular response, and perfusion reserve, based on the findings of cerebral circulation and metabolism study, are present. Indication and timing of RV surgery should be differentiated between typical bilateral MMD, unilateral MMD, and moyamoya syndrome (MMS).

In a study of unilateral intracranial arteriopathy in children, 94% (74/79 patients) with unilateral intracranial arteriopathy had transient cerebral arteriopathy (TCA) of the internal carotid artery bifurcation simulating unilateral MMD, even though the follow-up duration was short (mean 1.4 years). These patients with TCA had characteristics of preceding chickenpox

(44%) and most showed localized infarction in the basal ganglia [32]. In adults showing unilateral MMD (defined as none, equivocal, or mild involvement of the contralateral side), six of eight patients (75%) with equivocal or mild contralateral disease progressed, whereas only one of ten patients (10%) with no initial contralateral disease progressed to bilateral MMD [33]. Our recent study revealed that 24 of 53 (45%) of patients with unilateral pediatric MMD progressed to bilateral involvement during a mean follow-up of 23 months (range 0.5–150 months) [submitted, 2009].

For adult-onset MMD, the progression of the disease is not common; however, progression has been reported in the cerebral hemispheres in 6 of 47 (12.8%) patients who were followed up conservatively, after which RV surgery was conducted. Their surgical indications included: (1) presence of ischemic symptoms, (2) apparent flow compromise by SPECT, (3) independent activity of daily life, and (4) absence of major cerebral infarction [34]. The authors' surgical indication seemed more strict and narrow than the Committee guidelines indication.

These findings suggest that close imaging and hemodynamic as well as clinical follow-ups are essential in unilateral MMD before making surgical decisions. In addition, delayed surgery should be considered until repeated ischemic attacks and progressive hemodynamic compromise are confirmed.

In general, the timing of surgery follows the indication of surgery. The mean interval between clinical presentation and surgery was 28.3 months (range 0.5–168 months), from a large literature review [2]. The appropriate time of surgery should be differentiated according to the age of onset of MMD. For patients in whom the disease begins when they are 2–5 years of age, EDAS performed before the age of 9 years may result in a good outcome with regard to mental ability, as well as resolution of paroxysmal symptoms and cerebral RV. EDAS operations should be performed within 6 years from onset of the disease for good prognosis. If the onset of the MMD occurs in individuals younger than 2 years of age, the prognosis is very poor; however, slight hope remains if the operation is performed within 3 months of onset [35]. For the asymptomatic side of unilaterally symptomatic pediatric MMD, surgery can be delayed until the development of ischemic symptoms, such as frequent transient ischemic attacks [36]. However, surgical treatment is recommended as soon as possible, regardless of the severity of clinical symptoms [4]. In young children, especially those below 3–5 years of age, disease progression is often very rapid and infarction is very frequent initial manifestation, compared with older children; thus, the RV procedure should be considered on an emergency basis to avoid infarction [37]. This may be because of the high cerebral metabolic rate of oxygen coupled with high CBF in the young developing brain [38].

A hemodynamic metabolic study using ^{15}O-PET in MMD recommended good timing of RV (good candidates for bypass surgery) in patients who have no clinical signs of infarction and demonstrate a decreased rCBF, increased regional oxygen extraction fraction (rOEF), and regional cerebral blood volume (rCBV) without any regional cerebral metabolic rate for oxygen ($rCMRO_2$) changes [39].

Asymptomatic MMD is mostly treated surgically when symptomatic ischemic attacks appear with hemodynamic compromise (decreased vascular reserve on Diamox-challenge single photon emission computed tomography study). However, early diagnosis and RV procedures over as wide an area as possible may be essential to improve intellectual outcome [40].

In typical bilateral MMD, RV is usually conducted on the clinically more symptomatic hemisphere first. If there are no lateralizing signs or symptoms, the dominant hemisphere is usually selected as the first side on which to conduct surgery to prevent possible damage of speech and dominant extremity [4, 23]. However, one large study series favoring the direct

RV procedure, even in young children, recommended conducting the first RV on the non-dominant side because of an increased incidence of transient neurological episodes after surgery in the dominant hemisphere [7].

Comparison of the Outcomes of Various Revascularization Procedures

Most comparative studies on the outcomes of different RV procedures have been conducted in small series and without aged-matched controls or randomization [14, 15, 27, 29].

Literature reviews of the outcomes of surgical intervention for MMD are summarized in Table 1.

Comparison of Outcomes Among Indirect Procedures

There are too many indirect RV procedures to compare every procedure for outcomes, and so only a few early representative comparison studies of small patient numbers are presented here.

EDAS and EMS were compared in seven patients who received EDAS in one hemisphere and EMS in the other hemisphere. The results showed much more RV in the EDAS-treated side than the EMS-treated side on postoperative angiograms and rCBF studies. This study concluded that the EDAS procedure is superior to that of EMS for pediatric MMD [41].

A comparison of EDAS alone and EDAS plus bifrontal EGPS showed significantly better angiographic, hemodynamic, and ACA symptomatic results with multiple indirect procedures than with the single indirect procedure. Incidence of perioperative infarction and overall clinical outcomes were not significantly different between the two procedures [23].

EDAS was compared with EDAMS/EMS in angiographic RV, which consisted of 11 pediatric patients with MMD treated with EDAS (16 sides in 10 patients), EDAMS (5 sides in 4 patients), and EMS (1 side). These patients were followed for more than 8.3 years. The findings revealed that EDAS showed grade A in 12 of 13 sides (92%) and grade B in 1 of 13 sides (8%) using Matsushima's angiographic RV grading. EMS (1 side) or EDAMS (5 sides in 4 patients) showed well-developed RV in 3 out of 6 sides (50%), and the other 3 sides revealed poor collateral formation, which were markedly large infarct areas. It was concluded that EDAS might indicate a therapeutic alternative for the surgical treatment of pediatric MMD [9]. Infarction sites show poor RV in general, regardless of what procedure is used; therefore, direct comparison between EDAS and EDAMS requires the premise of the same preoperative clinical and angiographic types and stages of patient groups.

In indirect procedures, when the ischemic cortices are more widespread, multiple combined indirect surgeries may achieve a more extensive area of angiographic RV than a single indirect procedure. However, the adequate amount of RV required for ischemic areas is not known, and the angiographic RV is not accurately correlated with symptomatic improvement. In addition, variable indirect procedures show good symptomatic improvement after surgery even if the angiographic RV is different. An important point to clarify is the difference in the degree of angiographic RV and its effects on long-term cognitive function as well as on quality of life of the patient.

Table 1 Literature review of studies on outcomes of surgery for moyamoya disease

Author and Year	Intervention	Age	No of patients (no. of hemispheres)	F/U	Outcome
Matsushima et al. 1981 [19]	EDAS	Ped	65	6.4 y	No TIAs (74% within 1 y; 97% within 2 y)
					Preop IQ=83.6±30.0, Postop IQ=85.0±31.8
Matsushima et al. 1992 [14]	STA–MCA+EMS	Ped	13	NA	Combined: no TIA (all), better than EDAS;
	EDAS		7		EDAS: no TIA in 23%
Karasawa et al. 1992 [3]	STA–MCA+EMS	Ped	104	9.6 y	Clin: complete recovery (45%), marked improv (38%), slight improv (12%)
				(4.8–16.0)	Angio RV: excellent filling (63.3%), good filling (36.7%), normal IQ in 63.5%
					<Age 3 y: worst prognosis
Kinugasa et al. 1993 [20]	EDAMS	Ped	17	3.2 y	Clin: E(8),G(5),F(3),P(1)
Mizoi et al. 1996 [27]	STA–MCA+EMS	Ped (7)	7 (13)	3.4 y	Clin: E (all 23)
	±EDAS	Adult (16)	16 (28)		RV: good to mod Coll in all IR (ped); RV: high and med Coll In all DR (adult)
					Over age 30y; age-dependent RV
Ishikawa et al. 1997 [15]	STA–MCA+EDAMS(48)	Ped	34 (64)	6.6 y	Clin: periop ischemia (≤2 weeks) 13 vs 31% (NS)
	vs EDAMS alone (16)				Postop ischemia (>2 weeks) 10 vs 56% ($p<0.01$)
Suzuki et al. 1997 [4]	STA–MCA (or EDAS<5y)	Ped	36	–	TIAs completely disappeared in 81% within one year
	+EDAS+EMS+F. burr holes				All patients improved, STA–MCA patency=96%
Miyamoto et al. 1998 [44]	STA–MCA±EMS	–	113	14.4±5.8 y	Complete cessation of ischemic episodes in 97% within one year
				(3–24 y)	Independent ADL in 88.5%
Golby et al. 1999 [6]	STA–MCA; STA–MCA+EDAS	Ped	12 (21)	35 m (12–65 m)	No periop strokes, global reduction in preop Sx and improved CBF

(continued)

Table 1 (continued)

Author and Year	Intervention	Age	No of patients (no. of hemispheres)			F/U	Outcome		
	or MMA–MCA + EDAS								
Houkin et al. 2000 [16]	STA–MCA; or EDAMS alone	Ped	(34)			–	DR (28): patency = 53% at 3 m + postop angio; Indirect (6) RV in >90%		
		Adult	(22)			–	DR (22): patency in 17/18 sides angio (94%)		
Isono et al. 2002 [9]	EDAS	Ped	10 (16)			>100 m	EDAS, RV in 12/13 (92%) sides		
	EDAMS		4 (5)				EDAMS/EMS, RV in 3/6 (50%) sides		
	EMS		(1)						
Kim et al. 2002 [23]	EDAS alone; or	Ped	67/92			45 m	EDAS + biF EGPS compared w/ EDAS		
	EDAS + biF. EGPS		159 (314)			22 m	Led to more favorable outconmes (62 vs 36%, $p < 0.003$), RV (79 vs 16%) and hemodynamic improv on d-SPECT (70 vs 52%, <0.002)		
Scott et al. 2004 [45]	EDAS (pial synangiosis)	Ped	126			Median 4.7 y	5.6% late-onset ischemic attaks		
						Mean 5.1 y	94.4% ischemia free		
							RV: Gr A (65%), Gr B (25%), Gr C (10%), 11 strokes and 3 severe TIAs within 30 days after surgery		
Fung et al. 2005 [2]			Clin	Angio	QoL		Clinical Sx aSx/improv	Angio RV Good/Poor	QoL Indep/Partial dep
	Indirect vs	Ped	699	864	204		57/30%	83/17%	70/22%
	Direct vs	Ped	9	7	–		11/56%	86/14%	–
	Combined procedure	Ped	56	101	35		43/43%	96/4%	74/23%
	Overall comparison (Literature Review)	Ped	1156	1005	272		51/36%	85/13%	69/23%
Guzman et al. 2008 [7]	STA–MCA first choice	Ped	96(168)			4.9 y	TIA free in 82.5% at one month		
	If inadequate, indirect RV	Adult	233(389)				In 91.8% at 1y and over+		

					Overall mortality = 2.3% Postop ischemic stroke = 5.5% 71.2% significant improv in mRS (0.83) Anastomotic patency = 99%
Starke et al. 2009 [10]	EDAS alone 19 unilateral 24 bilateral	Adult	43	41 m (4–126 m)	Angio RV (+) in 98% Inc perfusion on SPECT in 82% Periop infarction (<48 h) in 3% of sides 88% improv or preserved mRS 5y infarction free survival: 94% in op; <36% in nonop
Narisawa et al. 2009 [34]	STA–MCA vs	Adult	49(63)	–	No cerebrovasc event since RV surg
	No surgery	Adult	15(27)	–	
	Conservative F/U		(48)	–	4(6)/(47): 12.8% hemispheres progressive steno-occlusion (RV surgery done)

EDAS encephaloduroarteriosynangiosis; *EMS* encephalomyosynangiosis; *STA–MCA* superficial temoral artey-middle meningeal artery anastomosis; *EDAMS* encephaloduroarteriomyosynangiosis; *EGPS* encephalogaleoperiosteal synangiosis; *MMA–MCA* middle meningeal artery-middle cerebral artery anastomosis, improve improvement or improved; *F/U* follow up, *Ped* pediatric, *Clin* clinical, *angio* angiographic; *TIA* transient ischemic attack; *y* year; *m* month; *h* hour; *periop* perioperative; *preop* preoperative; *postop* postoperative; *op* operation; *nonop* nonoperation; *E* excellent (grade); *G* good; *F* fair; *P* poor(grade); *inc* increased; *Coll* collateralization; *IQ* intelligence quotient; *F* frontal; *biF* bifrontal; *NS* not significant (statistically); *vs* versus; *Sx* symptom; *aSx* asymptomatic; *CBF* cerebral blood flow; *QoL* quality of life; *indep* independent; *dep* dependent; *med* medium; *d-SPECT* diamox SPECT, *ADL* activity of daily living; *mRS* modified Rankin Scale; *IR* indirect revascularization; *DR* direct revascularization; *RV* revascularization (Gr A more than 2/3 of MCA distribution, Gr B between 1/3 and 2/3 of MCA distribution; *Gr* C less than 1/3 of MCA distribution); *cerebrovasc* cerebrovascular; *surg* surgery

Comparison of Outcomes Between Indirect and Combined Procedures

A comparison between EDAS and STA–MCA anastomosis plus EMS showed that better collateral formation and clinical improvement occurred in children treated with STA–MCA anastomosis plus EMS [14]. A comparison of STA–MCA anastomosis plus EDAMS (48 sides) and EDAMS (16 sides) showed that perioperative ischemic events (≤2 weeks after surgery) were 13 and 31%, respectively (p = NS); however, postoperative ischemic events (>2 weeks after surgery) were significantly reduced in the combined group (10%) compared with the indirect group (56%; $p < 0.01$) in pediatric MMD [15].

Age-dependent differences in angiographic RV for different procedures were confirmed in one study. A total of 23 patients (7 children, 16 adults) were treated with STA–MCA plus indirect bypass (mostly EMS), and each patient was analyzed for the degree of RV of the STA–MCA and EMS in relation to age. In children (<20 years of age), indirect bypass (EMS) was superior to direct bypass for angiographic RV: 64% of patients were classified as "good," 36% as "moderate," and none as "poor." In adults, direct bypass was superior to the indirect procedure for angiographic RV results. Thus, age-dependent RV was shown; below 30 years of age showed better angiographic RV for the indirect procedure compared with the direct bypass. Clinical outcomes were excellent in children and adults during the mean follow-up of 3.4 years (range 1–6 years) [27]. Outcome comparisons among 24 pediatric patients with MMD were performed. EDAS was given on 16 sides in 12 patients, EDAMS on 8 sides in 5 patients, and combined STA–MCA and EDAMS on 12 sides in 7 patients. Angiographic RV was superior in EDAMS and the combined group than in EDAS alone; however, clinical outcomes were not statistically different in these modalities of surgery [17].

In a literature review of 57 studies (1,148 patients, 2,218 hemispheres), indirect procedures, direct procedures, and combined procedures were applied in 73, 4, and 23% of patients, respectively. This review revealed that clinical outcomes were "asymptomatic" in 57, 11 (one of nine patients), and 43%, respectively, and "improvement" occurred in 30, 56, and 43%, respectively. Postoperative angiographic RV showed collateralization of more than one-third of the MCA territory (good collateralization) in 83% of the indirect procedures (including in six of seven direct procedures) and in 96% of combined procedures. When the indirect-procedure group was compared with pooled data from the direct- and combined-procedure groups, good collateralization was seen significantly more often in the direct- and combined-procedure groups. However, there was no statistically significant difference in the rate of good clinical outcomes between the three different techniques [2].

Selection of Surgical Procedure

Direct, indirect, and combined direct and indirect RVs are three basic operative procedures for MMD and MMS. Many modifications of indirect RV procedures have been developed for pediatric MMD. The main goal for the extensive modification of the conventional indirect RV procedure is to attain a larger extent of angiographic RV and improved hemodynamic perfusion reserve, as well as symptomatic improvement. However, postoperative hemodynamic studies show that the degree of preoperative hemodynamic compromise is correlated with the postoperative extent of RV, CBF, and hemodynamic reserve [42]. This means that the area of normal vascular perfusion reserve does not form collateral channels, regardless of the extent of the procedure.

In pediatric MMD, a larger extent of angiographic RV may be accomplished by wider coverage of the ischemic brain surface with multiple donor tissues containing blood vessels. However, we do not know exactly how much and which donor tissue is adequate for the preoperative hemodynamically compromised brain. Accordingly, multiple combined indirect procedures, multiple EDAS, pan-synangiosis, and multiple burr holes covering whole bilateral hemispheres have been tried with success in pediatric MMD [24, 25, 30, 31]. Furthermore, a novel combined procedure using STA, dura mater, temporal muscle, and the pericranial flap as donor tissues for indirect bypass, called encephalo-duro-myo-arterio-pericranial synangiosis (EDMAPS) has been developed, and single or double STA–MCA anastomosis plus EDMAPS have been applied for over 10 years in 58 patients, with extensively improved cerebral hemodynamics as well as no ischemic or hemorrhagic strokes [43]. The main reason for this complex combined procedure is to take maximal advantage of direct and indirect procedures. It is also based on the fact that completed stroke and small craniotomy surgery are independent poor intellectual outcome factors in pediatric MMD on multivariate analysis [40]. It is questionable whether this complex combined procedure is indicated for all patients with MMD. Selection criteria for an appropriate surgical procedure should include efficacy factors for angiographic RV, risk factors of complications, and the goal of improved quality of life.

Coverage of the ischemic brain surface of ACA and MCA territories with multiple donor tissues is necessary, because both territories are involved simultaneously in MMD, and because of symptomatic improvement of ACA territory ischemia in addition to the improvement of MCA ischemia [23]. We do know the benefits of ACA RV on recovery of cognitive function. However, we do not know the effect of a postoperative chronic low-perfusion state without symptoms on long-term brain function, particularly on cognitive function.

In general, it has been shown that indirect techniques are less effective in the elderly population, possibly because of age-associated reduction in angiogenic capability, and the degree of RV has not been shown to definitively correlate with clinical outcome. Currently, there are no clear data to support direct or indirect RV techniques in pediatric populations with MMD [13].

In adult patients with MMD, the direct (STA–MCA) bypass procedure plus the indirect procedure is the preferred technique; however, surgery for hemorrhagic MMD remains controversial, and it is inconclusive whether surgery will prevent future rebleedings or not. In contrast, a study showed comparable clinical and angiographic outcomes by EDAS alone in adult patients with MMD [10].

Conclusion

The surgical management of MMD is effective in improving the clinical symptoms, angiographic RV, and hemodynamic perfusion reserve with resultant functional improvement. The selection of a surgical procedure for MMD depends on a patient's age of onset, extent of hemodynamic compromise, anatomic characteristics of donor/recipient arteries, and the surgeon's preference. The multiple combined indirect procedure in younger children or the combined direct and indirect procedure in older children are good treatment options for clinical symptomatic improvement and good long-term outcomes. The direct procedure with or without additional indirect bypass is the primary option for adults with MMD; however, for hemorrhagic MMD, the beneficial effect of surgery to prevent further bleeding remains controversial. A uniform standardized evaluation protocol is needed for exact long-term outcome analysis and comparison between the various procedures. In this regard, international cooperative networks are required.

References

1. Yoshida YK, Shirane R (2001) Indirect bypass procedure. In: Ikezaki K, Loftus CM (eds) Moyamoya disease. AANS Publication Committee, Rolling Meadows
2. Fung LW, Thompson D, Ganesan V (2005) Revascularization surgery for pediatric moyamoya: a review of the literature. Childs Nerv Syst 21:358–364
3. Karasawa J, Touho H, Ohnishi H et al (1992) Long-term follow-up study after extracranial-intracranial bypass surgery for anterior circulation ischemia in childhood moyamoya disease. J Neurosurg 77:84–89
4. Suzuki Y, Negoro M, Shibuya M et al (1997) Surgical treatment for pediatric moyamoya disease: use of the superficial temporal artery for both areas supplied by the anterior and middle cerebral arteries. Neurosurgery 40:324–330
5. Houkin K, Ishikawa T, Yoshimoto T et al (1997) Direct and indirect revascularization for moyamoya disease surgical techniques and peri-operative complications. Clin Neurol Neurosurg 99:S142–S145
6. Golby AJ, Marks MP, Thompson RC et al (1999) Direct and combined revascularization in pediatric moyamoya disease. Neurosurgery 45:50–60
7. Guzman R, Lee M, Achrol A et al (2009) Clinical outcome after 450 revascularization procedures for moymoy disease. J Neurosurg, doi: 10.3171/2009.4.JNS081649
8. Scott RM (1997) Comments in article of Suzuki Y. et al [4]
9. Isono M, Ishii K, Kamida T et al (2002) Long-term outcomes of pediatric moyamoya disease treated by encephalo-duro-arterio-synangiosis (EDAS). Pediatr Neurosurg 36:14–21
10. Starke RM, Komotar RJ, Hickman ZL et al (2009) Clinical features, surgical treatment, and long-term outcome in adult patients with moyamoya disease. J Neurosurg, DOI:10.3171/2009.3.JNS08837
11. Fujimura M, Kaneta T, Mugikura S et al (2007) Temporary neurologic deterioration due to cerebral hyperperfusion after superficial temporal artery-middle cerebral artery anastomosis in patients with adult-onset moyamoya disease. Surg Neurol 67(3):273–282
12. Kim JE, Oh CW, Kwon OK et al (2008) Transient hyperperfusion after superficial temporal artery/middle cerebral artery bypass as a possible cause of postoperative transient neurological deterioration. Cerebrovasc Dis 25:580–586
13. Veeravagu A, Guzman R, Path CG et al (2008) Moyamoya disease in pediatric patients: outcomes of neurosurgical interventions. Neurosurg Focus 24(2):1–9
14. Matsushima T, Inoue T, Suzuki SO et al (1992) Surgical treatment of moyamoya disease in pediatric patients-comparison the results of indirect and direct revascularization procedures. Neurosurgery 31:401–405
15. Ishikawa T, Houkin K, Kamiyama H et al (1997) Effects of surgical revascularization on outcome of patients with pediatric moyamoya disease. Stroke 27:1170–1173
16. Houkin K, Kuroda S, Ishikawa T et al (2000) Neovascularization(Angiogenesis) after revascularization in moyamoya disease. Which technique is most useful for moyamoya disease? Acta Neurochir (Wien) 142:269–276
17. Kim DS, Kang SG, Yoo DS et al (2007) Surgical results in pediatric moyamoya disease: Angiographic revascularization and clinical results. Clin Neurol Neurosurg 109:125–131
18. Han DH, Nam DH, Oh CW (1997) Moyamoya disease in adults: characteristics of clinical presentation and outcome after encephalo-duro-arterio-synangiosis. Clin Neurol Neurosurg 99(Suppl 2):S151–S155

19. Matsushima Y, Fukai N, Tanaka K et al (1981) A new surgical treatment of moyamoya disease in children: a preliminary report. Surg Neurol 15:313–320
20. Kinugasa K, Mandai S, Kamata I et al (1993) Surgical treatment of moyamoya disease: operative technique for encephalo-duro-arterio-myo-synangiosis, its follow-up, clinical results, and angiograms. Neurosurgery 50:88–96
21. Ikezaki K (2000) Rational approach to treatment of moyamoya disease in childhood. J Child Neurol 15:350–356
22. Karasawa J, Kikudhi H, Furuse S et al (1977) A surgical treatment of "moyamoya" disease "encephalo-myo-synangiosis". Neurol Med Chir 17:29–37
23. Kim SK, Wang KC, Kim IO et al (2002) Combined encephaloduroarteriosynangiosis and bifrontal encephalogaleo(periosteal)synangiosis in pediatric moyamoya disease. Neurosurgery 50:88–96
24. Matsushima T, Inoue T, Katsuta T et al (1998) An indirect revascularization method in the surgical treatment of moyamoya disease: various kinds of indirect procedure and a multiple combined indirect procedure. Neurol Med Chir(Tokyo) 38(Suppl):297–302
25. Ishikawa T, Kamiyama H, Kuroda S et al (2006) Simultaneous superficial temporal artery to middle cerebral or anterior cerebral bypass with pan-synangiosis for moyamoya disease covering both anterior and middle cerebral artery territories. Technical note. Neurol Med Chir(Tokyo) 46:462–468
26. Scott RM (2000) Moyamoya syndrome: a surgically treatable cause of stroke in pediatric patient. Clin Neurosurg 47:378–384
27. Mizoi K, Kayama T, Yoshimoto T et al (1996) Indirect revascularization for moyamoya disease: is there a beneficial effect for adult patients? Surg Neurol 45:541–549
28. Kinugasa K, Mandai S, Tokunaga K et al (1994) Ribbon encephalo-duro-arterio-myo-synangiosis for moyamoya disease. Surg Neurol 41:455–461
29. Nakashima H, Meguro T, Kawada S et al (1997) Long-term results of surgically treated moyamoya disease. Clin Neurol Neurosurg 99(Suppl 2):156–161
30. Tenjin H, Ueda S (1997) Multiple EDAS, additional EDAS using the frontal branch of the STA and the occipital artery for pediatric moyamoya patients in whom EDAS using the parietal branch of STA was insufficient. Child's Nerv Syst 13:220–224
31. Sainte-Rose C, Oliveira R, Puget S et al (2006) Multiple bur hole surgery for the treatment of moyamoya disease in children. J Neurosurg 105(Suppl 6):437–443
32. Braun KPJ, Bulder MMM, Chabrier S et al (2009) The course and outcome of unilateral intracranial arteriopathy in 79 children with ischemic stroke. Brain 132:544–557
33. Kelly ME, Bell-Stephens TE, Mark MP et al (2006) Progression of unilateral moyamoya disease: A clinical series. Cerebrov Dis 22:109–115
34. Narisawa A, Fujimura M, Tominaga T (2009) Efficacy of the revascularization surgery for adult-onset moyamoya disease with the progression of cerebrovascular lesions. Clin Neurol Neurosurg 111(2):123–126
35. Matsushima Y, Aoyagi M, Masaoka H et al (1990) Mental outcome following encephaloduroarterio-synangiosis in children with moyamoya disease with the onset earlier than 5 years of age. Childs Nerv Syst 6(8):440–443
36. Nagata S, Matsushima T, Morioka T et al (2006) Unilaterally symptomatic moyamoya disease in children: long-term following of 20 patients. Neurosurgery 59(4):830–836
37. Kim SK, Seol HJ, Cho BK et al (2004) Moyamoya disease among young patients: its aggressive clinical course and the role of active surgical treatment. Neurosurgery 54:840–844; discussion 844–846
38. Ogawa A, Yoshimoto T, Suzuki J et al (1990) Cerebral blood flow in moyamoya disease Part 1: Correlation with age and regional distribution. Acta Neurochir (Wien) 105:30–34
39. Ikezaki K, Matsushima T, Kuwabara Y et al (1994) Cerebral circulation and oxygen metabolism in childhood moyamoya disease: a perioperative positron emission tomography study. J Neurosurg 81:843–850
40. Kuroda S, Houkin K, Ishikawa T et al (2004) Determinants of intellectual outcome after surgical revascularization in pediatric moyamoya disease: a multivariate analysis. Childs Nerv Syst 20(5):302–308
41. Fujita K, Tamaki N, Matsumoto S (1986) Surgical treatment of moyamoya disease in children: which is more effective procedure, EDAS or EMS? Childs Nerv Syst 2:134–138

42. Nariai T, Suzuki R, Matsushima Y et al (1994) Surgically induced angiogenesis to compensate for hemodynamic cerebral ischemia. Stroke 25:1014–1021
43. Kuroda S, Houkin K (2008) Moyamoya disease: current concepts and future prospective. Lancet Neurol 7:1056–1066
44. Miyamoto S, Akiyama Y, Nagata I et al (1998) Long-term outcome after STA–MCA anastomosis for moyamoya disease. Neurosurg Focus 5(5):Article 5
45. Scott RM, Smith JL, Robertson RL et al (2004) Long-term outcome in children with moyamoya syndrome after cranial revascularization by pial synangiosis. J Neurosurg 100(2 Suppl Pediatrics):142–149

Risk Factors for Complication

Miki Fujimura and Teiji Tominaga

Introduction

Surgical revascularization for moyamoya disease prevents cerebral ischemic attacks by improving cerebral blood flow (CBF), and superficial temporal artery (STA)-middle cerebral artery (MCA) anastomosis and/or indirect pial synangiosis such as encephalo-myo-synangiosis (EMS) are generally accepted as the optimal surgical treatment for moyamoya disease [1–3]. Despite their favorable long-term outcome, perioperative cerebral ischemia and cerebral hyperperfusion are potential complications of these procedures [1, 4–6]. Patients with moyamoya disease are known to suffer from transient neurological deterioration in the acute stage after surgical revascularization at a substantial rate, and cerebral ischemia has been considered as the major reason for this deterioration [7]. Recent investigations of the time-sequential cerebral hemodynamics in the acute stage after revascularization surgery for moyamoya disease, however, revealed that cerebral hyperperfusion as well as cerebral ischemia could result in transient neurologic deterioration after surgical revascularization [4–6]. In this chapter, the author seeks to focus on perioperative cerebral ischemia and cerebral hyperperfusion as potential complications, and discuss their risk factors. Prediction and accurate diagnosis of these pathologies is clinically important because the management of each of these conditions is contradictory.

Perioperative Cerebral Ischemia

Ischemic complication can be due to the intraoperative hypotention, hyper/hypo-capnea, perioperative anemia, and dehydration [1, 7]. Patients of younger age and with preoperative frequent transient ischemic attack (TIA) or progressing stroke, or significant bilateral

M. Fujimura (✉)
Department of Neurosurgery, Kohnan Hospital, 4-20-1 Nagamachi-minami, Taihaku-ku, Sendai, 982-8523, Japan
e-mail: fujimur@kohnan-sendai.or.jp

T. Tominaga
Department of Neurosurgery, Tohoku University Graduate School of Medicine, Sendai, Japan

B.-K. Cho and T. Tominaga (eds.), *Moyamoya Disease Update*,
DOI 10.1007/978-4-431-99703-0_38, © Springer 2010

hemodynamic compromise are considered to have a higher risk of perioperative ischemic complication. To avoid this complication, we precede revascularization surgery on the hemisphere with more significant hemodynamic compromise, or operate on the dominant hemisphere. Indirect pial synangiosis has been reported to have substantial risk for cerebral ischemia owing to compression of the brain by swollen temporal muscle used for EMS [8, 9]. A 26-year-old woman, who had been suffering TIA, underwent STA-MCA anastomosis with EMS. The *N*-isopropyl-*p*-[^{123}I]iodoamphetamine single-photon emission computed tomography (^{123}I-IMP-SPECT) 1 day after surgery demonstrated an improvement of CBF on the operated hemisphere (Fig. 1a), but she suffered fluctuating aphasia 2 days later when CT scan revealed marked swelling of the temporal muscle used for EMS (arrow in Fig. 1b). The ^{123}I-IMP-SPECT 4 days after surgery showed significant decrease in CBF by compression of the brain (arrows in Fig. 1b). We then performed revision of EMS for decompression, which resolved her symptoms. The CBF normalized 7 days after surgery (Fig. 1c). These results indicate that surgical revascularization including EMS has a substantial risk for cerebral ischemia owing to compression of the brain by temporal muscle swelling [9].

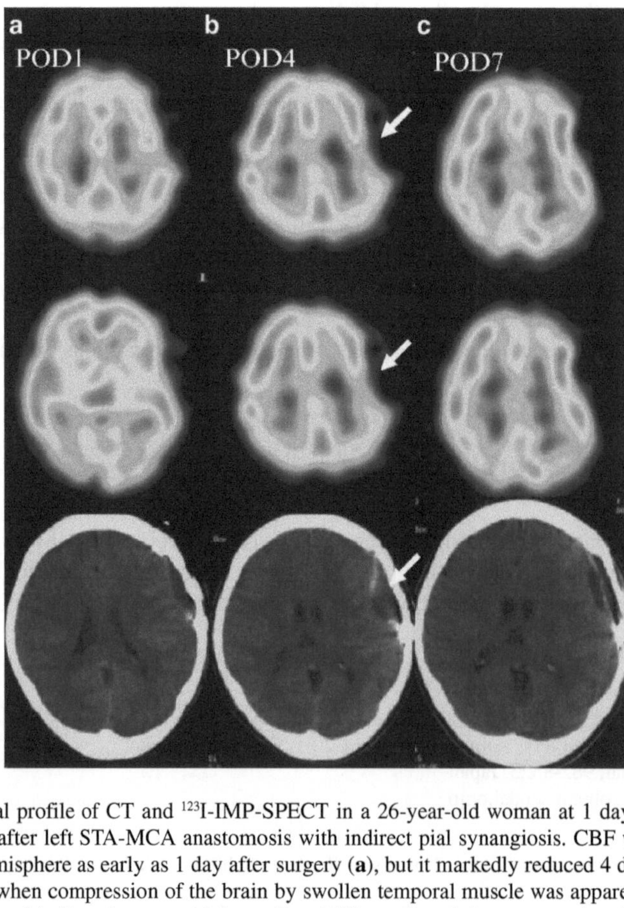

Fig. 1 Temporal profile of CT and ^{123}I-IMP-SPECT in a 26-year-old woman at 1 day (**a**), 4 days (**b**), and 1 week (**c**) after left STA-MCA anastomosis with indirect pial synangiosis. CBF was increased on the operated hemisphere as early as 1 day after surgery (**a**), but it markedly reduced 4 days after surgery (*arrows* in (**b**)) when compression of the brain by swollen temporal muscle was apparent by CT (*arrow* in (**b**)). Revision of indirect bypass with bone flap drilling relieved the compression (**c**), and CBF was significantly increased after decompression (**c**)

Cerebral Hyperperfusion

Recent evidence supports not only cerebral ischemia but symptomatic cerebral hyperperfusion as a potential complication of STA-MCA anastomosis for moyamoya disease [4–6]. Based on our recent results of postoperative CBF measurement by ^{123}I-IMP-SPECT in the acute stage after STA-MCA (M4) anastomosis, the patients with moyamoya disease showed significantly higher risk for symptomatic cerebral hyperperfusion compared to other patients with steno-occlusive cerebrovascular diseases such as atherosclerotic carotid artery occlusion (Table 1). Accurate and early diagnosis of postoperative cerebral hyperperfusion is clinically important because its treatment is contradictory to that for ischemia [4, 6]. A 55-year-old woman, presenting with right putaminal hemorrhage, underwent bilateral STA-MCA anastomosis with EMS. She suffered from dysarthria and numbness on her left hand from 7 to 15 days after successful revascularization surgery on the right hemisphere. Time-sequential ^{123}I-IMP-SPECT before and after surgery revealed focal intense increase in CBF at the site of the anastomosis 6 days after surgery (arrow in Fig. 2c), suggesting cerebral hyperperfusion. Postoperative magnetic resonance imaging showed no evidence of ischemic change, and magnetic resonance angiography demonstrated the thick high signal of

Table 1 Incidence of symptomatic cerebral hyperperfusion after STA-MCA (M4) anastomosis: prospective study using ^{123}I-IMP-SPECT in the acute stage

	Moyamoya disease	Others
Number of operated hemispheres (number of patients)	105 (73)	21 (21)
Age (mean)	2~67 (34.9)	12~67 (55.9)
Sex (M/F)	19/54	19/2
Symptomatic cerebral hyperperfusion	25 (24.8%)*	0 (0%)

*P=0.0105

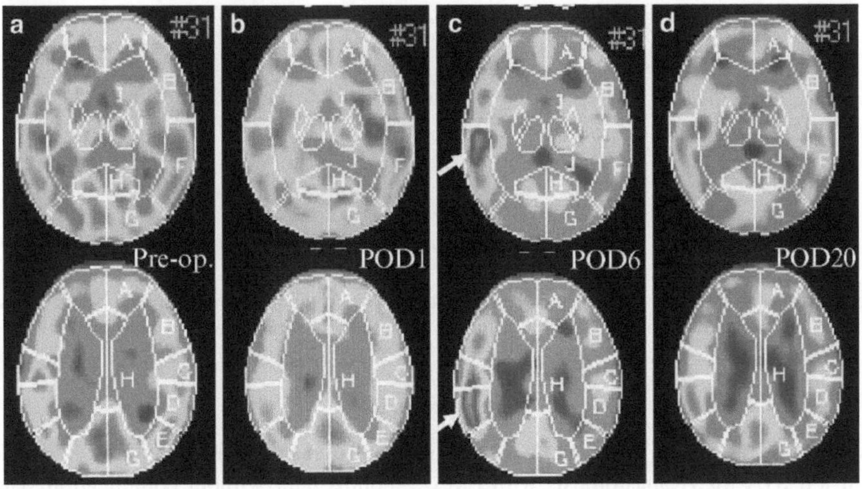

Fig. 2 Time-sequential ^{123}I-IMP-SPECT in a 55-year-old woman before (**a**) and after surgery (**b**–**d**) revealed focal intense increase in CBF at the site of the anastomosis 6 days after surgery (*arrows* in (**c**)), which normalized at postoperative day 20 (**d**)

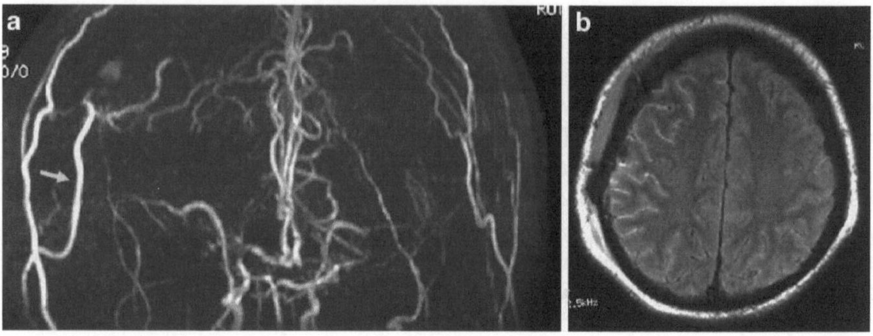

Fig. 3 Postoperative MRI demonstrating no evidence of ischemic change, and magnetic resonance angiography demonstrated the thick high signal of ipsilateral STA

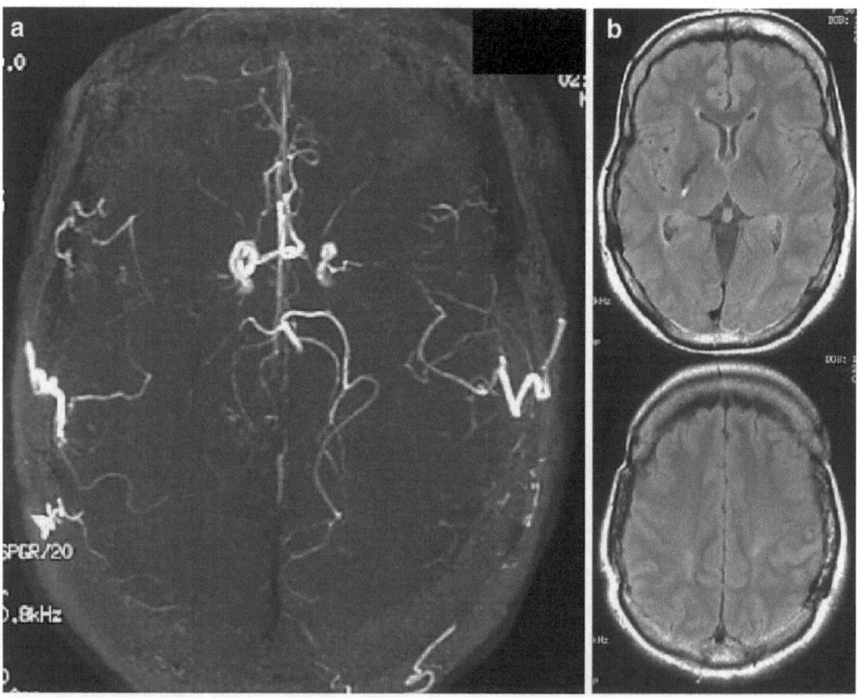

Fig. 4 MRA (**a**) and fluid attenuated inversion recovery (**b**) 4 years after bilateral STA-MCA bypasses demonstrating apparently patent STA-MCA bypass without cortical damage

ipsilateral STA (Fig. 3). Intensive blood pressure control relieved her symptoms. She underwent left STA-MCA anastomosis with EMS 2 months later without complication. There was no cerebrovascular event during the follow-up period of 4 years. Bilateral STA-MCA bypasses were apparently patent 4 years after surgery, and there was no delayed cortical damage (Fig. 4). Based on our data from prospective performance of postoperative CBF

Table 2 Correlation between each factor and symptomatic hyperperfusion in moyamoya disease

	χ^2 value	*P* value
Age	6.1919	0.0128*
Adult-onset (16 years old or older)		
Sex	1.3444	0.2462
Onset-type		
Hemorrhage	4.9079	0.0267*
Cerebral infarction	0.8868	0.3463

$^*p<0.05$

measurement in the acute stage, the incidence of symptomatic cerebral hyperperfusion was as high as 27.5% in moyamoya disease, including mild focal neurologic deficit, among 80 consecutive surgeries [6]. Final outcomes of these patients were favorable with intensive blood pressure control, while one patient manifested an intracerebral hemorrhage due to hyperperfusion [10].

Risk Factors for Cerebral Hyperperfusion Syndrome

Risk factors for cerebral hyperperfusion syndrome after carotid endarterectomy has been well described, while that after revascularization surgery for moyamoya disease has been described only in a single report [6]. Adult-onset ($P=0.013$) or hemorrhagic-onset patients ($P=0.027$) were shown to have significantly higher risk for symptomatic hyperperfusion (Table 2), while there was no difference in intraoperative temporary occlusion time [6]. The correlation between preoperative hemodynamic compromise and postoperative hyperperfusion is undetermined. Based on these findings, routine CBF measurement for adult-onset and/or hemorrhagic-onset patients is recommended, because the management of hyperperfusion is contradictory to that for ischemia. Alternatively, it would be of great value to develop intraoperative techniques to detect hyperperfusion. Using a novel infrared imaging system, the intraoperative monitoring of the brain surface tempreture has been attempted to predict postoperative cerebral hyperperfusion [11]. Temperature rise around the site of the anastomosis during surgery has been suggested as an indicator of postoperative hyperperfusion [11].

References

1. Houkin K, Ishikawa T, Yoshimoto T et al (1997) Direct and indirect revascularization for moyamoya disease: surgical techniques and peri-operative complications. Clin Neurol Neurosurg 99 (Suppl 2):S142–145
2. Okada Y, Shima T, Nishida M et al (1985) Effectiveness of superficial temporal artery-middle cerebral artery anastomosis in adult moyamoya disease: cerebral hemodynamics and clinical course in ischemic and hemorrhagic varieties. Stroke 29:625–630
3. Shirane R, Yoshida Y, Takahashi T et al (1997) Assessment of encephalo-galeo-myo-synangiosis with dural pedicle insertion in childhood moyamoya disease: characteristics of cerebral blood flow and oxygen metabolism. Clin Neurol Neurosurg 99 (Suppl 2):S79–85
4. Fujimura M, Kaneta T, Mugikura S et al (2007) Temporary neurologic deterioration due to cerebral hyperperfusion after superficial temporal artery-middle cerebral artery anastomosis in patients with adult-onset moyamoya disease. Surg Neurol 67:273–282

5. Kim JE, Oh CW, Kwon OK et al (2008) Transient hyperperfusion after superfisial temporal artery/ middle cerebral artery bypass surgery as a possible cause of postoperative transient neurological deterioration. Cerebrovasc Dis 25:580–586
6. Fujimura M, Mugikura S, Kaneta T et al (2009) Incidence and risk factors for symptomatic cerebral hyperperfusion following superficial temporal artery-middle cerebral artery anastomosis in patients with moyamoya disease. Surg Neurol 71:442–447
7. Sakamoto T, Kawaguchi M, Kurehara K et al (1997) Risk factors for neurologic deterioration after revascularization surgery in patients with moyamoya disease. Anesth Analg 85:1060–1065
8. Touho H (2007) Cerebral ischemia due to compression of the brain by and hypertrophied muscle used for encephalomyosynangiosis in childhood moyamoya disease. Surg Neurol [Epub ahead of print]
9. Fujimura M, Kaneta T, Shimizu H et al (2009) Cerebral ischemia owing to compression of the brain by swollen temporal muscle used for encephalo-myo-synangiosis in moyamoya disease. Neurosurg Rev 32:245–249
10. Fujimura M, Mugikura S, Shimizu H et al (2009) Delayed intracerebral hemorrhage after superficial temporal artery-middle cerebral artery anastomosis in a patient with moyamoya disease: possible involvement of cerebral hyperperfusion and increased vascular permeability. Surg Neurol 71:223–227
11. Nakagawa A, Fujimura M, Arafune T et al (2009) Clinical implications of intraoperative infrared brain surface monitoring during superficial temporal artery-middle cerebral artery anastomosis in patients with moyamoya disease. J Neurosurg [Epub ahead of print]

Cognition and Quality of Life

Satoshi Kuroda

Introduction

Moyamoya disease is an uncommon cerebrovascular disorder that is characterized by progressive stenosis of the supraclinoid internal carotid arteries (ICA) and its main branches within the circle of Willis. This occlusion results in the formation of a fine vascular network (the moyamoya vessels) at the base of the brain. Moyamoya vessels are dilated perforating arteries and function as collateral pathways. It is well known that pediatric patients with moyamoya disease often develop transient ischemic attacks (TIA) or cerebral infarction, while adult patients also suffer intracranial bleeding. Surgical revascularization such as superficial temporal artery to middle cerebral artery (STA-MCA) anastomosis and indirect bypass improves their cerebral hemodynamics and prevents further ischemic attacks [1]. With regard to stroke recurrence and activity of daily living (ADL), postoperative long-term outcome is favorable in both pediatric and adult patients [2–5]. However, it is also known that intellectual development is impaired in a certain subgroup of pediatric patients [6, 7]. Even after surgical revascularization, intellectual impairment has been reported to disturb an independent social life in more than 20% of the patients [3, 5, 8, 9]. In this chapter, the author reviews neuropsychological aspects in patients with moyamoya disease and discusses the strategies to improve their intellectual outcome.

Pediatric Patients

Based on previous reports, the natural course of intellectual outcome is poor in pediatric patients with moyamoya disease. Cognitive function is reported to decline within 5–10 years after the onset [10]. The older patients have a more marked reduction of intelligence quotient (IQ). Lower IQ is closely associated with cerebral blood flow reduction [11]. More than one-third of them

S. Kuroda (✉)
Department of Neurosurgery, Hokkaido University Graduate School of Medicine,
North 15 West 7, Kita-ku, Sapporo, 060-8638, Japan
e-mail: skuroda@med.hokudai.ac.jp

B.-K. Cho and T. Tominaga (eds.), *Moyamoya Disease Update*,
DOI 10.1007/978-4-431-99703-0_39, © Springer 2010

were poorly educated [6, 7]. Kurokawa et al. (1985) evaluated the natural course of pediatric patients with moyamoya disease, and reported that mild intellectual and/or motor impairment was observed in 26% of them, with special schools or care by parents/institutions in teenage years in 11%, and total 24-h care in 7% [7]. According to these studies, poor intellectual outcome was correlated with early onset, completed stroke (CS), or a longer diseased period [6, 7].

Surgical revascularization may improve cognitive function in pediatric patients with moyamoya disease. Thus, Ishii et al. (1984) reported that performance IQ markedly improved in ten patients, remained unchanged in three and deteriorated in two [11]. Bowen et al. (1998) have also reported gradual improvement of cognitive function after surgical revascularization in two pediatric patients with moyamoya disease [12]. Although surgical revascularization is known to resolve TIA and ischemic stroke very effectively, intellectual delay is still serious problem for a certain subgroup of pediatric patients and their families even after surgery. Thus, previous studies have clarified that about 10–30% of the patients had difficulties in social or school life because of intellectual impairment [3–5, 9, 13]. These reports have suggested that CS, cerebral infarction, and early onset (<5 years) may have significant effects on intellectual outcome. It has also been suggested that the procedures of surgical revascularization may have some influence on intellectual outcome [3]. Previously, however, significant predictors of poor intellectual outcome after surgery have not been fully analyzed.

Using a univariate analysis model, Matsushima et al. (1997) reported that there was no significant factor for intellectual outcome after encephalo-duro-arterio-synangiosis (EDAS) [13]. However, their study had some bias in their patient selection, because they excluded the patients with a Full Scale IQ below 70, and they did not perform a multivariate analysis probably because of the small sample size ($n=20$) [13]. Recently, Kuroda et al. (2004) assessed significant predictors for poor intellectual outcome in a total of 52 pediatric patients who underwent surgical revascularization, using multivariate analysis. They found that CS and "small craniotomy" surgery were independent predictors of poor intellectual outcome in pediatric patients with moyamoya disease. Odds ratios of each factor were 33.4 [95% confidential interval (CI), 2.4–474] and 19.6 (95% CI, 1.8–215), respectively [14]. In their study, contrary to previous reports, age of the onset, preoperative diseased period, and cerebral infarction were not significant factors. Most of the CS-type patients already had hemiparesis or tetraparesis before surgical revascularization, indicating that poor intellectual outcome is closely related to the impairment of motor function. Previous studies have clarified that the incidence of CS-type patients is very much higher in a subgroup of patients who develop ischemic attacks in very early childhood (<2 years) or who did not undergo surgical treatment for a long time [3, 7, 8, 15].

Kuroda et al. (2004) also showed that "small craniotomy" surgery was another independent predictor of poor intellectual outcome [14]. There were no reports that clearly defined the effect of surgical procedures on intellectual outcome. Indirect procedures such as EDAS and encephalo-myo-synangiosis (EMS) are very easy, and have been widely performed for patients with moyamoya disease [15]. However, one of the disadvantages is the fact that the revascularized area is limited and is confined to the craniotomy field after these procedures [16–18]. Previous reports have pointed out that, regardless of the disappearance of ischemic attacks, intellectual outcome was poor in a majority of the patients who underwent these procedures [17]. Thus, Sato et al. (1990) reported that intellectual outcome was poor in 9 of 13 children who underwent EMS or EDAS, although none of them suffered recurrent ischemic attacks. Using SPECT, they also showed that blood flow improved in a limited area around the surgical field, and that blood flow reduction was persistent in the frontal lobe even after EDAS or EMS [17]. It is not fully understood why the "small craniotomy" group was proved to be an independent predictor of poor intellectual outcome. However, a wide range of craniotomy and indirect synangiosis extending to the frontal region may play a crucial role in improving their intellectual outcome. In fact, Isobe et al. (1992) also measured blood flow and cerebrovascular reactivity after bypass surgery, and showed that there was a marked impairment in cerebral hemodynamics in the frontal lobe in the patients who underwent indirect synangiosis through "small craniotomy" [19]. On the other hand, STA-MCA anastomosis and EDAMS through "large craniotomy" can normalize rCBF distribution and cerebrovascular reactivity to acetazolamide in the frontal lobe [19, 20]. Furthermore, using cerebral angiography, Takahashi et al. (1994) reported that collateral development was confined to the parietal region in the patients who underwent "small craniotomy" surgery, whereas extensive collaterals were developed in the frontal, temporal, and parietal lobes in those who underwent "large craniotomy" surgery [18]. Ohtaki et al. (1998) also reported that deterioration of intellectual functions and quality of life (QOL) in pediatric moyamoya patients can be prevented by extensive omental transplantation spread over both frontal lobes combined with STA-MCA anastomosis [21].

Based on these results, therefore, it is essential to identify pediatric patients with moyamoya disease as early as possible and to surgically treat them through "large" craniotomy covering the frontal lobes in order to reduce the incidence of CS and to improve their intellectual outcome.

Adult Patients

There are few studies that denote the impact of moyamoya disease on cognitive function in adult patients. Bornstein et al. (1985) reported an adult case with moyamoya disease who had essentially normal performance on a wide range of neuropsychological tasks [22]. Cognitive function may be related to cerebral hemodynamics in each patient [23]. Very recently, Karzmark et al. (2008) evaluated the cognitive function in a total of 36 adult patients with moyamoya disease [24]. They identified cognitive impairment in 11 (31%) of the patients, of which a Full Scale IQ was less than 80 in 4 patients (11%). They concluded that adult moyamoya disease had a significant impact on cognition but that this effect is not severe or pervasive. However, clinical conditions of the subjects were unclear in their study. Further intense evaluations would be necessary to shed the light on cognitive function in adult moyamoya disease.

Conclusions

The impact of moyamoya disease on cognition is still unclear. Further clinical studies should be focused on a wide range of neuropsychological testing and cerebral blood flow and metabolism measurements in a large series.

References

1. Kuroda S, Houkin K (2008) Moyamoya disease: current concepts and future perspectives. Lancet Neurol 7:1056–1066
2. Houkin K, Kamiyama H, Takahashi A et al (1997) Combined revascularization surgery for childhood moyamoya disease: STA-MCA and encephalo-duro-arterio-myo-synangiosis. Childs Nerv Syst 13:24–29

3. Ishikawa T, Houkin K, Kamiyama H et al (1997) Effects of surgical revascularization on outcome of patients with pediatric moyamoya disease. Stroke 28:1170–1173
4. Karasawa J, Touho H, Ohnishi H et al (1992) Long-term follow-up study after extracranial-intracranial bypass surgery for anterior circulation ischemia in childhood moyamoya disease. J Neurosurg 77:84–89
5. Miyamoto S, Akiyama Y, Nagata I et al (1998) Long-term outcome after STA-MCA anastomosis for moyamoya disease. Neurosurg Focus 5:e5
6. Fukuyama Y, Umezu R (1985) Clinical and cerebral angiographic evolutions of idiopathic progressive occlusive disease of the circle of Willis ("moyamoya" disease) in children. Brain Dev 7:21–37
7. Kurokawa T, Tomita S, Ueda K et al (1985) Prognosis of occlusive disease of the circle of Willis (moyamoya disease) in children. Pediatr Neurol 1:274–277
8. Imaizumi T, Hayashi K, Saito K et al (1998) Long-term outcomes of pediatric moyamoya disease monitored to adulthood. Pediatr Neurol 18:321–325
9. Matsushima Y, Aoyagi M, Masaoka H et al (1990) Mental outcome following encephaloduroarteriosynangiosis in children with moyamoya disease with the onset earlier than 5 years of age. Childs Nerv Syst 6:440–443
10. Imaizumi C, Imaizumi T, Osawa M et al (1999) Serial intelligence test scores in pediatric moyamoya disease. Neuropediatrics 30:294–299
11. Ishii R, Takeuchi S, Ibayashi K et al (1984) Intelligence in children with moyamoya disease: evaluation after surgical treatments with special reference to changes in cerebral blood flow. Stroke 15:873–877
12. Bowen M, Marks MP, Steinberg GK (1998) Neuropsychological recovery from childhood moyamoya disease. Brain Dev 20:119–123
13. Matsushima Y, Aoyagi M, Nariai T et al (1997) Long-term intelligence outcome of post-encephalo-duro-arterio-synangiosis childhood moyamoya patients. Clin Neurol Neurosurg 99:S147–S150
14. Kuroda S, Houkin K, Ishikawa T et al (2004) Determinants of intellectual outcome after surgical revascularization in pediatric moyamoya disease: a multivariate analysis. Childs Nerv Syst 20:302–308
15. Fukui M (1997) Current state of study on moyamoya disease in Japan. Surg Neurol 47:138–143
16. Matsushima T, Inoue T, Suzuki S et al (1992) Surgical treatment of moyamoya disease in pediatric patients – comparison between the results of indirect and direct revascularization procedures. Neurosurgery 31:401–405
17. Sato H, Sato N, Tamaki N et al (1990) Chronic low-perfusion state in children with moyamoya disease following revascularization. Childs Nerv Syst 6:166–171
18. Takahashi A, Kamiyama H, Houkin K et al (1995) Surgical treatment of childhood moyamoya disease – comparison of reconstructive surgery centered on the frontal region and the parietal region. Neurol Med Chir (Tokyo) 35:231–237
19. Isobe M, Kuroda S, Kamiyama H et al (1992) Cerebral blood flow reactivity to hyperventilation in children with spontaneous occlusion of the circle of Willis (moyamoya disease). No Shinkei Geka 20:399–407
20. Kuroda S, Houkin K, Kamiyama H et al (1995) Regional cerebral hemodynamics in childhood moyamoya disease. Childs Nerv Syst 11:584–590
21. Ohtaki M, Uede T, Morimoto S et al (1998) Intellectual functions and regional cerebral haemodynamics after extensive omental transplantation spread over both frontal lobes in childhood moyamoya disease. Acta Neurochir (Wien) 140:1043–1053; discussion 1052–1053
22. Bornstein RA (1985) Neuropsychological performance in moya moya disease: a case study. Int J Neurosci 26:39–46
23. Jefferson AL, Glosser G, Detre JA et al (2006) Neuropsychological and perfusion MR imaging correlates of revascularization in a case of moyamoya syndrome. Am J Neuroradiol 27:98–100
24. Karzmark P, Zeifert PD, Tan S et al (2008) Effect of moyamoya disease on neuropsychological functioning in adults. Neurosurgery 62:1048–1051; discussion 1051–1052

Part XII
Special Consideration I

Overview: Issues in Young Children and Adults

Teiji Tominaga and Miki Fujimura

Introduction

Moyamoya disease is a chronic, occlusive cerebrovascular disease with unknown etiology which has two peaks in age distribution, a first peak in children and the second peak in young adults [1]. The most recent epidemiological national survey in Japan estimates that the annual number of the patients with moyamoya disease is 7,700 with the incidence rate of 5.4 per million populations, with the female/male ratio of 1.8:1 [2]. The peaks in age distribution of moyamoya disease consist of a first peak in children and the second peak in young adults. The incidence of patients with family history was 12.1% among definitive moyamoya patients [2]. In this chapter, the authors seek to overview the characteristics of moyamoya disease in children and young adults.

Common Genetic Background of Childhood and Adult-Onset Moyamoya Disease

It has been controversial whether childhood moyamoya disease and adult-onset moyamoya disease belong to the same entity, since their clinical presentations are distinct from each other. Recent advances in genetic analysis of moyamoya disease have given clues to answer this question. Although the etiology of moyamoya disease is still undetermined, increasing evidence from the genetic analysis of familial moyamoya disease suggests its linkage on chromosome 3p24-26, 8q23, 6q25, and 17q25 [3–5]. The most recent linkage analysis on familial cases of moyamoya disease indicates that there is a major gene locus for autosomal dominant moyamoya disease on chromosome 17q25.3 [6]. The common genetic characteristics

T. Tominaga (✉)
Department of Neurosurgery, Tohoku University Graduate School of Medicine,
1-1 Seiryo-machi, Aoba-ku, Sendai 980-8574, Japan
e-mail: tomi@nsg.med,tohoku.ac.jp

M. Fujimura
Department of Neurosurgery, Kohnan Hospital, Sendai, 982-8523, Japan

B.-K. Cho and T. Tominaga (eds.), *Moyamoya Disease Update*,
DOI 10.1007/978-4-431-99703-0_40, © Springer 2010

between pediatric and adult-onset moyamoya disease, or between definitive and unilateral moyamoya disease, strongly suggest that they could be classified into the same entity. Histopathological characteristics include multilayered eccentric intimal fibrous thickening and medial thinness of the major cerebral arteries both in pediatric and adult-onset moyamoya disease [7].

Clinical Presentation of Childhood and Adult-Onset Moyamoya Disease

Clinical presentation of moyamoya disease includes transient ischemic attack, cerebral infarction, intracerebral hemorrhage, seizure, and headache [8]. Transient ischemic attack is one of the most common clinical presentations of moyamoya disease both in pediatric and adult cases [8], while intracerebral hemorrhage is mostly seen among adult cases [9]. Children are known to present with ischemic symptoms including transient ischemic attack and cerebral infarction, while half the adult patients manifest as hemorrhage [8]. Patients with repeated hemorrhage, or with younger onset-age (2 years or younger), are shown to have poorer outcome [9]. The recent advance in noninvasive diagnostic modalities such as magnetic resonance (MR) imaging and MR angiography has led to the realization that the incidence of asymptomatic moyamoya disease, both in children and adults, could be higher than previously thought. The recent multicenter, nationwide, survey of asymptomatic moyamoya disease in Japan revealed that the annual risk for any stroke was 3.2% in asymptomatic patients with the disease [10].

Diagnosis

The definitive diagnosis of moyamoya disease can be made by the angiographic finding of bilateral steno-occlusive changes at the terminal portion of the internal carotid artery and an abnormal vascular network at the base of the brain [1]. Besides cerebral angiography, MR imaging is a useful noninvasive modality for the diagnosis of moyamoya disease, especially in children. Bilateral steno-occlusive changes at the terminal portion of internal carotid arteries (arrows in Fig. 1a) and the presence of more than two flow voids in each basal ganglia (arrows in Fig. 1b) lead to the definitive diagnosis of moyamoya disease according to the diagnostic criteria of the Research Committee on Spontaneous Occlusion of the Circle of Willis, of the Ministry of Health, Labor, and Welfare, Japan [11]. Children with moyamoya disease have a progressive nature in their symptoms and angiographic stage [1], while the progression of occlusive lesions in the major intracranial arteries was believed to be very rare in adult patients with the disease. A recent report by Kuroda and colleagues, however, demonstrated that the incidence of disease progression in adult moyamoya disease is much higher than recognized before, accounting for 23.8% during several years of follow-up [12]. Positron emission tomography and/or single-photon emission computed tomography is useful to evaluate cerebral hemodynamics and determine surgical indication for ischemic-onset moyamoya disease in both children and adults [13, 14], while the use of acetazolamide should be carefully conducted for children to avoid ischemic complication during the examination. The representative figure of *N*-isopropyl-*p*-[^{123}I]iodoamphetamine single-photon

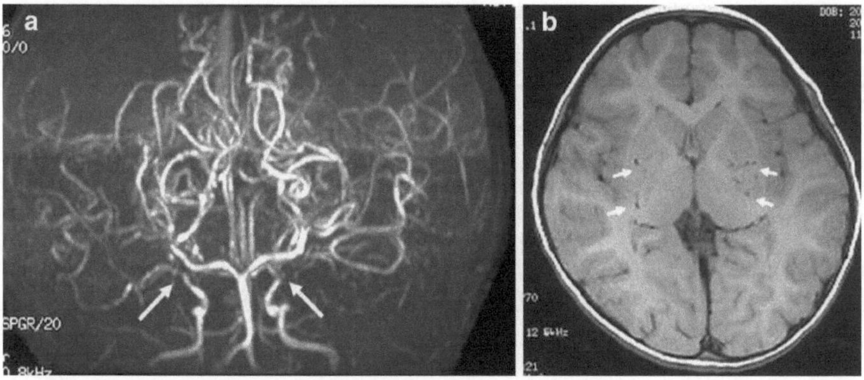

Fig. 1 Magnetic resonance (MR) imaging is useful noninvasive modality for the diagnosis of moyamoya disease, especially in children. Bilateral steno-occlusive changes at the terminal portion of internal carotid arteries [*arrows* in (**a**)] and the presence of more than two flow void in each basal ganglia [*arrows* in (**b**)] lead to the definitive diagnosis of moyamoya disease

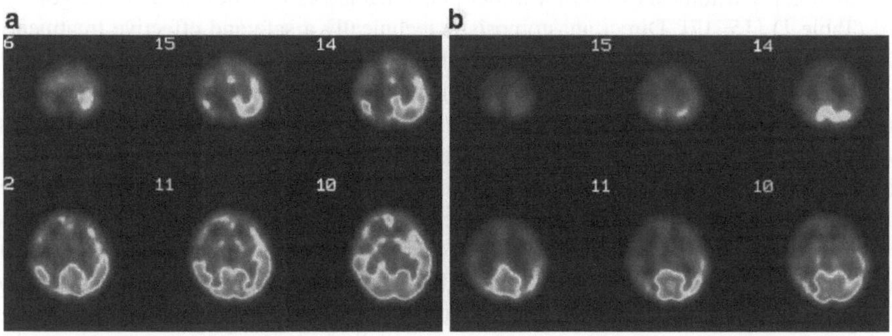

Fig. 2 *N*-isopropyl-*p*-[^{123}I]iodoamphetamine single-photon emission computed tomography in 4-year-old children presenting with crescendo transient ischemic attack. (**a**) At rest; (**b**) acetazolamide stress, indicating her cerebral blood flow and cerebrovascular reactivity are markedly compromised bilaterally

emission computed tomography in 4-year-old children presenting with crescendo transient ischemic attack (Fig. 2) indicates that cerebral blood flow and cerebrovascular reactivity are markedly compromised bilaterally.

Revascularization Surgery for Moyamoya Disease in Children and Adults

Surgical revascularization for moyamoya disease prevents cerebral ischemic attacks by improving cerebral blood flow, and superficial temporal artery-middle cerebral artery anastomosis and indirect pial synangiosis such as encephalo-myo-synangiosis (EMS) are generally

Table 1 Preoperative diagnosis, surgical procedure and surgical complication in moyamoya disease (MMD)

	Childhood MMD	Adult-onset MMD
Preoperative evaluation	MRI/MRA SPECT; rest, (acetazolamide)	Angiography MRI/MRA SPECT; rest and acetazolamide
Surgical procedure	Indirect pial synangiosis Direct/indirect combined surgery Direct revascularization	Direct/indirect combined surgery Direct revascularization
Surgical complication	Cerebral ischemia (cerebral hyperperfusion)	Cerebral hyperperfusion Cerebral ischemia

accepted as the optimal surgical treatment for the disease [15–17]. For children, both direct and indirect revascularization surgeries are known to be effective for preventing future stroke and improving long-term cognitive function. On the other hand, indirect pial synangiosis was shown to have a limited effect for adult cases [18], and the superficial temporal artery-middle cerebral artery anastomosis with or without pial synangiosis is believed to be the gold standard (Table 1) [15, 17]. Direct anastomosis is technically a safe and effective treatment for childhood moyamoya disease despite the small diameter of the recipient artery in young children (Fig. 3). The efficacy of revascularization surgery for hemorrhagic-onset patiens to prevent rebleeding is still undetermined [19]. A 38-year-old woman underwent successful revascularization surgeries on both hemispheres, which resolved her ischemic symptoms (Fig. 4). Three years later, however, she manifested as right thalamic hemorrhage, when cerebral angiography ruled out the presence of cerebral aneurysm and revascularization from both direct and indirect bypass was well visualized (Fig. 4), indicating the limitation of revascularization surgery to prevent future hemorrhage. To address this issue, a prospective randomized trial for direct revascularization surgery for hemorrhagic-onset moyamoya disease in adults has been conducted in Japan [19].

Difference in the Risk of Surgical Complication Between Children and Adult Patients

Despite their favorable long-term outcome, perioperative cerebral ischemia and cerebral hyperperfusion are potential complications of these revascularization procedures both in children and adult patients with moyamoya disease [20–22]. Ischemic complication, especially in children, could be due to the intraoperative hypotention and hyper/hypo-capnea, perioperative anemia and dehydration, and the mechanical compression by temporal muscle used for EMS. On the other hand, adult patients with moyamoya disease are known to have potential risk for cerebral hyperperfusion syndrome such as transient neurologic deficit, seizure, and hemorrhagic complication in the acute stage after direct revascularization surgery (Table 1) [21, 22]. Adult-onset and/or hemorrhagic-onset moyamoya patients are reported to have a higher risk for symptomatic cerebral hyperperfusion after STA-MCA anastomosis, and routine postoperative CBF measurement is recommended in these patients [23]. A 42-year-old woman suffered from progressive headache and subarachnoid hemorrhage 2 days after successful

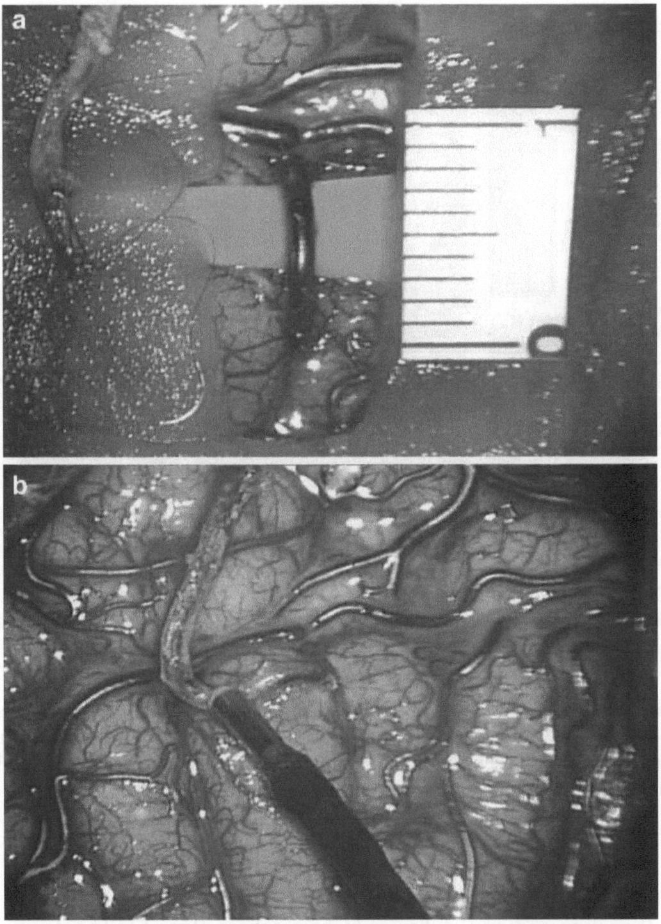

Fig. 3 Intraoperative view in a 4-year-old girl. Despite the small diameter of the recipient artery, superficial temporal artery middle cerebral artery anastomosis with pial synangiosis is technically a safe and effective treatment for childhood moyamoya disease

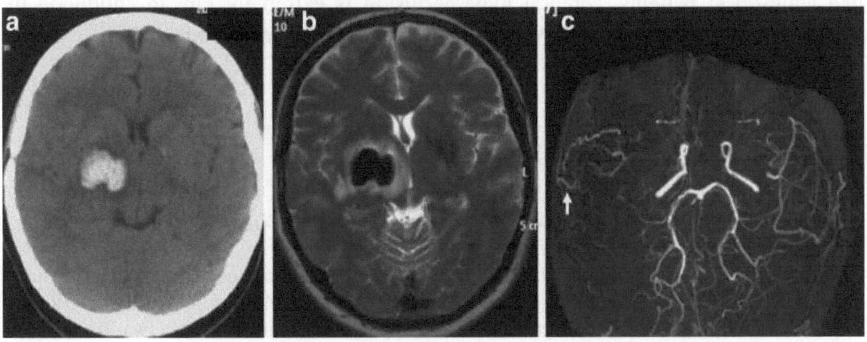

Fig. 4 Plain CT (**a**), T2-weighted MRI (**b**), and MRA (**c**) in a 38-year-old woman 3 years after successful revascularization surgeries on both hemispheres, indicating right thalamic hemorrhage. Cerebral angiography ruled out the presence of cerebral aneurysm, and revascularization from both direct [*arrow* in (**c**)] and indirect bypass was well visualized

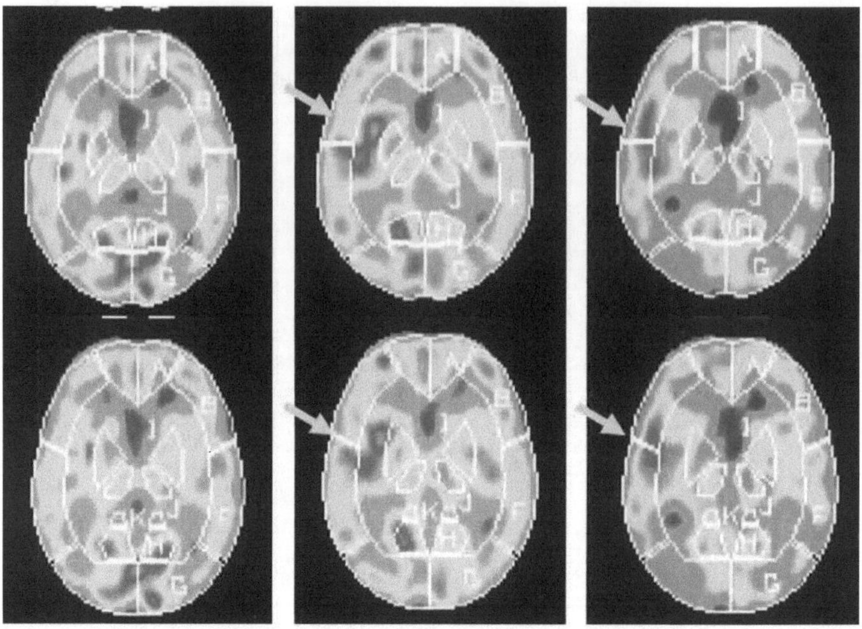

Fig. 5 Temporal change of *N*-isopropyl-*p*-[^{123}I] iodoamphetamine single-photon emission computed tomography in 42-year-old woman demonstrating focal intense increase in CBF on the hemisphere operated on (*arrows*), which was responsible for progressive headache with subarachnoid hemorrhage at postoperative day 2. Intensive blood pressure control relieved her symptom

direct revascularization surgery on her right hemisphere (Fig. 5). The *N*-isopropyl-*p*-[^{123}I] iodoamphetamine single-photon emission computed tomography before and after surgery indicated cerebral hyperperfusion on the operated hemisphere (Fig. 5). Intensive blood pressure control relieved her symptoms and she was discharged without neurologic deficit. Unlike adult-onset patients, cerebral hyperperfusion is extremely rare in childhood moyamoya disease following STA-MCA anastomosis, only being reported in a single case [24].

References

1. Suzuki J, Takaku A (1969) Cerebrovascular 'moyamoya' disease. Disease showing abnormal net-like vessels in base of brain. Arch Neurol 20:288–299
2. Kuriyama S, Kusaka Y, Fujimura M, et al. (2008) Prevalence and clinicoepidemiological features of moyamoya disease in Japan: findings from a nationwide epidemiological survey. Stroke 39:42–47
3. Ikeda H, Sasaki T, Yoshimoto T, et al. (1999) Mapping of a familial moyamoya disease gene to chromosome 3q24-p26. Am J Hum Genet 64:533–537
4. Sakurai K, Horiuchi Y, Ikeda H, et al. (2004) A novel susceptibility locus for moyamoya disease on chromosome 8q23. J Hum Genet 49:278–281
5. Yamaguchi T, Tada M, Houkin K, et al. (2000) Linkage of familial moyamoya disease to chromosome 17q25. Stroke 31:930–935

6. Mineharu Y, Liu W, Inoue K, et al. (2008) Autosomal dominant moyamoya disease maps to chromosome 17q25.3. Neurology 70:2357–2363
7. Oka K, Yamashita M, Sadoshima S, et al. (1981) Cerebral hemorrhage in moyamoya disease at autopsy. Virchows Arch Pathol Anat Histol 392:247–261
8. Oki K, Suzuki N (2007) In: Hashimoto N (ed) Report by the Research Committee on Spontaneous Occlusion of the Circle of Willis (Moyamoya Disease), pp 4–5
9. Yoshida Y, Yoshimoto T, Shirane R, et al. (1999) Clinical course, surgical management, and long-term outcome of moyamoya patients with rebleeding after an episode of intracerebral hemorrhage: a extensive follow-up study. Stroke 30:2272–2276
10. Kuroda S, Hashimoto N, Yoshimoto T, et al. (2007) Radiological findings, clinical course, and outcome in asymptomatic moyamoya disease. Results of multi-center survey in Japan. Stroke 38:1430–1435
11. Fukui M (1997) Guidelines for the diagnosis and treatment of spontaneous occlusion of the circle of Willis ('moyamoya disease'). Research Committee on Spontaneous Occlusion of the Circle of Willis (Moyamoya Disease) of the Ministry of Health and Welfare, Japan. Clin Neurol Neurosurg 99 Suppl 2:S238–240
12. Kuroda S, Ishikawa T, Houkin K, et al. (2005) Incidence and clinical features of disease progression in adult moyamoya disease. Stroke 36:2148–2153
13. Ikezaki K, Matsushima T, Kuwabara Y, et al. (1994) Cerebral circulation and oxygen metabolism in childhood moyamoya disease: a perioperative positron emission tomography study. J Neurosurg 81:843–850
14. Saito N, Nakagawara J, Nakamura H, et al. (2004) Assessment of cerebral hemodynamics in childhood moyamoya disease using a quantitative and a semiquantitative IMP-SPECT study. Ann Nucl Med 18:323–331
15. Ishikawa T, Houkin K, Kamiyama H, et al. (1997) Effects of surgical revascularization on outcome of patients with pediatric moyamoya disease. Stroke 28:1170–1173
16. Scott RM, Smith JL, Robertson RL, et al. (2004) Long-term outcome in children with moyamoya disease after cranial revascularization by pial synangiosis. J Neurosurg 100:142–149
17. Morimoto M, Iwama T, Hashimoto N, et al. (1999) Efficacy of direct revascularization in adult moyamoya disease: haemodynamic evaluation by positron emission tomography. Acta Neurochir (Wien) 141:377–384
18. Mizoi K, Kayama T, Yoshimoto T, et al. (1996) Indirect revascularization for moyamoya disease: is there a benefical effect for adult patients? Surg Neurol 45:541–548
19. Miyamoto S, Japan Adult Moyamoya Trial Group. (2004) Study design for a prospective randomized trial of extracranial-intracranial bypass surgery for adults with moyamoya disease and hemorrhagic onset: the Japan Adult Moyamoya Trial Group. Neurol Med Chir (Tokyo) 44:218–219
20. Houkin K, Ishikawa T, Yoshimoto T, et al (1997) Direct and indirect revascularization for moyamoya disease: surgical techniques and peri-operative complications. Clin Neurol Neurosurg 99 Suppl 2:S142–145
21. Fujimura M, Kaneta T, Mugikura S, et al. (2007) Temporary neurologic deterioration due to cerebral hyperperfusion after superficial temporal artery-middle cerebral artery anastomosis in patients with adult-onset moyamoya disease. Surg Neurol 67:273–282
22. Kim JE, Oh CW, Kwon OK, et al. (2008) Transient hyperperfusion after superfisial temporal artery/middle cerebral artery bypass surgery as a possible cause of postoperative transient neurological deterioration. Cerebrovasc Dis 25:580–586
23. Fujimura M, Mugikura S, Kaneta T, et al. (2009) Incidence and risk factors for symptomatic cerebral hyperperfusion following superficial temporal artery-middle cerebral artery anastomosis in patients with moyamoya disease. Surg Neurol 71:442–447
24. Fujimura M, Kaneta T, Shimizu H, et al. (2007) Symptomatic hyperperfusion after superficial temporal artery-middle cerebral artery anastomosis in a child with moyamoya disease. Childs Nerv Syst 23:1195–1198

Moyamoya Disease in Young Children

Kyu-Chang Wang, Seung-Ki Kim, Ho-Jun Seol, and Byung-Kyu Cho

Introduction

Moyamoya disease (MMD) is characterized by the progressive occlusion of the bilateral distal internal carotid arteries or of the proximal portions of the middle and anterior cerebral arteries (MCAs and ACAs), which is accompanied by extensive collateral vessel formation at the base of the brain. In children, MMD frequently manifests itself as a transient ischemic attack (TIA) that is provoked by hyperventilation. As the cerebral perfusion gradually decreases, the frequency, extent, and duration of TIAs increase, which leads to cerebral infarction. The benefits of revascularization surgery, either direct or indirect, have been well established in patients with slow progression of ischemia, as this type of surgery is effective for the elimination of TIA and the prevention of cerebral infarction.

In some children (especially young children), however, the initial MMD presentation may be a rapidly progressing cerebral infarction with neurological deficits or seizure, which are sometimes associated with a subsequent attack of cerebral infarction on the contralateral cerebral hemisphere shortly after disease onset [1–6]. Because of the rapid progression of disease and of the critically compromised cerebral perfusion, these patients may also be vulnerable to postoperative ischemic complications [7]. The natural course of rapid progression and the high rate of perioperative ischemic complications warrant special consideration for these patients regarding diagnosis, timing of surgery, initial site of surgery, etc. The development of screening methods for MMD patients will be valuable for the management of young children affected by this disease, as it may preserve these children from major stroke via the performance of preventive revascularization surgery.

K.-C. Wang (✉), S.-Ki Kim, and B.K. Cho
Division of Pediatric Neurosurgery, Pediatric Clinical Neuroscience Center, Seoul National University Children's Hospital, Seoul National University College of Medicine,
101 Daehang-no, Jongno-gu, Seoul 110-744, Republic of Korea
e-mail: kcwang@snu.ac.kr

S.-Ki Kim
Research Center for Rare Disease, Seoul, Republic of Korea

H.-J. Seol
Department of Neurosurgery, Kangwon National University Hospital, Kangwon-do, Republic of Korea

B.-K. Cho and T. Tominaga (eds.), *Moyamoya Disease Update*,
DOI 10.1007/978-4-431-99703-0_41,

Illustrative Case

A 13-month-old boy displayed seizure and sudden right hemiplegia after irritability and crying. The initial magnetic resonance imaging (MRI), which was acquired at the onset of the first symptoms, revealed the presence of wide infarction in the left cerebral hemisphere. In addition, magnetic resonance angiography (MRA) showed occlusion of the left MCA (Fig. 1). One month after the manifestation of initial symptoms, the boy's father visited our hospital for the management of the child's MMD. We recommended early indirect revascularization surgery on the right (noninfarcted side) superficial temporal artery area and bifrontal areas (MCA and both ACA territories). However, the father rejected the surgery and followed the opinion of a doctor at the local hospital, who recommended a conservative treatment that included medication and rehabilitation. One and a half months after the onset of initial symptoms, the patient had seizure recurrence, which was accompanied by left weakness, lethargy, irritability, intermittent general rigidity, loss of head control, and swallowing difficulty. The MRI acquired at the second attack revealed widespread infarction in the right cerebral hemisphere, and MRA showed bilateral occlusion or severe stenosis of the ACAs and MCAs (Fig. 2). Despite indirect revascularization surgery, the patient's condition did not improve significantly, and he died from asphyxia in a car, 8 months after the initial manifestation of MMD symptoms.

Rapid Progression of Disease

The rapid progression of MMD in young children has been emphasized by several investigators [1–6]. Karasawa et al. [3] reported that 36% of MMD patients who are younger than 3 years of age have major stroke before surgical treatment resulting in poor outcomes. Kuroda et al. [8] divided the patients into infantile (younger than 6 years of age, $n=32$) and schoolchild (6 years or older, $n=23$) groups. The infantile group showed significantly more frequent complete stroke, cerebral infarction, and posterior cerebral artery stenosis/occlusion and significantly lower cerebral blood flow (CBF) values than the schoolchild group.

In general, collateral formation in young children with MMD is not extensive, as shown in the illustrative case presented in this chapter. The rapid progression of disease does not allow extensive collateral formation, which leads to cerebral infarction and stroke rather than TIA.

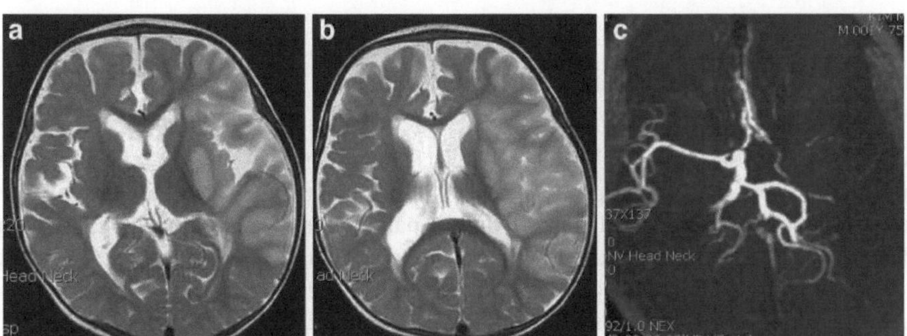

Fig. 1 Magnetic resonance imaging findings of a 13-month-old infant, which were acquired at the initial onset of symptoms (i.e., seizure and sudden right hemiplegia). Diffuse left cerebral hemispheric infarction and occlusion of the left MCA are noted

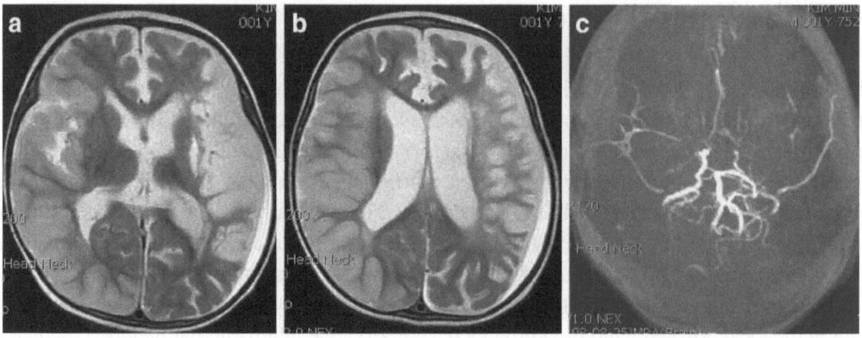

Fig. 2 Magnetic resonance images acquired at the second seizure and developmental regression one and a half months after the initial presentation reveal the presence of new extensive cerebral infarction on the right side (i.e., the previously noninfarcted side) and bilateral occlusion or severe stenosis of the ACAs and MCAs, with faint visualization of basal collaterals

According to our previous study [5], infarctions were significantly more frequent as the initial presentation in children younger than 3 years (group A: $n=23$; 87%) and in those between the ages of 3 and 6 (group B: $n=50$, 58%) than in patients older than 6 (group C: $n=131$, 46%). Subsequent preoperative infarctions (often on the contralateral cerebral hemisphere) were significantly more frequent in group A (39%; seven contralateral infarctions in nine patients, which occurred within 7 months of the onset of initial symptoms, and two ipsilateral infarctions in nine patients, which occurred 7 and 14 months after the onset of initial symptoms, respectively) than in groups B (6%) and C (0.8%), and the median interval between the initial symptoms and subsequent preoperative infarction was 3 months (range, 1–14 months). The median interval between the onset of initial symptoms and the first surgery was 5 months (range, 1–24 months). The delay of surgery implied a greater number of subsequent infarctions.

It is well known that the prognosis of bilateral cerebral hemispheric infarction of significant size is poor. Cognition, intelligence, emotional stability, and brain stem functions may be seriously deteriorated. The diagnosis of MMD with cerebral infarction in a young child implies that the patient is subject to a subsequent contralateral cerebral hemispheric infarction within a short period, which results in a serious impact on the quality of life of the patient.

Surgery-Related Ischemic Complication

Revascularization surgery for MMD may cause perioperative surgery-related ischemic complications, because of compromised cerebral perfusion and increased vulnerability to hyperventilation and disturbed hemodynamic parameters, which include hypovolemia and anemia. Young children with MMD who show rapid disease progression may be more vulnerable to surgery-related ischemic complications. Therefore, special attention should be paid in young MMD patients, to avoid hyperventilation, hypovolemia, anemia, etc.

Kim et al. [7] reported a higher surgery-related ischemic risk in patients who are younger than 3 years and in patients who have a preoperative cerebral infarction. In contrast, Kuroda et al. [8] described satisfactory effects of surgery on TIA in groups of children younger and older than 6. Our previous study [5] also did not find a significant difference in the rates of surgery-related infarction between the groups younger and older than 3, even though this rate was slightly higher in the younger group (4/23 in the younger group vs 24/181 in the older group). Considering the high risk of subsequent cerebral infarction before surgery in the younger group, the increased rate of surgery-related perioperative infarction is not purely caused by surgery; rather, it is a summation of surgical effects and the natural course of rapid disease progression. The rate of permanent neurological deficits caused by surgery-related perioperative cerebral infarction was not different between the groups. The performance of surgery within 3 months of the onset of symptoms tended to result in a lower rate of surgery-related perioperative cerebral infarction. We also found that surgery-related perioperative cerebral infarction occurred within 1 week of surgery.

Overall Management Outcome

Natural history and surgical risk should be weighed when deciding on the appropriate time of operation, to define the benefits and risks of early or delayed revascularization surgery. The assessment of the overall management outcome is more important than the risk of perioperative complications alone.

Regarding the natural history of the disease, as described above, it is well known that, in the majority of young children, the initial MMD symptoms are caused by cerebral infarction and that subsequent infarction may be expected within a few months [1–6]. Even though the results of our previous study stemmed from the limited observation of patients who had to wait for surgery for various reasons (upper respiratory infection, parents' hesitation, misinformation from other medical institutes, etc.), more than one-third of the young children showed subsequent infarction, which frequently happened on the contralateral noninfarcted cerebral hemisphere within a median of 3 months [5]. Because the initial disease presentation in the majority of young children is cerebral infarction, subsequent contralateral infarction leads to bilateral cerebral dysfunction, which leads to devastating consequences for the patients.

Regarding the surgery-related ischemic complications, young patients are more vulnerable to these perioperative problems [7]. However, the data of Kuroda et al. [8] and our previous study [5] failed to demonstrate a significant increase in perioperative complications in cases where the surgery is performed with great caution. About 17% of patients experienced perioperative complications, which usually occurred within 1 week of the surgery.

According to the literature, many investigators regard preoperative ischemic injury as the main reason for poor outcome in young-age MMD, rather than surgery-related ischemic complications [2, 3, 5]. These reports also strongly support the performance of revascularization surgery before major cerebral infarction.

The rate of the increase in postoperative CBF after indirect revascularization depends on the degree of ischemia on the noninfarcted brain region, recruitment of collateral flow through other routes, and the progression of the disease. According to reports on blood flow time course after indirect revascularization surgery, the increase in CBF begins 2 weeks after surgery, becomes well developed 3 months after surgery, and surpasses preoperative levels within 6 months of surgery [9–12]. Because there is slow recruitment, or none, of other collateral channels and rapid disease progression in young children, the postoperative beneficial effects of surgery may manifest themselves faster than in older children, even though these same factors render the young patients more vulnerable to surgery-related ischemic complications. If surgery can halt the progression of the disease within a few months (or preferably within a few weeks), then the overall management outcome will be better in cases treated with early surgery.

As emphasized in our previous study, we recommend early surgery for young MMD patients (i.e., younger than 3 years of age), to improve the overall management outcome [5]. Matsushima et al. [2] also stated that in children younger than 2 years of age, there is still a slight chance of preserving mental function if the surgery is performed within 3 months of the onset of symptoms. This warrants further verification via a large-scale comparative study.

Site of the First Surgery: Infarcted Hemisphere Versus Contralateral Noninfarcted Hemisphere

It is well known that, in general, bilateral widespread cerebral hemispheric damage has a great adverse impact on neurological outcome. In addition, the fact that preoperative subsequent cerebral infarction tends to occur in the contralateral noninfarcted cerebral hemisphere within a few months after the onset of symptoms [5] constitutes important background information that should be taken into consideration when choosing the site of the first surgery.

The manifestation of MMD as a sizable cerebral infarction and stroke in young children implies a very limited possibility of surgically saving the ipsilateral infarcted cerebral hemisphere. Instead, every effort should be focused on the preservation of the contralateral noninfarcted cerebral hemisphere to avoid bilateral widespread brain damage. For this reason, we recommend early indirect revascularization surgery on the contralateral noninfarcted side. The simultaneous performance of surgery on the infarcted side or the performance of a bifrontal procedure will provide the concerted bilateral reinforcement of CBF. If one side has to be chosen for the first surgery, the contralateral noninfarcted cerebral hemisphere has definite priority.

Future Perspectives: Rapid Revascularization and Screening of High-Risk Patients

In young children, MMD commonly manifests itself as a sizable cerebral infarction and stroke. Symptoms can be easily overlooked, even in cases presenting with TIA. Therefore, young-age MMD patients are rarely identified before cerebral infarction occurs. As preinfarction revascularization surgery is essential for good disease prognosis, the early identification of patients at high risk of developing young-age MMD using imaging tools or molecular markers will have great value for the prevention of devastating cerebral infarction.

MMD has a familial tendency. About 10–15% of MMD patients have a family history of the disease [13, 14]. The probability of having MMD increases remarkably if a blood relative has MMD [15].

Based on current knowledge, a young child or a young sibling of an MMD patient may be a candidate for MMD screening, preferably MRA, even in the absence of symptoms suggestive of MMD. However, a single MRA examination is not sufficient. Theoretically, several examinations are required before the age of 3 years. The practical feasibility and the cost-effectiveness of performing serial MRA examinations are questionable. The identification of a specific molecular marker for early-childhood MMD will render the pre-onset screening practical and cost-effective. This presymptomatic screening may save the cerebral hemispheres of young MMD patients.

References

1. Maki Y, Enomoto T (1988) Moyamoya disease. Childs Nerv Syst 4:204–212
2. Matsushima Y, Aoyagi M, Masaoka H et al (1990) Mental outcome following encephaloduroarterio-synangiosis in children with moyamoya disease with the onset earlier than 5 years of age. Childs Nerv Syst 6:440–443
3. Karasawa J, Touho H, Ohnishi H et al (1992) Long-term follow-up study after extracranial-intracranial bypass surgery for anterior circulation ischemia in childhood moyamoya disease. J Neurosurg 77:84–89
4. Imaizumi T, Hayashi K, Saito K et al (1998) Long-term outcomes of pediatric moyamoya disease monitored to adulthood. Pediatr Neurol 18:321–325
5. Kim SK, Seol HJ, Cho BK et al (2004) Moyamoya disease among young patients: its aggressive clinical course and the role of active surgical treatment. Neurosurgery 54:840–844
6. Kuroda S, Houkin K (2008) Moyamoya disease: current concepts and future perspectives. Lancet Neurol 7:1056–1066
7. Kim SH, Choi JU, Yang KH et al (2005) Risk factors for postoperative ischemic complications in patients with moyamoya disease. J Neurosurg 103:433–438
8. Kuroda S, Nanba R, Ishikawa T et al (2003) Clinical manifestations of infantile moyamoya disease. No Shinkei Geka 31: 1073–1078 (in Japanese)
9. Karasawa J, Kikuchi H, Kuriyama Y et al (1981) Cerebral hemodynamics in "moyamoya" disease – II. Measurements of cerebral circulation and metabolism by use of the argon desaturation method in pre- and post-neurosurgical procedures. Neurol Med Chir (Tokyo) 21:1161–1168 (in Japanese)
10. Suzuki R, Matsushima Y, Takada Y et al (1989) Changes in cerebral hemodynamics following encephalo-duro-arterio-synangiosis (EDAS) in young patients with moyamoya disease. Surg Neurol 31:343–349
11. Kinugasa K, Mandai S, Kamata I et al (1993) Surgical treatment of moyamoya disease: operative technique for encephalo-duro-arterio-myo-synangiosis, its follow-up, clinical results, and angiograms. Neurosurgery 32:527–531
12. Ishikawa T, Houkin K, Kamiyama H et al (1997) Effects of surgical revascularization on outcome of patients with pediatric moyamoya disease. Stroke 28:1170–1173
13. Wakai K, Tamakoshi A, Ikezaki K et al (1997) Epidemiological features of moyamoya disease in Japan: findings from a nationwide survey. Clin Neurol Neurosurg 99:S1–5
14. Yamauchi T, Houkin K, Tada M et al (1997) Familial occurrence of moyamoya disease. Clin Neurol Neurosurg 99:S162–167
15. Hamada JI, Yoshioka S, Nakahara T et al (1998) Clinical features of moyamoya disease in sibling relations under 15 years of age. Acta Neurochir (Wien) 140:455–458

Moyamoya Disease in Adult: Management of Hemorrhage

Susumu Miyamoto and Jun C. Takahashi

Overview of Intracranial Hemorrhage in Moyamoya Disease

It is well known that more than one-half of all adult patients with moyamoya disease suffer intracranial hemorrhage, whereas most nonadult patients present with cerebral ischemia [1]. Typically, the hemorrhage involves the thalamus and basal ganglia, and it frequently involves perforation to the ventricles (Fig. 1); in rare instances, subcortical or subarachnoid hemorrhage can also be observed. Such bleeding attacks, which are potentially fatal, seriously affect the patient's prognosis [2]. It is speculated that chronic and exceptionally high hemodynamic stress might induce vascular wall pathologies such as microaneurysms or vessel fragility, which lead to hemorrhagic attacks (Fig. 2a). On occasion, subarachnoid hemorrhage is caused by rupture of saccular aneurysms located on the circle of Willis, especially on the posterior cerebral artery, which acts as the collateral pathway to the anterior circulation (Fig. 2b).

It is reported that, following a hemorrhagic attack, the rate of a rebleeding attack is quite high [3, 4]. A survey by Nishimoto et al. revealed that 33% of 175 patients with hemorrhagic moyamoya disease experienced a rebleeding attack [3]. Moreover, Kobayashi et al. reported the annual rebleeding rate as 7.09% [4]. Therefore, management of hemorrhagic moyamoya disease presents a serious challenge (Fig. 3).

Management of Hemorrhagic Moyamoya Disease During the Acute Period

Intracranial hemorrhage can be easily diagnosed with computed tomography (CT). If the bleeding does not resemble typical hypertensive intracerebral hemorrhage, the cerebral vessels should be evaluated with magnetic resonance (MR) angiography or conventional angiography

S. Miyamoto (✉) and J.C. Takahashi
Department of Neurosurgery, Kyoto University,
54 Shogoin Kawahara-cho Sakyo-ku, Kyoto 606-8507, Japan
e-mail: miy@kuhp.kyoto-u.ac.jp

B.-K. Cho and T. Tominaga (eds.), *Moyamoya Disease Update*,
DOI 10.1007/978-4-431-99703-0_42,

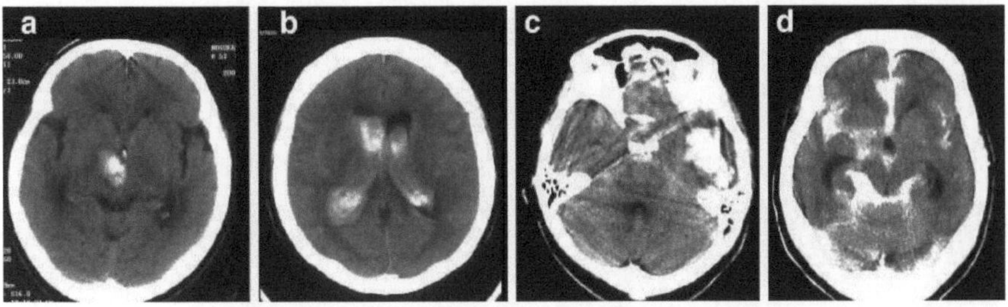

Fig. 1 Various patterns of intracranial hemorrhage in patients with moyamoya disease (**a**) thalamic hemorrhage, (**b**) intraventricular hemorrhage, (**c**) subcortical hemorrhage, (**d**) subarachnoid hemorrhage

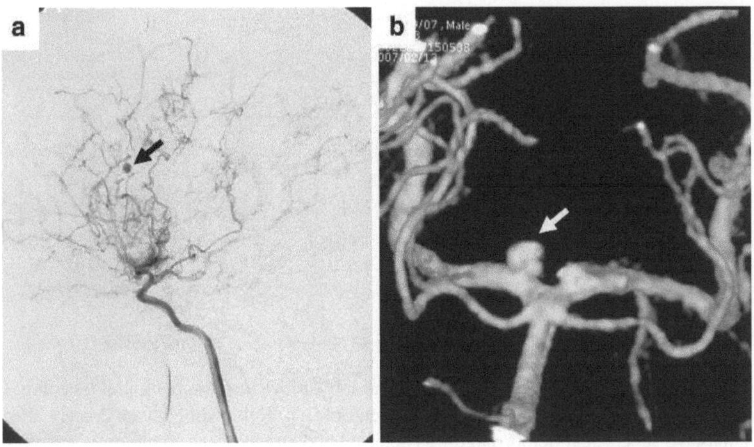

Fig. 2 Vascular lesions arising from collateral vessels in moyamoya disease (**a**) microaneurysms on the dilated lenticulostriate artery (*arrow*) (**b**) saccular aneurysm on the posterior cerebral artery (*white arrow*)

in order to detect vascular lesions. If the diagnosis is hemorrhagic moyamoya disease, the patient should be treated with special consideration for the pathophysiology of that disease. Blood pressure should be strictly controlled to prevent rebleeding during the acute period. However, excessive reduction of blood pressure and dehydration must be avoided in those patients with hemodynamic failure, such as those with ischemic moyamoya disease [5]. When acute hydrocephalus is in evidence, emergent ventricular drainage is indicated to reduce the intracranial pressure and maintain adequate cerebral perfusion pressure. Although a small intracerebral hematoma can be treated conservatively, massive intracerebral bleeding requires removal of the hematoma through a craniotomy. A ruptured saccular aneurysm on the circle of Willis (basilar tip or posterior cerebral artery) should be treated with aneurismal neck clipping or intravascular embolization. Ruptured microaneurysms in tiny collateral vessels are, however, usually treated conservatively because direct excision and intravascular treatment are both difficult procedures.

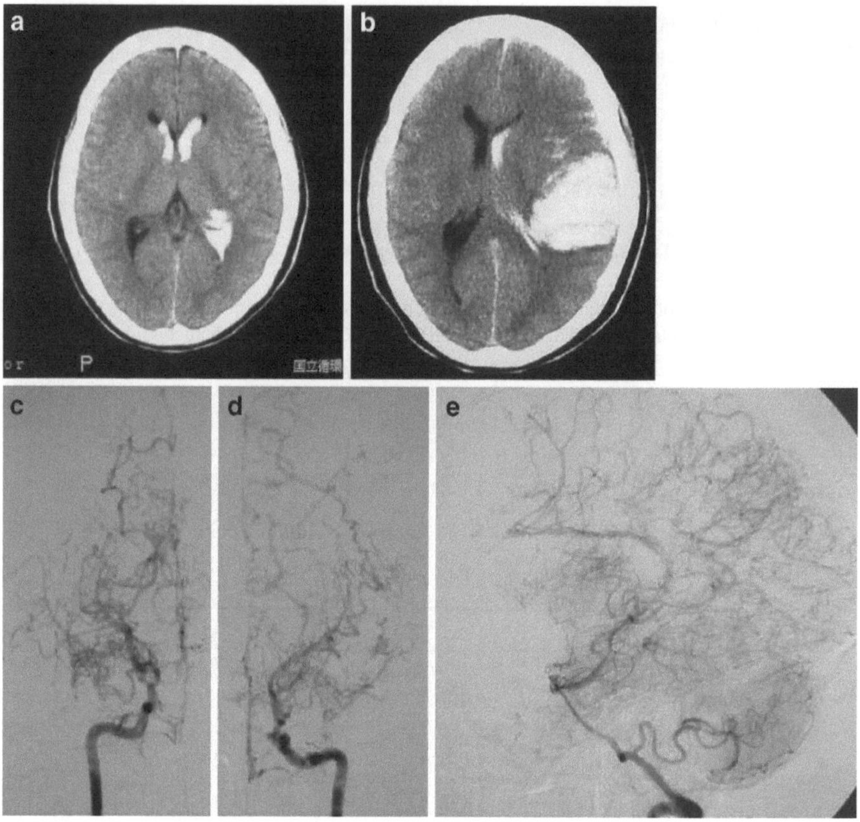

Fig. 3 Rebleeding attack in a 31-year-old female with moyamoya disease. (**a**) Initial bleeding: CT reveals a small hematoma near the trigon of the left lateral ventricle. (**b**) Rebleeding attack 2 years after the initial bleeding: a massive subcortical hemorrhage was detected and an emergent craniotomy was needed

Prevention of Rebleeding in the Chronic Stage

Although hemorrhagic attacks cause serious permanent neurological deficits and the massive bleeding is potentially fatal, no therapeutic method for preventing rebleeding attacks has been established. No evidence exists that treatment of hypertension reduces the rebleeding rate in hemorrhagic moyamoya disease. At present, the only promising strategy is revascularization surgery. It is well known that, in ischemic moyamoya disease, reductions in moyamoya vessels can often be detected by angiography after bypass surgery (Fig. 4) [6]. Because the source of the bleeding is the tiny moyamoya vessels present in most patients with hemorrhagic moyamoya disease, the rate of hemorrhagic attacks can possibly be decreased by reducing this hemodynamic stress and consequently reducing the moyamoya vessels. As a result, a hypothesis has emerged that bypass surgery prevents bleeding; in fact, some authors have reported the effectiveness of direct anastomotic bypass for hemorrhagic moyamoya disease [6, 7]. Additionally, these reports emphasize that a direct bypass is preferable to the indirect procedure.

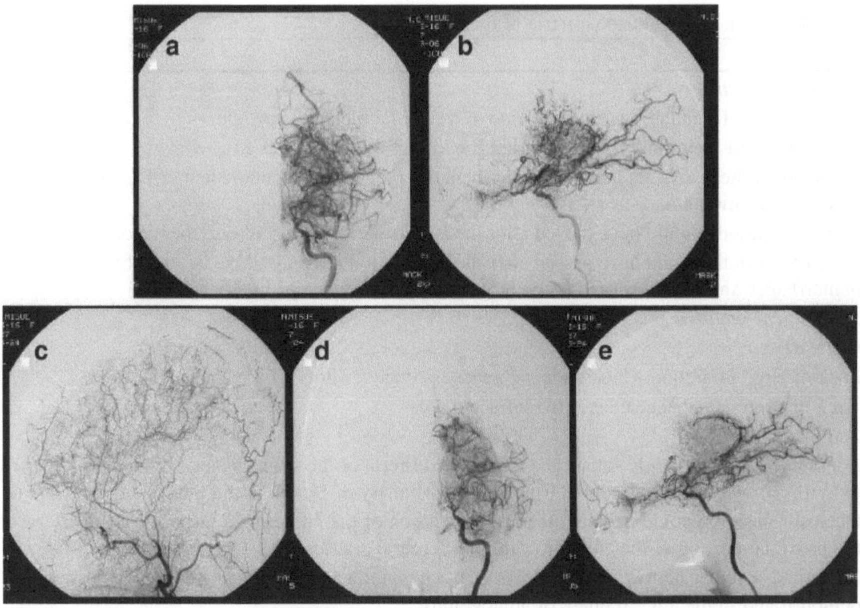

Fig. 4 Reduction of moyamoya vessels after STA-MCA bypass in adult patients. (**a**) and (**b**) Left internal carotid angiograms obtained before surgery. The moyamoya vessels are remarkably well developed. (**c**) A left internal carotid angiogram obtained after STA-MCA anastomosis. The collateral blood flow via the direct bypass covers approximately two-thirds of the outer surface of the left hemisphere. (**d**) and (**e**) Left internal carotid angiograms obtained after surgery. The reduced size of the moyamoya vessels is evident

On the other hand, some reports indicate no significant reduction in the rebleeding rate following revascularization surgery [2, 8]. Clearly, surgical treatment of adult hemorrhagic moyamoya disease remains controversial.

To resolve these issues, the Japan Adult Moyamoya (JAM) Trial was developed and has been under way in Japan since 2001 [9]. This randomized controlled trial seeks to determine whether direct bypass surgery affects the prognosis for and incidence of recurrent bleeding attacks. This trial does not deal with indirect bypass procedures alone, as direct bypass treatments such as STA-MCA anastomosis are considered essential for adult patients [10].

Design of the JAM Trial

Patient Eligibility and Randomization

The inclusion and exclusion criteria are summarized in Table 1. Patients must fulfill all the clinical and radiological requirements. In addition, patients undergo single photon emission CT (SPECT) with *N*-isopropyl-4-[123I] iodoamphetamine. Quantitative measuring of cerebral

Table 1 Inclusion and exclusion criteria of the JAM trial

Patient eligibility
1. Clinical requirements
(1) Age: between 18 and 60 years at the time of the initial bleeding episode
(2) Independent in their daily lives (modified Rankin disability scale 0–2)
(3) Intracerebral hemorrhage, intraventricular hemorrhage, or subarachnoid hemorrhage within the preceding 12 months
(4) At least 1 month should have passed after the last stroke episode, either ischemic or hemorrhagic
(5) At least 1 month should have passed after the completion of acute phase treatment for the hemorrhages and for the related secondary pathophysiology (e.g., hydrocephalus)
2. Radiological requirements
(1) CT/MRI
(a) Lack of large infarction which widely spreads over the territory of a main arterial trunk
(b) Lack of contrast enhancement in the infracted area
(2) Angiography
Angiographic findings should satisfy the diagnostic criteria of the spontaneous occlusion of the Circle of Willis (moyamoya disease) published by the Ministry of Health, Labor and Welfare of Japan:
(a) Occlusive lesions should exist in the terminal portion of the intracranial internal carotid artery, or in the proximal portion of the anterior or middle cerebral arteries
(b) Abnormal vascular network in the region of basal ganglia and thalamus (moyamoya vessels) is demonstrated in the arterial phase of angiography
(c) These findings should be demonstrated on both sides
3. Exclusion criteria
(1) Not independent in daily lives (modified Rankin disability 3–5)
(2) Atherosclerotic carotid disease, or cardiac arrhythmia which may cause thromboembolic complications
(3) Malignant tumors or organ failure of the heart, liver, kidney, or lung
(4) Unstable angina or has had a myocardial infarction within the past 6 months
(5) Hematological abnormality showing bleeding diathesis
(6) Uncontrolled diabetes showing a serum fasting blood glucose level of more than 300 mg/dl, or requires insulin
(7) Hypertension with the diastolic blood pressure of more than 110 mm Hg
(8) Treated with EC–IC bypass surgery before enrollment
(9) Pregnancy

blood flow at a resting state and after acetazolamide loading must be performed. After informed consent is obtained, a computer-generated randomization scheme is applied and the patient is assigned to receive either the best medical care alone to modify risk factors or the best medical care plus extracranial–intracranial (EC–IC) bypass.

Treatment and Follow-Up

EC–IC bypass, if assigned, is performed on both sides (with an appropriate interval between procedures). As the operative maneuver, a direct bypass procedure such as STA-MCA anastomosis is essential. A surgeon can combine an indirect bypass procedure with a direct bypass; however, the use of an indirect bypass alone or a high-flow bypass graft such as a venous graft or radial artery graft is not permitted. All patients, either surgical or medical, are followed up for more than 5 years after enrollment, and their medical, neurological, and functional status is reported.

Outcome Events

The following items constitute the primary end points after enrollment: (1) recurrent bleeding; (2) completed stroke causing significant morbidity in daily life activities; (3) significant morbidity or mortality from other causes; or (4) the performance of an additional EC–IC bypass at the discretion of the participating neurologist, as in the case of progressive stroke or crescendo TIA. The following items constitute the secondary end point in the prevention of recurrent bleeding: (1) recurrent bleeding; or (2) related death or severe disability (modified Rankin disability scale 3–5).

Status of the JAM Trial

Eighty patients were enrolled in the JAM trial and registration was closed in June 2008. These patients are now under close follow-up. The results of the trial will be disclosed in 2013, and expectations are high that this trial will establish a guiding principle for treatment of hemorrhagic moyamoya disease.

References

1. Nishimato A (1979) Moyamoya disease. Neurol Med Chir (Tokyo) 19:221–228
2. Yoshida Y, Yoshimoto T, Shirane R et al (1999) Clinical course, surgical management, and long-term outcome of moyamoya patients with rebleeding after an episode of intracerebral hemorrhage: an extensive follow-up study. Stroke 30:2272–2276
3. Nishimoto A, Ueda K, Honma Y (1983) Follow-up study on outcome of the occlusion of the circle of Willis. In: Gotoh S (ed) (1982) Proceedings of the Research Committee on Spontaneous Occlusion of the Circle of Willis (in Japanese). Ministry of Health and Welfare, Tokyo, Japan, pp 66–74
4. Kobayashi E, Saeki N, Oishi H et al (2000) Long-term natural history of hemorrhagic moyamoya disease in 42 patients. J Neurosurg 93:976–980
5. Okada Y, Shima T, Nishida M et al (1998) Effectiveness of superficial temporal artery-middle cerebral artery anastomosis in adult moyamoya disease: cerebral hemodynamics and clinical course in ischemic and hemorrhagic varieties. Stroke 29:625–630
6. Houkin K, Kamiyama H, Abe H et al (1996) Surgical therapy for adult moyamoya disease. Can surgical revascularization prevent the recurrence of intracranial hemorrhage? Stroke 27:1342–1346
7. Kawaguchi S, Okuno S, Sakaki T (2000) Effect of direct arterial bypass on the prevention of future stroke in patients with the hemorrhagic variety of moyamoya disease. J Neurosurg 93:397–401
8. Fujii K, Ikezaki K, Irikura K et al (1997) The efficacy of bypass surgery for the patients with hemorrhagic moyamoya disease. Clin Neurol Neurosurg 99:S194–S195
9. The Japan Adult Moyamoya (JAM) Trial Group (2004) Study design for a prospective randomized trial of extracranial-intracranial (EC-IC) bypass surgery for adults with moyamoya disease with hemorrhagic onset. Neurol Med Chir (Tokyo) 44:218–219
10. Mizoi K, Kayama T, Yoshimoto T et al (1996) Indirect revascularization for moyamoya disease: is there a beneficial effect for adult patients? Surg Neurol 45:541–548

Moyamoya Disease in Adult: Post-Bypass Symptomatic Hyperperfusion

Jeong Eun Kim and Chang Wan Oh

Introduction

Physicians have tried various nonsurgical treatments for moyamoya disease (MMD), but none has so far proven effective [1]. Surgical revascularization, by contrast, increases collateral irrigation and improves cerebral hemodynamics in MMD, thereby reducing the risk of subsequent ischemic insult by improving cerebral hemodynamics in MMD [2]. The various revascularization techniques used with MMD can be roughly classified into three categories according to the use of arterial anastomosis: (1) indirect nonanastomotic revascularization surgery; (2) direct anastomotic bypass surgery, usually superficial temporal artery (STA)-middle cerebral artery (MCA) bypass; and (3) combined surgery. Many kinds of indirect revascularization are effectively used for pediatric MMD [3], but surgical options for adult MMD are quite different. The two situations differ for the following reasons: (1) adults have less fragile cortical branches with larger diameter than children, so direct bypass is technically less challenging [4, 5]; and (2) direct bypass theoretically provides more immediate resolution of ischemic conditions by improving cerebral hemodynamics shortly after surgery [6]. Postoperative changes in cerebral hemodynamics are both marked and abrupt, however, and often induce symptomatic hyperperfusion, particularly in MMD patients with preoperative chronic sustained profound ischemia [7, 8]. Consequently, patients should be carefully managed after direct bypass surgery. In this chapter, the authors review the pertinent literature and relate their personal experience, paying special attention to hyperperfusion after direct bypass in the treatment of adult MMD.

J.E. Kim (✉)
Department of Neurosurgery, Seoul National University Hospital,
Seoul National University College of Medicine, 28 Yeongeon-dong,
Jongno-gu, Seoul 110-744, Republic of Korea
e-mail: eunkim@snu.ac.kr

C.W. Oh
Division of Cerebrovascular Surgery, Department of Neurosurgery,
Seoul National University Bundang Hospital, Seoul National University College of Medicine,
Gyeonggi-do, Republic of Korea

B.-K. Cho and T. Tominaga (eds.), *Moyamoya Disease Update*,
DOI 10.1007/978-4-431-99703-0_43, © Springer 2010

Direct Bypass in Adult MMD

Because a large portion of adult MMD patients do not make collateral pathways following indirect surgery, direct bypass is the preferred method for treating them [9–11]. By contrast, most pediatric MMD patients respond to indirect revascularization by developing extensive collateral vessels. In a study of 16 adult MMD patients treated by direct and indirect bypass surgery, Mizoi et al. [11] found that the effectiveness of indirect bypass declines after the age of 30, falling dramatically after age 40. Among those patients treated by direct bypass, however, excellent filling of cortical branches by anastomosis on cerebral angiography was observed. Based on their study, Houkin et al. [10] reported on the nature of revascularization in 22 adult MMD patients who had undergone direct and indirect surgeries. Among persons treated by indirect surgery, revascularization occurred by STA in 9%, by the middle meningeal artery in 36%, and by the deep temporal artery in 45%. Direct STA-MCA anastomosis resulted in good revascularization of the MCA territory in 94% of cases. Drawing on their study of 11 adult MMD patients examined by postoperative angiography, Kawaguchi et al. [9] reported that none of the five persons treated by encephalo-duro-arterio-synangiosis (EDAS) showed good revascularization. Those who had an STA-MCA bypass exhibited a substantially greater decrease of moyamoya vessels. As stated above, an additional disadvantage of indirect revascularization is the inherent delay in providing collaterals. Immediate improvement in cerebral blood flow (CBF) following direct bypass is distinctly advantageous over the situation seen with indirect bypass [4, 6, 10]. Recent reports indicate that the combined use of direct and indirect procedures is more effective than is the single use of either one [12, 13]. In the light of the complementary effects of the two sorts of surgery, this observation is not surprising. Consequent upon direct surgery, anastomosis helps form immediate collaterals around the anastomotic site. Moreover, in the aftermath of indirect surgery, the tissue volume that is revascularized includes territory outside the distribution of a single recipient arterial division.

Post-Bypass Symptomatic Hyperperfusion in Adult MMD

Definition

Cerebral hyperperfusion is the substantial increase in ipsilateral CBF above the metabolic demands of brain tissue as occurs after surgical revascularization of arterial stenosis or occlusion [14, 15]. Carotid endarterectomy (CEA), carotid angioplasty with stenting, or STA-MCA bypass in patients with cerebral atherosclerotic occlusive diseases (ASDs), and other cerebral revascularization surgeries are frequently followed by a rapid restoration of normal perfusion pressure. Such regional hyperperfusion is a consequence of impaired autoregulation of CBF that occurs in the context of chronic ischemia [14, 15]. "Cerebral hyperperfusion syndrome," a complication secondary to cerebral edema or intracerebral hemorrhage (ICH), is characterized by unilateral headache, face and eye pain, seizures, and focal symptoms [14–16]. The postoperative transient neurologic deterioration (TND) reported to follow STA-MCA bypass treatment for MMD [7, 8, 17] may bear a relationship to cerebral hyperperfusion syndrome. In particular, cerebral hyperperfusion may contribute to postoperative TND. It must be noted that STA-MCA bypass surgery for MMD impacts arteries with a relatively small diameter. Upon revascularization, the restored blood flow is

Table 1 Reports on symptomatic hyperperfusion syndrome after direct bypass in MMD

Author	No. patients (Incidence)	Patient	Sex		Mean age (years)	Laterality		Preop symptoms	Indirect bypass	Presentation			Treatment	Outcome
			Male	Female		Right	Left			Symptom	Mean onset (day)	Mean duration (day)		
Furuya (2004) [20]	case report	adult only	1	0	39	0	1	TIA/Inf	–	speech difficulty	2	5	BPC, antiplatelet, hemodilution, hypervolemia	fully recovered
Ogasawara (2005) [25]	case report	adult only	1	0	48	1	0	Inf	–	headache, delirium	4	5	BPC, clonidine, nicardipine	fully recovered
Fujimura (2007) [8][a]	13/34 (38.2%)	adult only	4	9	40 (26–62)	9	4	6 TIA, 4 Inf, 3 Hmr, 1 TIA/Sz	±	7 senseD, 6 aphasia, 5 dysarthria, 2 FP, 2 Sz, 2 SAH	3.7 (2–9)	8.3 (1–23)	BPC, edavarone	no PND for all
Fujimura (2008) [22][a]	2/17 (11.8%)	child only	1	1	4, 8	2	0	5 TIA, 4 TIA/Inf	+	1 FP, 1 MP	5, 9	5, 3 months	BPC, edavarone	no PND for all
Fujimura (2009) [18][a]	22/80 (27.5%)	adult/ child	ND		39.8	ND		ND	±	18 FND, 3 SAH, 1 ICH	2–7 for FND, 1–2 for SAH, 4 for ICH	ND	BPC, edavarone, pedicle ligation for 1 SAH	no PND for all
Ohue (2008) [17][b]	8/24 (33.3%)	adult only	4	4	24 (18–37)	3	5	6 ischemia, 2 Hmr	+	5 aphasia, 4 HP, 2 senseD, 1 Sz, 1 dysarthria	5.1 (0–14)	5.1 (0–14)	ND	no PND for all
Kim (2008) [7]	9/61 (14.8%)	adult only	3	6	33 (19–60)	5	4	5 TIA, 3 TIA/Inf, 1 Inf	+	3 aphasia, 3 hand weakness, 2 dysarthria, 1 senseD, 1 Sz	3.4 (1–6)	6.7 (2–12)	BPC, anticon vulsant, steroid, citicoline	no PND for all

BPC Strict blood pressure control, *FND* focal neurologic deficit, *FP* facial palsy, *Hmr* hemorrhage, *HP* hemiparesis, *ICH* intracerebral hemorrhage, *Inf* cerebral infarction, *MP* monoparesis, *ND* no data, *PND* permanent neurologic deficit, *SAH* subarachnoid hemorrhage, *senseD* sensory deficit, *Sz* seizure, *TIA* transient ischemic attack, *TIA/Inf* transient ischemic attack with cerebral infarction, *TIA/Sz* transient ischemic attack with seizure

[a] Some data are overlapped between the reports.

[b] The results of this report are actually based on postoperative temporary neurological deficits. Three of them were proven to be hyperperfusion syndrome by SPECT. One case with indirect bypass is omitted from the data in the original report.

proportionally low. Nevertheless, there are many recent reports concerning hemodynamics that suggest that STA-MCA bypass *can* result in symptomatic cerebral hyperperfusion in MMD (Table 1) [3–6, 12, 14]. According to these data, post-bypass symptomatic hyperperfusion (PBSH) after direct bypass has similar clinical features, and may be defined if the following issues are included [7, 18].

The commonest clinical manifestations of PBSH are transient and focal neurologic deficits or seizures. In severe cases, PBSH can also cause intracranial hemorrhage such as ICH or subarachnoid hemorrhage (SAH). Some patients, however, have an asymptomatic period that follows full postoperative recovery. In all cases, hemodynamic study including brain SPECT shows the presence of the significant increase in CBF at the site of the anastomosis, the condition responsible for neurological symptoms. There is apparent visualization of patent anastomosis by angiography with the absence of any ischemic changes on diffusion-weighted MRI. It is unusual to observe other pathologies, e.g., compression of the brain surface by the temporal muscle inserted for indirect revascularization or subdural hematoma as observed by MRI.

Incidence

TND occurs after STA-MCA bypass surgery for ischemic cerebral diseases. Some patients suffer transient ischemic attacks or reversible focal neurological deficits that last up to a few days or weeks even if they are normal by CT, MRI or angiography. In a study of 134 consecutive such operations, Heros et al. [19] found that all but 5 patients without CT or angiography abnormalities exhibited postoperative TND different from the preoperative symptoms. In fact, postoperative TND occurs in about 4–20% of patients [19, 20]. In our study of 120 procedures, 20 (17%) of adult patients suffered from post-bypass TND with chronic ischemic cerebral diseases (e.g., ASD and MMD) [7]. This frequency is far higher than the reported incidence of cerebral hyperperfusion syndrome following CEA and stenting (0–3%) [7, 21]. In our experience with adult MMD patients, the incidence of post-bypass TND was 14.8% (9 out of 61), an outcome attributable to hyperperfusion [7]. Ohue et al. [22] report a 27% incidence of post-bypass TNDs in adult MMD. The incidence of PBSH is substantially greater among adult that pediatric MMD patients. Fujimura et al. report that the symptomatic hyperperfusion syndrome occurs in 27.5% surgeries for adult MMD [18] but only 11.8% for pediatric ones.

Pathophysiology

The underlying mechanism by which PBSH and other symptoms of MMD become manifest is not yet understood. Cerebral ischemia causes resistant vessels to dilate, thereby accommodating the increase in local CBF. After a long period of such dilation, the vessels may become atonic and lack autoregulation, resulting in hyperperfusion and consequent local cerebral edema. These processes culminate in transient localized cortical dysfunction [23]. Indeed, ipsilateral CBF increases to 20–40% over baseline in most patients immediately after CEA. Although this syndrome typically lasts for several hours, it is generally asymptomatic [21]. In severe cases, long-lasting hyperperfusion may increase CBF to as much as 100–200% over baseline, reaching a maximal 3–4 days after surgery. Though it falls to a steady

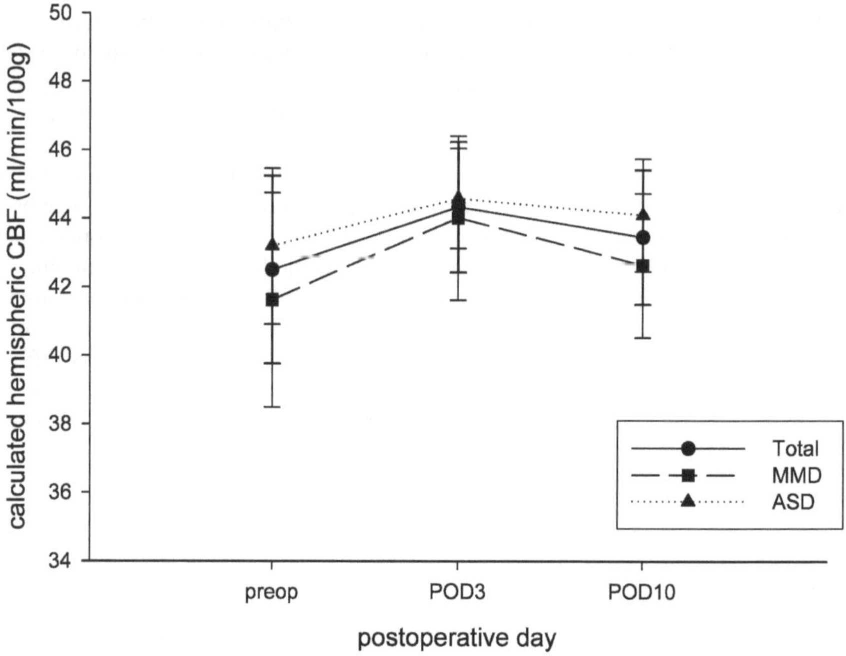

Fig. 1 Twenty-five basal SPECT taken on the preoperative and the third and tenth postoperative days using statistical parametric mapping (SPM) and a probabilistic brain atlas (from [7], with permission). The cerebral blood flow (CBF) increases on the third postoperative day ($p<0.001$) and then decreases on the tenth day ($p=0.006$). The mean values of calculated hemispheric CBF are 42.5 ml/min/100 g preoperatively, 44.3 on the third day, and 43.5 on the tenth day (*solid line*). Such a change of CBF is more exaggerated in moyamoya disease (*long dashed line*) than in atherosclerotic disease (*dotted line*). *preop* Preoperative, *POD3* the third postoperative day, *POD10* the tenth postoperative day, *MMD* moyamoya disease, *ASD* atherosclerotic disease

state by the sixth or seventh postoperative day, elevated blood flow can last 1–2 weeks [21]. In such extreme situations, patients suffer from the symptomatic cerebral hyperperfusion syndrome after CEA. In our experience with chronic ischemic cerebral diseases, the change of CBF in one hemisphere after STA-MCA bypass was much less than after CEA when measured by a hemisphere-based SPECT examination (Fig. 1) [7]. In SPECT images, however, the hyperperfused area appeared as a very bright focal spot around the anastomosis site [7, 8, 17, 18, 20, 24, 25]. Though we were unable to measure the changes in focal CBF in the area closest to the anastomotic site, we speculate that their focal characteristics explain post-bypass TND after STA-MCA bypass. Supporting that hypothesis, we note that focal lesions shown on the SPECT images correlated with clinical symptoms exhibited by those patients [7, 8, 20, 24, 25].

In our experience, relative hyperperfusion on the third versus tenth postoperative day is greater in MMD than in ASD (Fig. 1) [7]. The difference can be explained by postulating different mechanisms of hyperperfusion syndrome in the two diseases. MMD is characterized by bilateral steno-occlusive changes at the terminal portion of the internal carotid artery. Unlike in ASD, of which the angioarchitecture is typically normal in vessels other than the occluded one, the angioarchitecture in MMD causes the territory irrigated by major branches of the internal carotid artery to be sequestered and compartmentalized. Once focal hyperperfusion in MCA territories occurs following STA-MCA bypass, it is buffered against spreading into other vascular territories. Consequently, focal cerebral edema caused by such focal hyperperfusion is more severe in MMD than in ASD. The molecular biology of surrounding brain tissue presumably also contributes to the etiology of MMD. Among proteins implicated in the pathogenesis of MMD are bFGF [26], HGF [27], VCAM-1 [28], ICAM-1, CRABP-1 [28], and MMP-9 [29]. In their capacity as growth factors and cell adhesion molecules, these proteins contribute to angiogenesis but at the same time also affect vascular permeability in the chronically ischemic cortex. The incidence of tissue hyperperfusion in MMD may make the ischemic cortex more vulnerable to the adverse effects of these proteins. Because reactive oxygen species (ROS) probably contribute to reperfusion injury in the ischemic brain [30, 31], formation of such reactive molecules upon vascular reconstruction is also apt to exacerbate tissue damage in the chronically ischemic brain. The pathologies associated with this syndrome may result from an abnormal spectrum of ROS, an increase in tissue vulnerability to these molecules, and/or a change in the expression of antioxidant enzymes consequent upon vascular reconstruction [30, 31].

Clinical Manifestation

Episodes of PBSH in MMD are characterized by their new-onset, transient, and focal nature [7, 8, 17, 20, 24, 25]. Such neurological deterioration differs from preexisting, preoperative neurologic symptoms and is sometimes more severe. The attributes listed above differentiate hyperperfusion syndrome from persisting transient ischemic attacks or aggravation of unrelated preexisting symptoms. The neurological deterioration from PBSH has a definite period without neurological deficits after recovery from anesthesia. According to the literature, defining symptoms are first observed between the 1st and 11th postoperative day and persist during 0–14 days. In rare instances, symptoms continue for longer periods (up to 3 months) (Table 1) [7, 8, 17, 18, 20, 22, 25]. These findings are consistent with the hemodynamic data from CEA (see the *Pathophysiology* section). It must be noted that the symptoms of hyperperfusion syndrome are also focal and well correlated with cortical dysfunctions around the site of anastomosis. In many cases, the recipient vessel is the M4 branch of MCA. Consequently, physiological deficit relates to perisylvian cortical function, e.g., motor dysfunction of the tongue, hands, and arms, as well as aphasia (Table 1) [7, 8, 17, 18, 20, 22, 25].

Imaging

Imaging techniques usually reveal phenomena secondary to hyperperfusion. Nevertheless, they can provide information enabling the diagnosis of PBSH. Brain CT and MRI often detect focal effacement of gyri around the anastomotic site, a hallmark of brain edema. They can also reveal hemorrhages (e.g., ICH and SAH) distant from locus of surgery. The latter sort of lesion is most frequently observed at the site of an earlier infarction or in an area with decreased basal perfusion as determined by preoperative SPECT [8, 18]. By contrast, diffusion-weighted MRI does not clearly reveal infarction around and adjacent to the anastomotic site [7, 8, 18, 20, 24, 25]. CT and MRI scans often reveal such malformations as the mass effect of a swollen muscle flap for indirect revascularization [32], a subdural hematoma [12], or a definite infarction around the anastomotic site. These pathologies are typically not a direct result of PBSH. A prominently greater signal from the donor over the contralateral STA as detected by MR angiography is a signature of PBSH [8, 18, 24]. Another telltale image sometimes seen by MR angiography is increased branching of the MCA around the site of anastomosis when compared to the preoperative formation [8]. One must be cautious when interpreting such information, however, as PBSH is not the only known cause of the aforementioned findings. Moreover, surgical manipulation of the STA can affect the results of MR angiography [8]. The rapid filling and washout of contrast material in the MCA territory as imaged by MR digital subtraction angiography has also been cited as a confounding variable [20]. Detection by SPECT of abnormal cerebral hemodynamics is indispensable to firmly diagnose PBSH. The syndrome is invariably associated with a large increase in CBF around the anastomotic site relative to the preoperative situation. If SPECT is not available, the physician can substitute perfusion CT or perfusion MRI as a means of evaluating cerebral hemodynamics [8, 20, 25].

Exemplary Case

A 24-year-old man with no marked risk factors for atherosclerosis was admitted to our hospital with a 1-month history of recurrent episodes of right hemiparesis. Each such episode lasted 5–10 min. Cerebral angiography revealed complete occlusion of the bilateral distal internal carotid artery bifurcation, and a system of diffuse fine basal collateral vessels. On the basis of these observations, he was diagnosed with MMD (Fig. 2a). Preoperative T2-weighted MRI revealed bilateral occipital infarctions and diffuse brain atrophy, particularly in the left temporoparietal area (Fig. 2b). Consistent with these findings, we noted decreased basal CBF in the left temporo-parieto-occipital lobe as determined by SPECT (Fig. 3a, 36.0 ml/min/100 g of calculated hemispheric CBF) and decreased cerebrovascular reserve capacity (Fig. 3b). Recognizing symptoms characteristic of the left hemisphere being in a misery perfusion state, we undertook an STA-MCA bypass surgery with indirect encephalo-duro-galeo-synangiosis (EDGS). The operation was completed without complications. Moreover, the patient was free of neurological deficits upon awaking from anesthesia. We began postoperative antiplatelet therapy immediately. On the second postoperative day, speech disturbance began to appear and progressed to complete aphasia within several hours despite the absence of other neurological deficits. Neither CT nor diffusion MRI revealed intracranial hemorrhage or any other acute infarction (data not shown). SPECT performed on the third postoperative day revealed an increase in basal perfusion in the left superior temporal and inferior parietal lobes around the anastomosis site as compared to preoperative basal perfusion (Fig. 3c). The calculated hemispheric CBF was 41.2 ml/min/100 g. Because this finding suggested post-bypass hyperperfusion, the patient's blood pressure was strictly controlled within the preoperative range. The patient's aphasia passed spontaneously over the next few days, and his verbal ability returned to normal levels by the seventh postoperative day. On the tenth postoperative day, SPECT revealed that focal intense accumulation of tracer in the left superior temporal and inferior parietal lobe around the anastomosis site was no longer present (Fig. 3d). In addition, hemispheric CBF was determined to be 40.5 ml/min/100 g. Upon discharge, the patient exhibited no neurological deficits and returned to work. Cerebral angiography performed 6 months postsurgery confirmed that blood was flowing to the left hemisphere through the direct STA-MCA anastomosis and the indirect EDGS.

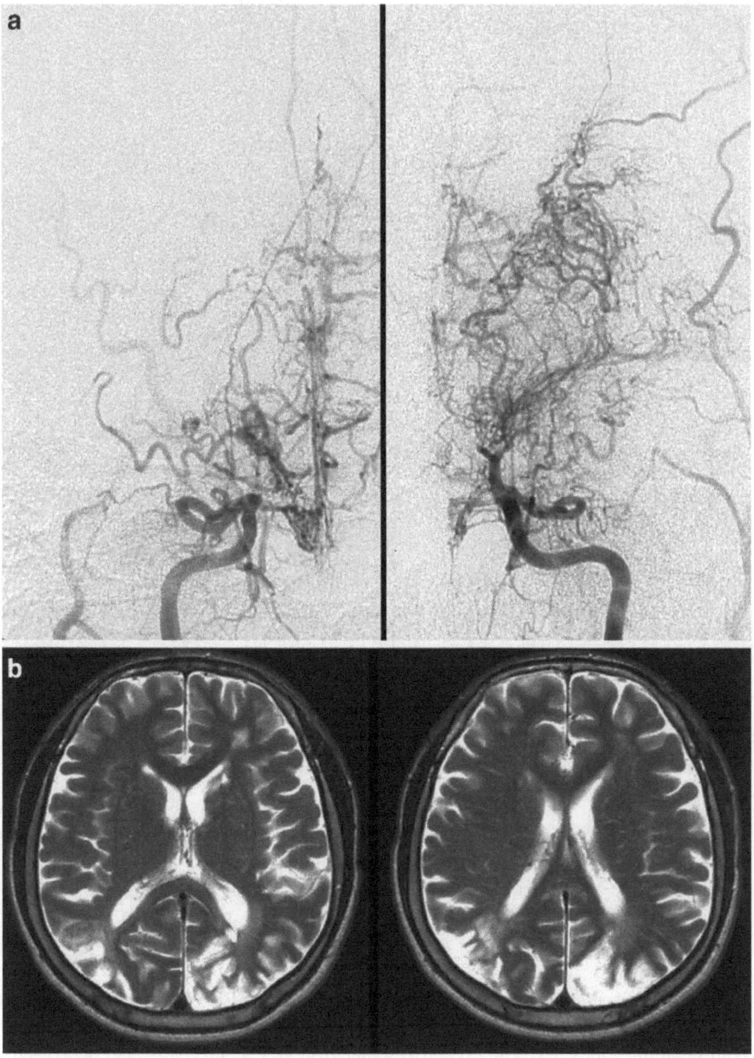

Fig. 2 (**a**) Internal carotid angiography demonstrates the complete occlusion of the terminal internal carotid artery and the profuse basal collateral vessels, which is compatible with the diagnosis of moyamoya disease. (**b**) Preoperative MRI shows an old infarction in both occipital lobes and in the left temporal lobe, resulting in cerebromalacia and brain atrophy in those regions

Preoperative Prognostics (Table 2)

There have been three reports concerning prognostics for PBSH. The most important risk factors are advanced age, hemorrhagic onset, diminished basal cerebral perfusion, and cerebrovascular reserve as measured by preoperative SPECT [7, 17, 18]. The patients at the greatest risk of developing PBSH are older individuals in whom preoperative CBF is reduced and cerebrovascular reserve is diminished.

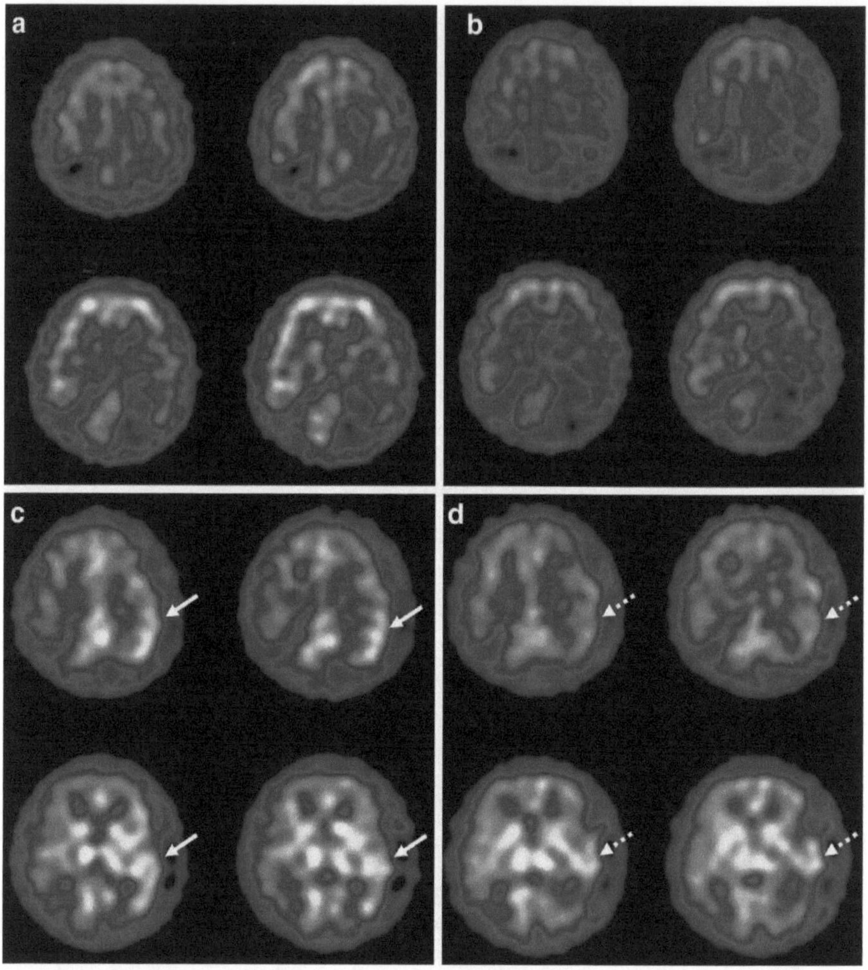

Fig. 3 (**a**) Preoperative acetazolamide-challenged brain perfusion SPECT images showing that the basal cerebral blood flow (CBF) was decreased in the left temporoparietal lobe and that there was a perfusion defect in both occipital lobes. (**b**) The cerebrovascular reserve capacity was also decreased in the left temporoparietal lobe. (**c**) The third postoperative day basal brain perfusion SPECT images showing the hyperperfusion in the left superior temporal lobe and the left inferior parietal lobe around the anastomosis site (*solid arrow*). (**d**) This hyperperfusion had decreased in brain SPECT images taken on the tenth postoperative day (*broken arrow*)

Treatment

The treatment for PBSH is opposite to that for ischemia. The commonest procedure is strict control of blood pressure. Since its cerebral autoregulation is impaired, excessive CBF must be prevented by limiting diastolic pressure. At the same time, systolic pressure must be kept high enough to prevent ischemic insult to brain tissue that is potentially ischemic in MMD. The most successful strategy is to rigidly maintain the mean arterial pressure within 20–30 mm Hg from the preoperative level throughout the first 7 days after surgery. In our facility, all high-risk

Table 2 Reports on the predictors for symptomatic hyperperfusion syndrome after direct bypass in MMD

			p-value	
Author	Predictors		Univariate	Multivariate
Fujimura (2009) [18]	age		0.0134*	–
		Adult-onset, age (≥16)	0.0128*	–
	sex		0.2462	–
	onset-type	Hemorrhage	0.0267*	–
		Cerebral infarction	0.3463	–
	side of the operated hemisphere		0.2506	–
	temporary occlusion time		0.6217	–
Ohue (2008) [17][a]	sex		NS	–
	age		<0.01*	–
	onset		NS	–
	side		NS	–
	angiographic staging		0.07	–
	CBF	Preoperative rest rCBF	NS	–
		Preoperative ΔCBF	<0.05*	–
		Postoperative rest rCBF	NS	–
		Postoperative ΔCBF	NS	–
Kim (2008) [7][b]	age		0.415	0.197
	sex		0.556	0.988
	hypertension		0.065	0.283
	diabetes mellitus		0.209	0.505
	hypercholesterolemia		0.296	0.194
	smoking		0.392	0.298
	family history		0.542	0.396
	presentation		0.26	0.252
	diagnosis		0.81	0.857
	decrease in both basal perfusion and cerebrovascular reserve on preop SPECT		<0.000*	<0.000*
	operative site		0.454	0.685
	double bypass		0.282	0.223
	co-indirect revascularization		0.325	0.988
	recipient artery		0.714	0.75
	postoperative perfusion ratio		0.312	0.586

rCBF Regional cerebral blood flow, ΔCBF = (acetazolamide rCBF-rest rCBF)/rest rCBF × 100

[a] The results of this report are actually based on postoperative temporary neurological deficits. Three of them were proven to be hyperperfusion syndrome by SPECT.

[b] This unpublished data include the STA-MCA bypass for atherosclerotic disease.

*Statistically significant

patients are kept in the ICU for the first 3 postoperative days and their bodily functions are monitored continually. While various medications are administered to MMD patients, there is little decisive information concerning their relative benefits for PBSH. Common pharmacologic agents and their mode of actions are as follows: clonidine, a centrally acting α2-agonist; nicardipine, a calcium channel blocker; edaravone, a free radical scavenger; citicoline, a cell membrane stabilizer; anticonvulsants and steroids (Table 1). It is noteworthy that antioxidant agents have been found to prevent hyperperfusion syndrome following CEA in patients with ASD. Moreover, they markedly affect cerebrovascular reserve capacity [33].

Conclusion

Direct bypass is an effective and relatively safe treatment for adult MMD. Unfortunately, postoperative TND due to hyperperfusion occurs with substantial frequency. Consequently, surgery must be preceded by accurate diagnosis, and appropriate management for this symptomatic hyperperfusion and other postoperative procedures must be meticulously conducted in order to avoid symptomatic hyperperfusion.

References

1. Kuroda S, Houkin K (2008) Moyamoya disease: current concepts and future perspectives. Lancet Neurol 7:1056–1066
2. Mesiwala AH, Sviri G, Fatemi N et al (2008) Long-term outcome of superficial temporal artery-middle cerebral artery bypass for patients with moyamoya disease in the US. Neurosurg Focus 24:E15
3. Robertson RL, Burrows PE, Barnes PD et al (1997) Angiographic changes after pial synangiosis in childhood moyamoya disease. Am J Neuroradiol 18:837–845
4. Veeravagu A, Guzman R, Patil CG et al (2008) Moyamoya disease in pediatric patients: outcomes of neurosurgical interventions. Neurosurg Focus 24:E16
5. Zipfel GJ, Fox DJ Jr, Rivet DJ (2005) Moyamoya disease in adults: the role of cerebral revascularization. Skull Base 15:27–41
6. Ishikawa T, Kamiyama H, Kuroda S et al (2006) Simultaneous superficial temporal artery to middle cerebral or anterior cerebral artery bypass with pan-synangiosis for moyamoya disease covering both anterior and middle cerebral artery territories. Neurol Med Chir (Tokyo) 46:462–468
7. Kim JE, Oh CW, Kwon OK et al (2008) Transient hyperperfusion after superficial temporal artery/middle cerebral artery bypass surgery as a possible cause of postoperative transient neurological deterioration. Cerebrovasc Dis 25:580–586
8. Fujimura M, Kaneta T, Mugikura S et al (2007) Temporary neurologic deterioration due to cerebral hyperperfusion after superficial temporal artery-middle cerebral artery anastomosis in patients with adult-onset moyamoya disease. Surg Neurol 67:273–282
9. Kawaguchi S, Okuno S, Sakaki T (2000) Effect of direct arterial bypass on the prevention of future stroke in patients with the hemorrhagic variety of moyamoya disease. J Neurosurg 93:397–401
10. Houkin K, Kuroda S, Ishikawa T et al (2000) Neovascularization (angiogenesis) after revascularization in moyamoya disease. Which technique is most useful for moyamoya disease? Acta Neurochir (Wien) 142:269–276
11. Mizoi K, Kayama T, Yoshimoto T et al (1996) Indirect revascularization for moyamoya disease: is there a beneficial effect for adult patients? Surg Neurol 45:541–548; discussion 548–549
12. Houkin K, Ishikawa T, Yoshimoto T et al (1997) Direct and indirect revascularization for moyamoya disease surgical techniques and peri-operative complications. Clin Neurol Neurosurg 99 (Suppl 2):S142–145
13. Matsushima T, Inoue T, Suzuki SO et al (1992) Surgical treatment of moyamoya disease in pediatric patients – comparison between the results of indirect and direct revascularization procedures. Neurosurgery 31:401–405
14. Hosoda K, Kawaguchi T, Shibata Y et al (2001) Cerebral vasoreactivity and internal carotid artery flow help to identify patients at risk for hyperperfusion after carotid endarterectomy. Stroke 32:1567–1573
15. Piepgras DG, Morgan MK, Sundt TM Jr et al (1988) Intracerebral hemorrhage after carotid endarterectomy. J Neurosurg 68:532–536

16. Ogasawara K, Yukawa H, Kobayashi M et al (2003) Prediction and monitoring of cerebral hyperperfusion after carotid endarterectomy by using single-photon emission computerized tomography scanning. J Neurosurg 99:504–510
17. Ohue S, Kumon Y, Kohno K et al (2008) Postoperative temporary neurological deficits in adults with moyamoya disease. Surg Neurol 69:281–286; discussion 286–287
18. Fujimura M, Mugikura S, Kaneta T et al (2009) Incidence and risk factors for symptomatic cerebral hyperperfusion after superficial temporal artery-middle cerebral artery anastomosis in patients with moyamoya disease. Surg Neurol 71:442–447
19. Heros RC, Scott RM, Kistler JP et al (1984) Temporary neurological deterioration after extracranial-intracranial bypass. Neurosurgery 15:178–185
20. Furuya K, Kawahara N, Morita A et al (2004) Focal hyperperfusion after superficial temporal artery-middle cerebral artery anastomosis in a patient with moyamoya disease. Case report. J Neurosurg 100:128–132
21. van Mook WN, Rennenberg RJ, Schurink GW et al (2005) Cerebral hyperperfusion syndrome. Lancet Neurol 4:877–888
22. Fujimura M, Kaneta T, Tominaga T (2008) Efficacy of superficial temporal artery-middle cerebral artery anastomosis with routine postoperative cerebral blood flow measurement during the acute stage in childhood moyamoya disease. Childs Nerv Syst 24:827–832
23. Higashi S, Matsuda H, Fujii H et al (1989) Luxury perfusion syndrome confirmed by sequential studies of regional cerebral blood flow and volume after extracranial to intracranial bypass surgery: case report. Neurosurgery 25:85–89
24. Fujimura M, Kaneta T, Shimizu H et al (2007) Symptomatic hyperperfusion after superficial temporal artery-middle cerebral artery anastomosis in a child with moyamoya disease. Childs Nerv Syst 23:1195–1198
25. Ogasawara K, Komoribayashi N, Kobayashi M et al (2005) Neural damage caused by cerebral hyperperfusion after arterial bypass surgery in a patient with moyamoya disease: case report. Neurosurgery 56:E1380; discussion E1380
26. Houkin K, Yoshimoto T, Abe H et al (1998) Role of basic fibroblast growth factor in the pathogenesis of moyamoya disease. Neurosurg Focus 5:e2
27. Nanba R, Kuroda S, Ishikawa T et al (2004) Increased expression of hepatocyte growth factor in cerebrospinal fluid and intracranial artery in moyamoya disease. Stroke 35:2837–2842
28. Soriano SG, Cowan DB, Proctor MR et al (2002) Levels of soluble adhesion molecules are elevated in the cerebrospinal fluid of children with moyamoya syndrome. Neurosurgery 50:544–549
29. Fujimura M, Watanabe M, Narisawa A et al (2009) Increased expression of serum matrix metalloproteinase-9 in patients with moyamoya disease. Surg Neurol [in press, available online]
30. Chan PH (1996) Role of oxidants in ischemic brain damage. Stroke 27:1124–1129
31. Fujimura M, Tominaga T, Chan PH (2005) Neuroprotective effect of an antioxidant in ischemic brain injury: involvement of neuronal apoptosis. Neurocrit Care 2:59–66
32. Fujimura M, Kaneta T, Shimizu H et al (2009) Cerebral ischemia owing to compression of the brain by swollen temporal muscle used for encephalo-myo-synangiosis in moyamoya disease. Neurosurg Rev 32:245–249
33. Ogasawara K, Inoue T, Kobayashi M et al (2004) Pretreatment with the free radical scavenger edaravone prevents cerebral hyperperfusion after carotid endarterectomy. Neurosurgery 55:1060–1067

Part XIII
Special Consideration II

Moyamoya Syndrome: Pial Synangiosis

Edward R. Smith and R. Michael Scott

Introduction

Moyamoya syndrome is an arteriopathy characterized by progressive stenosis at the apices of the intracranial internal carotid arteries associated with cerebral ischemia. As the internal carotids undergo this reduction in flow, the brain compensates through the development of smaller collateral vessels. This alternative blood supply provides circulation to the region formerly supplied by the internal carotids, and this fine network of vessels arises from the carotid apex, the leptomeninges, and branches of the external carotid artery supplying the dura and skull base. Although usually limited to the anterior circulation, there are rare cases where the process encompasses the posterior circulation as well, including the basilar and posterior cerebral arteries. The appearance of this collateral network on angiogram has been compared to a puff of smoke; in Japanese, "moyamoya."

Diagnosis is made on the basis of radiographic evidence of these typical angiographic changes and, when present, clinical evidence of ischemia. There is a distinction between moyamoya *syndrome* and moyamoya *disease*. Individuals with a well-recognized associated condition (Table 1) are categorized as having moyamoya syndrome while those idiopathic cases with no known risk factors have moyamoya disease. By definition, the pathognomic arteriographic findings must be found bilaterally in moyamoya disease (although the severity can vary between sides). Those patients with angiographic findings only on one side are considered to have moyamoya syndrome, even if no other conditions are present [1]. When used alone, the term moyamoya refers solely to the distinctive findings on arteriogram, independent of etiology.

E.R. Smith and R.M. Scott (✉)
Department of Neurosurgery, Children's Hospital, Harvard Medical School,
300 Longwood Avenue, Boston, MA 02115, USA
e-mail: edward.smith@childrens.harvard.edu; michael.scott@childrens.harvard.edu

B.-K. Cho and T. Tominaga (eds.), *Moyamoya Disease Update*,
DOI 10.1007/978-4-431-99703-0_44, © Springer 2010

Table 1 Associated conditions, risk factors, or syndromes

Syndrome	Number
No associated conditions (idiopathic)	66
Neurofibromatosis type I (NF 1)	16
Asian	16
Cranial therapeutic radiation	15
Hypothalamic-optic system glioma	8
Craniopharyngioma	4
Medulloblastoma, with Gorlin's Syndrome	1
Acute lymphocytic leukemia, intrathecal chemotherapy	2
Down syndrome	10
Congenital cardiac anomaly, previously-operated	7
Renal artery stenosis	4
Hemoglobinopathy (2 sickle cell, 1 "Bryn Mawr")	3
Other hematologic (1 spherocytosis, 1 ITP)	2
Giant cervico-facial hemangiomas	3
Shunted hydrocephalus	3
Idiopathic hypertension requiring medication	3
Hyperthyroidism (one with Graves syndrome)	2

Other syndromes, one patient each: Reyes (remote), Williams, Alagille, cloacal extrophy, renal artery fibromuscular dysplasia, and congenital cytomegalic inclusion virus infection (remote). Two patients had unclassified syndromic presentations. There were four African Americans, two of whom had sickle cell disease [4].

Incidence and Epidemiology

First described in Japan and once considered a condition primarily limited to individuals of Asian ancestry, it has now been reported in all ethnicities around the world. Incidence peaks in two age groups; the first at around 5 years of age and the second in the mid-40s. Females are affected about twice as commonly as males. Moyamoya is the most common pediatric cerebrovascular disease in Japan with a prevalence of approximately 3/100,000. The European incidence appears to be about 1/10th of that observed in Japan. Results from a recent American review suggest an incidence of 0.086/100,000 persons. Ethnicity-specific incidence rate ratios compared to whites were 4.6 for Asian-Americans, 2.2 for African-Americans, and 0.5 for Hispanics [1].

Clinical Features and Presentation

Patients with moyamoya become symptomatic secondary to decreased flow to the regions of the brain supplied by the internal carotid arteries. In general, there are two major etiologic categories of patient symptoms: those due to cerebral ischemia [stroke, transient ischemic attacks (TIAs), seizures] and those due to the deleterious consequences of the compensatory mechanisms responding to the ischemia (hemorrhage from fragile collateral vessels, headache from dilated transdural collaterals). Individual variation in degrees of arterial involvement, rates of progression, regions of ischemic cortex, and response to the reduction in blood supply help to explain the wide range of clinical presentations. Approximately 14% of all patients with moyamoya will have unilateral arteriopathy at the time of diagnosis [2].

In the United States, the majority of affected adults and children present with ischemic symptoms. Notably, the rate of hemorrhage is approximately seven times greater in adults than in children (20 vs 2.8%) [3, 4]. Manifestations of the condition vary in different geographic regions. Reports from Asian populations indicate that adults have much higher rates of hemorrhage as a presenting symptom (42%) as compared to US patients. In contrast, it is extremely rare for children to present with hemorrhage (2.8%); they generally present with TIAs or ischemic strokes (68%) [4]. Children have a higher rate of completed strokes, a circumstance considered to be secondary to immature verbal and reporting skills, making them unable to communicate TIA symptoms clearly and thus delaying diagnosis and increasing the likelihood that completed a stroke will occur [1].

Once identified, the natural history of moyamoya is variable. Disease progression can be slow with rare, intermittent events or fulminant with rapid neurological decline [4]. However, regardless of the course, moyamoya inevitably progresses in the majority of patients [5, 6].

Rationale for Treatment

The prognosis of moyamoya syndrome is difficult to predict because the natural history of this disorder has not yet been elucidated. Overall prognosis of patients with moyamoya syndrome depends on the rapidity and extent of vascular occlusion, the patient's ability to develop effective collateral circulation, the age at onset of symptoms, the severity of presenting neurological deficits and degree of disability, and the extent of infarction seen on computed tomography or magnetic resonance imaging studies at the time of initial presentation [7]. In general, neurological status at time of treatment, more so than age of the patient, predicts long-term outcome [4, 8].

A recent report indicated that the rate of disease progression is high, even in asymptomatic patients, and that medical therapy alone does not halt disease progression [9]. It has been estimated that up to two-thirds of patients with moyamoya have symptomatic progression over a 5-year period; outcome is poor without treatment [1]. In contrast, the estimated rate of symptomatic progression is only 2.6% following surgery according to a recent meta-analysis of 1,156 patients [10]. Importantly, if surgical revascularization is performed prior to disabling infarction in moyamoya syndrome, even if severe angiographic changes are present, the prognosis tends to be excellent [1]. However, if left untreated, both the angiographic process and the clinical syndrome invariably progress, producing clinical deterioration with potentially irreversible neurological deficits over time [1]. Thus, early diagnosis of moyamoya coupled with expeditious institution of therapy is of paramount importance.

Surgical Treatment: Overview

There are a number of studies in the literature that support a role for surgical management of moyamoya disease, and surgery is generally recommended for the treatment of patients with recurrent or progressive cerebral ischemic events and associated reduced cerebral perfusion reserve [1]. Many different operative techniques have been described, all with the main goal of preventing further ischemic injury by increasing collateral blood flow to hypoperfused areas of cortex, using the external carotid circulation as a donor supply [11, 12].

Various bypass procedures have been performed in the treatment of moyamoya disease which can generally be divided into direct and indirect types. Direct anastomosis procedures [most commonly superficial temporal artery (STA) to middle cerebral artery (MCA) bypasses] may achieve instant improvement in focal cerebral perfusion, but these procedures are often technically difficult to perform because small pediatric patients often do not have a large enough donor scalp artery or recipient MCA to allow for a anastomosis large enough to supply a significant amount of additional collateral blood supply. Because of proximal stenoses, new blood supply provided to a single MCA branch may not allow wide redistribution of the newly available collateral. Temporary occlusion of a middle cerebral branch during the anastomosis may interfere with leptomeningeal collateral pathways already present and lead to an increased incidence of perioperative stroke.

A variety of indirect anastomotic procedures have been described: encephaloduroarterio-synangiosis (EDAS) whereby the STA is dissected free over a course of several inches and then sutured to the cut edges of the opened dura; encephalomyosynangiosis in which the temporalis muscle is dissected and placed onto the surface of the brain to encourage collateral vessel development; and the combination of both: encephalo-myo-arterio-synangiosis. There are multiple variations of these procedures including only drilling burr holes without vessel anastomosis and craniotomy with inversion of the dura in hopes of enhancing new dural revascularization of the brain. Cervical sympathectomy and omental transposition or omental pedicle grafting have also been described [1].

Pial Synangiosis: Technique

At Children's Hospital Boston, we utilize a modification of the EDAS procedure to treat moyamoya syndrome in both children and adults termed "pial synangiosis" which has demonstrated superb induction of new collateral vessels in the patient with chronic ischemia due to moyamoya [12]. The technique involves the following steps: (1) a scalp donor artery (most commonly, the parietal branch of the STA) is dissected from distal to proximal along with a cuff of galea and surrounding soft tissue (Fig. 1); (2) a large craniotomy is turned in the region that is subjacent to the artery; (3) the dura is opened into at least six flaps in order to increase the surface area of dura exposed to the pial surface and thereby enhance formation of collateral vessels from the dural vascular supply; (4) the arachnoid is opened widely over the surface of brain exposed by the dural opening (Fig. 2); and (5) the intact donor artery is sutured directly to the pial surface using four to six interrupted 10-0 nylon sutures placed through the donor vessel adventitia and the underlying pia (Figs. 1 and 2). The bone flap is replaced over a gel-foam cover of the dura which is left widely open and carefully secured to avoid compression of the donor artery (Fig. 3). The temporal muscle and skin edges are carefully closed with absorbable sutures to similarly avoid compression of the donor vessel. The rationale behind this procedure is that opening the arachnoid removes a barrier to the in-growth of new blood vessels into the brain while also facilitating access of growth factors within the CSF to the donor vessel. Furthermore, the donor vessel's adventitia is sutured to the pial surface to maintain its contact with the brain in areas where the arachnoid has been cleared; providing a stable site for collateral development.

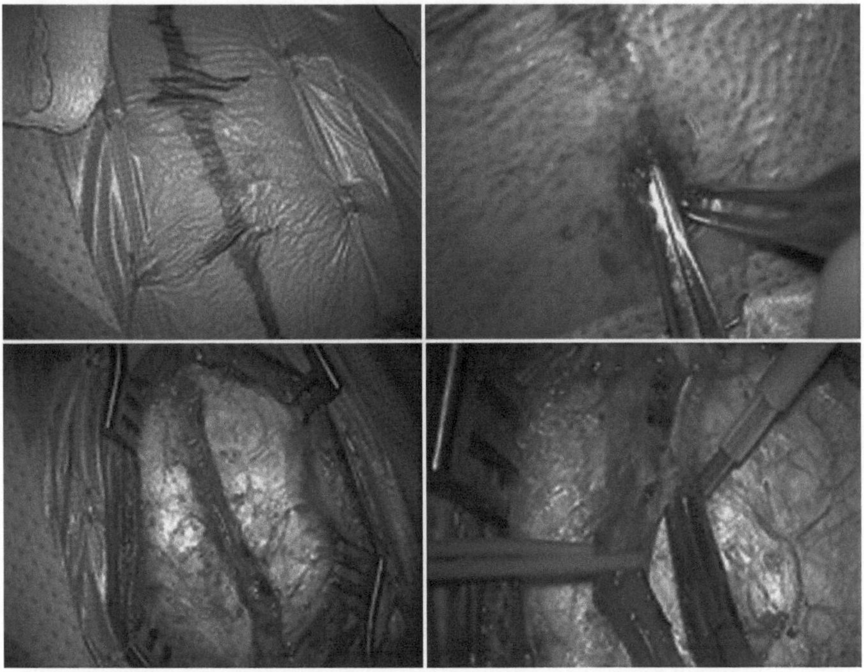

Fig. 1 Extracranial dissection of the superficial temporal artery. (**a**) The course of the artery is marked following mapping with Doppler. (**b**) Using the microscope the artery is dissected along its course, (**c**) revealing a length prepared for synangiosis. (**d**) An adventital cuff is prepared

Pial Synangiosis: Indications

Indications for operative revascularization in moyamoya are broad, given the contrast between the poor response to medical therapy and the documented success of surgery [10]. Two large studies with long-term follow-up demonstrated a good safety profile for surgical treatment of moyamoya (approximately 4% risk of stroke within 30 days of surgery per hemisphere) with a 96% probability of remaining stroke-free over a 5-year follow-up period [4, 13]. A recent meta-analysis of 1,156 moyamoya patients treated with surgery concluded that 87% (1,003 patients) derived symptomatic benefit from surgical revascularization [10]. Given the data supporting the clear and durable benefit of surgery, coupled with the unpredictable but unrelentingly progressive course of the disease, we have adopted a proactive approach to surgical intervention at our institution.

If the diagnosis of moyamoya is made, we will commonly recommend surgery, and the technique of pial synangiosis allows its application to all ages. However, we may defer intervention in the setting of very early (Suzuki stage I) or indeterminate disease. Our data suggest that a substantial number (up to 70%) of unilateral patients may not progress on the contralateral side, making the risk of second-side surgery unnecessary [2]. Careful monitoring with MRI and clinical follow-up in patients with unilateral disease or in patients with unclear diagnoses may help to identify appropriate candidates while avoiding unwarranted operations. Furthermore, patients who are systemically ill or who have had recent large infarcts may not be safe operative candidates, requiring a delay in treatment, often 4–6 weeks.

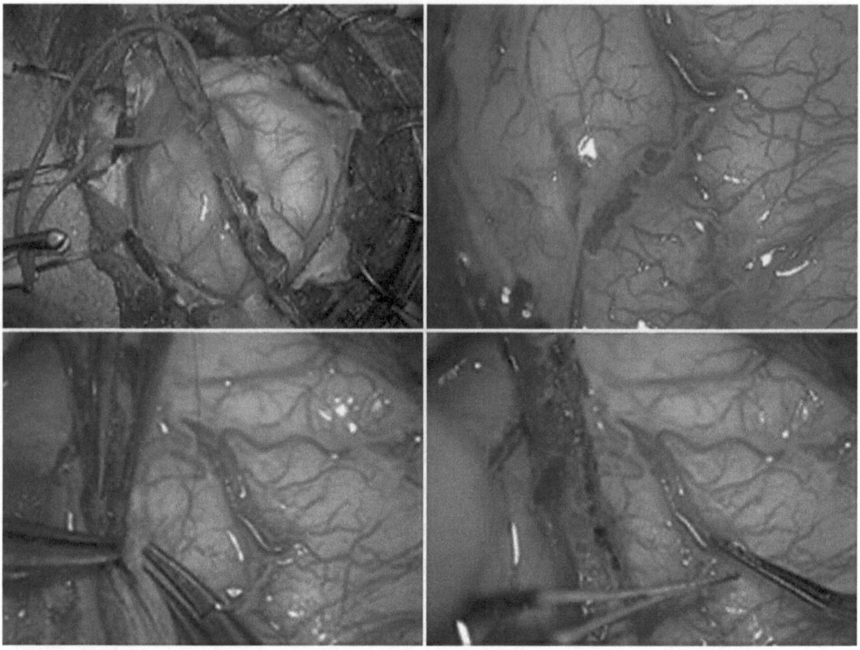

Fig. 2 Intracranial aspects of the pial synangiosis. (**a**) The course of the artery laid out over the exposed region of cortex. (**b**) Using the microscope arachnoid is opened widely and (**c**) the adventital cuff is sutured to the cortex with a pial stitch. (**d**) Once affixed in place, the open arachnoid and stay sutures facilitate ingrowth of new collaterals

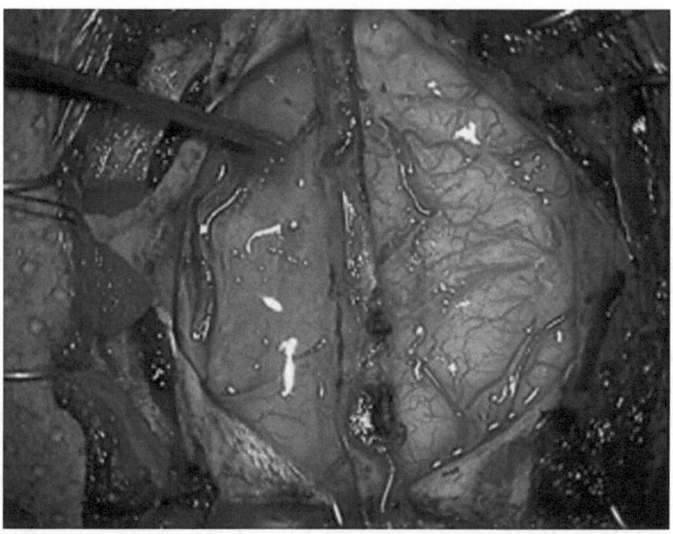

Fig. 3 Final appearance of the synangiosis prior to folding the dura down, laying on Gelfoam and closing the craniotomy

Perioperative Considerations

Once the decision for surgical therapy has been made, several perioperative considerations need to be addressed. In addition to the general issues regarding surgery in children, moyamoya patients are at particular risk of ischemic events in the perioperative period. Risks of surgery are more often related to neurological instability of the patient at the time of surgery and to the risks of anesthesia rather than to actual surgical manipulations. The administration of general anesthesia can result in transient, but significant, physiologic changes which can affect cerebral blood flow. Blood pressure, blood volume, and $PaCO_2$ require careful monitoring because moyamoya patients have a diminished cerebral perfusion reserve, and deviation from normal levels can result in stroke.

To reduce the risk of intraoperative and perioperative neurologic morbidity, meticulous management of the patient is required to avoid hypotension, hypovolemia, hyperthermia, and hypocarbia both intraoperatively as well as perioperatively [12]. To help prevent hypovolemia during surgery, we admit patients the evening prior to surgery for aggressive intravenous hydration. A further perioperative consideration is the use of monitoring, such as intraoperative EEG or near-infrared spectroscopy used to identify and ameliorate ischemic events detected while the patient is under general anesthesia [14, 15]. At our institution, we have been using full scalp EEG monitoring during procedures where both hemispheres will be operated on during the same anesthetic. It has helped us identify situations in which continuing with the second side was felt to be unsafe for the patient, but its definitive role is yet to be established and EEG changes are often observed. We have noted that the addition of thrombin to our gelfoam pledget covering the brain at the time of closure is associated with almost invariable EEG slowing, and we have since omitted the use of thrombin at this stage of the operation, with a marked reduction in the occurrence of this phenomenon.

Postoperatively, the patients are hydrated with intravenous fluids at one and one-half the normal maintenance rate based on weight for 48–72 h. Aspirin is given on the first postoperative day. Crying and hyperventilation, common occurrences in children at times during hospitalization, can lower pCO_2 and induce ischemia secondary to cerebral vasoconstriction. Any techniques to reduce pain – including the use of perioperative sedation, painless wound dressing techniques, and absorbable wound suture closures – helped to reduce the incidence of strokes, TIAs, and length of stay in a recent study [16].

Management Considerations for Subgroups of Patients with Moyamoya Syndrome Which Differ from Moyamoya Disease

There are a number of conditions that are found in association with moyamoya syndrome that require special consideration. In particular, patients with Down syndrome, sickle cell disease, and unilateral moyamoya syndrome can present specific challenges to the treating surgeon. Although the operative technique remains unchanged, there are differences in the preoperative and postoperative management of these complex patients that can profoundly influence outcomes.

Patients with Down syndrome can have cognitive impairments that can limit their ability to communicate changes in their neurological status. These patients require careful perioperative monitoring to identify new symptoms that may herald a TIA or seizure.

These communication issues seem to contribute to a delay in diagnosis in this population; resulting in operative candidates that are older and with higher Suzuki scores than non-Down syndrome moyamoya patients [17]. In addition, these patients have a higher incidence of cardiac anomalies and cervical spine instability, both of which mandate careful consideration to determine if further preoperative evaluation or perioperative alterations in management are needed.

The presence of sickle cell disease in a patient with moyamoya presents a number of significant challenges to the treating surgeon. These children can be quite fragile medically and often have a number of co-morbid conditions that can complicate their hospital stay. They are prone to acute chest syndrome, can have a high tolerance to narcotics secondary to previous exposure during treatments for sickle crises (making pain control difficult), and can have renal impairment which can complicate angiograms or fluid management. We have summarized our experience and described our guidelines for treating these patients previously [18]. Close collaboration with hematology (including scheduled preoperative transfusions and in-hospital consultation when necessary) and anesthesia (for both intraoperative management and postoperative pain control) is very important in the successful treatment of these patients. Long-term, we have found that it may be possible to wean selected patients dependent on exchange transfusions from this requirement

Unilateral moyamoya syndrome prompts questions about treatment strategy (operate on one side or two?) and follow-up (what is the natural history and how should follow-up be done?). If disease is present only on one side, it has been our practice to operate only on the single hemisphere. As discussed previously, up to 70% of unaffected hemispheres will remain unchanged (at least over a 5-year period), making the risk of surgery on the nondiseased side probably unjustified. In addition, it has been our experience that revascularization procedures do not exhibit a significant response when performed on nonischemic hemispheres.

Regarding follow-up, it appears that younger patients are more likely to progress to develop moyamoya on the unaffected hemisphere at a faster rate than do older children. In particular, approximately one-third of children with unilateral moyamoya under the age of 7 years – especially those with any type of angiographic abnormality on the nonaffected side – will develop disease within 1 year from initial diagnosis on average [2]. All children with unilateral moyamoya should be considered for routine follow-up, both clinically and radiographically. Although annual studies and visits may be adequate, one should give consideration to more frequent evaluation for younger children (especially under age 7) or for those with risk factors that may suggest a higher likelihood of progression (such as previous cranial radiation, angiographic abnormalities, cardiac anomalies or a familial history of moyamoya) [2].

Complications and Follow-Up

Potential complications associated with surgical treatment of moyamoya syndrome include postoperative stroke, subdural hematoma (both following trauma and spontaneous), and intracerebral hemorrhage. Although a CSF leak can occur after any cranial procedure, we have only two such complications in our pial synangiosis series – which now numbers over 300 pediatric patients – despite the fact that the dura is left widely open following the synangiosis.

Postoperative angiograms are usually obtained 12 months after surgery and typically demonstrate excellent MCA collateralization from both the donor STA and the meningeal arteries (Fig. 4). A review of 143 children with moyamoya syndrome treated with pial synangiosis had marked reductions in their stroke frequency after surgery, especially after the first year postoperatively. In this group, 67% had strokes preoperatively, 7.7% had strokes in the perioperative period, and only 3.2% had strokes after at least 1 year of follow-up. The long-term results are excellent with a stroke rate of 4.3% (2 patients in a group of 46) in patients with a minimum of 5 years of follow-up [12]. This work supports the premise that pial synangiosis provides a significant protective effect against new strokes in this patient population.

We endeavor to provide long-term follow-up for all our moyamoya patients, utilizing a centralized computer database, and performing annual or biennial MRI/MRA studies and office visits. While this is important for all patients, it is especially useful for those with unilateral disease to monitor for contralateral progression. It has been our practice to keep patients on aspirin permanently.

Conclusions

Moyamoya syndrome is an increasingly recognized entity associated with cerebral ischemia. Diagnosis is made on the basis of clinical and radiographic findings; including a characteristic stenosis of the internal carotid arteries in conjunction with abundant collateral vessel development. Treatment is predicated on revascularization of the ischemic brain which can be direct (STA–MCA bypass) or indirect (including pial synangiosis). Certain groups of patients with moyamoya syndrome have specific issues that require careful attention pre-, peri-, and postoperatively to maximize the likelihood of a good outcome. The use of pial synangiosis is a safe, effective, and durable method of cerebral revascularization in moyamoya syndrome and should be considered as a primary treatment for moyamoya, especially in the pediatric population.

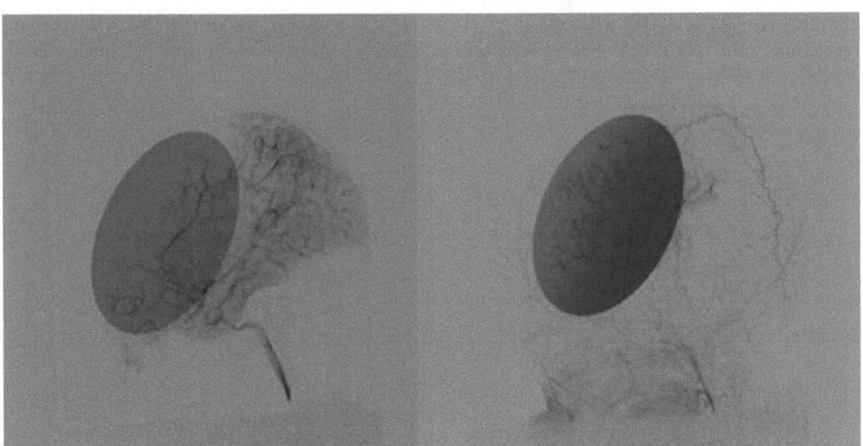

Fig. 4 Matsushima grade A collaterals 1 year following synangiosis. (**a**) Internal carotid injection with poor supply to the cortex denoted in *gray*. (**b**) External carotid injection demonstrating new supply to the cortex from the synangiosis

References

1. Scott RM, Smith ER (2009) Moyamoya disease and moyamoya syndrome. N Engl J Med. doi: 360/12/1226 [pii] 10.1056/NEJMra0804622
2. Smith ER, Scott RM (2008) Progression of disease in unilateral moyamoya syndrome. Neurosurg Focus 24:E17
3. Hallemeier CL, Rich KM, Grubb RL Jr et al (2006) Clinical features and outcome in North American adults with moyamoya phenomenon. Stroke 37:1490–1496
4. Scott RM, Smith JL, Robertson RL et al (2004) Long-term outcome in children with moyamoya syndrome after cranial revascularization by pial synangiosis. J Neurosurg Spine 100:142–149
5. Suzuki J, Takaku A (1969) Cerebrovascular "moyamoya" disease: disease showing abnormal net-like vessels in base of brain. Arch Neurol 20:288–299
6. Imaizumi T, Hayashi K, Saito K et al (1998) Long-term outcomes of pediatric moyamoya disease monitored to adulthood. Pediatr Neurol 18:321–325
7. Maki Y, Enomoto T (1988) Moyamoya disease. Childs Nerv Syst 4:204–212
8. Fukuyama Y, Umezu R (1985) Clinical and cerebral angiographic evolutions of idiopathic progressive occlusive disease of the circle of Willis ("moyamoya" disease) in children. Brain Dev 7:21–37
9. Kuroda S, Ishikawa T, Houkin K et al (2005) Incidence and clinical features of disease progression in adult moyamoya disease. Stroke 36:2148–2153
10. Fung LW, Thompson D, Ganesan V (2005) Revascularisation surgery for paediatric moyamoya: a review of the literature. Childs Nerv Syst 21:358–364
11. Ohaegbulam C, Magge S, Scott RM (2001) Moyamoya syndrome. In: McLone DG (ed) Pediatric neurosurgery: surgery of the developing nervous system. Saunders, New York
12. Scott RM, Smith JL, Robertson RL et al (2004) Long-term outcome in children with moyamoya syndrome after cranial revascularization by pial synangiosis. J Neurosurg 100:142–149
13. Choi JU, Kim DS, Kim EY et al (1997) Natural history of moyamoya disease: comparison of activity of daily living in surgery and non surgery groups. Clin Neurol Neurosurg 99 Suppl 2:S11–18
14. Lin Y, Yoshiko K, Negoro T et al (200) Cerebral oxygenation state in childhood moyamoya disease: a near-infrared spectroscopy study. Pediatr Neurol 22:365–369
15. Fujiwara J, Nakahara S, Enomoto T et al (1996) The effectiveness of O2 administration for transient ischemic attacks in moyamoya disease in children. Childs Nerv Syst 12:69–75
16. Nomura S, Kashiwagi S, Uetsuka S et al (2001) Perioperative management protocols for children with moyamoya disease. Childs Nerv Syst 17:270–274
17. Jea A, Smith ER, Robertson R (2005) Moyamoya syndrome associated with Down syndrome: outcome after surgical revascularization. Pediatrics 116:e694–701
18. Smith ER, McClain CD, Heeney M et al (2009) Pial synangiosis in patients with moyamoya syndrome and sickle cell anemia: perioperative management and surgical outcome. Neurosurg Focus, doi:10.3171/2009.01.FOCUS08307

Pregnancy and Delivery in Moyamoya Disease

Jun C. Takahashi

Introduction

Moyamoya disease is more prevalent in females than in males [1]. Moreover, this disease occurs most frequently during childhood and early adulthood; thus, it is not uncommon for patients to become pregnant and give birth. Although serious vascular events in pregnant patient of moyamoya disease have been reported, no guidelines have been established on managing the pregnancies of such patients (Fig. 1). In this chapter, this problem is discussed in light of a review of the literature and a recent nationwide survey on pregnancy, delivery, and moyamoya disease.

Pregnancy and Cerebrovascular Diseases

Pregnancy induces various physiological changes. During the third trimester, blood volume is known to increase by 40–50% and cardiac output increases by 30–50% compared with the impregnant state. During vaginal delivery, blood pressure increases in the wake of labor pains, and pregnant women are encouraged to begin hyperventilating. Moreover, in the case of pregnancy-induced hypertension (PIH) and eclampsia, blood pressure increases to a hazardous level; this hypertension is difficult to control medically. Previously, it was believed that pregnancy increases intracranial hemorrhagic and ischemic attacks [2, 3]. However, some authors have pointed out that the risk increases only during puerperium, at least in developed countries [4]. Nevertheless, serious cerebrovascular accidents (CVAs) do occur during the perinatal period, and intracranial hemorrhage has been proved to be the second most frequent cause of perinatal death of women in Japan following massive obstetrical bleeding [5].

J.C. Takahashi (✉)
Department of Neurosurgery, Kyoto University,
54 Shogoin Kawahara-cho, Sakyo-ku, Kyoto, 606-8507, Japan
e-mail: juntak@kuhp.kyoto-u.ac.jp

B.-K. Cho and T. Tominaga (eds.), *Moyamoya Disease Update*,
DOI 10.1007/978-4-431-99703-0_45, © Springer 2010

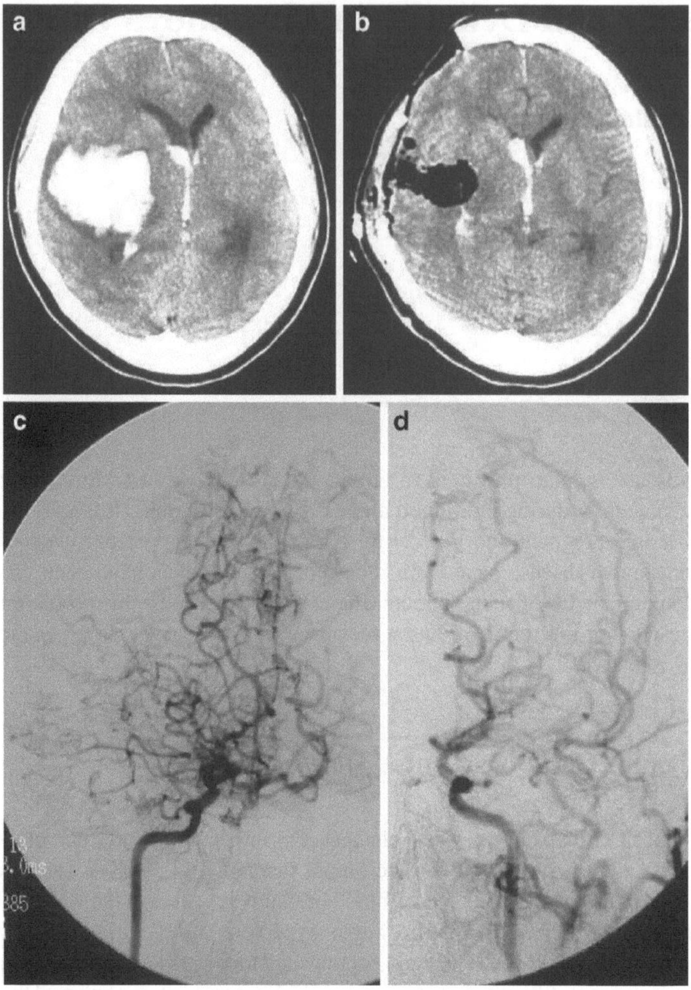

Fig. 1 Intracerebral hemorrhage in a 30-year-old woman at 36 weeks of pregnancy. (**a**) CT on admission. Massive hematoma is demonstrated in the right temporal lobe. The patient was in a semicomatose state and her right pupil had dilated. (**b**) CT after the emergent Caesarian section and craniotomy, the hematoma was completely removed. Right (**c**) and left (**d**) carotid angiograms. Occlusion of the bilateral internal carotid artery with development of basal moyamoya vessels is demonstrated. These angiograms led to the patient first being diagnosed with moyamoya disease

Moyamoya Disease and Pregnancy

No evidence exists that the risk of ischemic or hemorrhagic stroke increases during pregnancy in patients with moyamoya disease. Moreover, no guidelines have been issued for managing pregnancy in patients diagnosed with moyamoya disease, and even the selection of the delivery method (natural labor, painless labor with spinal epidural anesthesia, or Caesarian section) seems to differ from one hospital to the next. Since the 1970s, there have been sporadic case reports of pregnant patients with moyamoya disease presenting with ischemic or hemorrhagic stroke. In 1998, Komiyama et al. extensively reviewed the management of pregnancy and delivery in patients with moyamoya disease by analyzing these case reports [6]. This review determined that 31 cases of pregnancy in women diagnosed with moyamoya disease have been reported. Caesarian section was selected in 81% of the cases, and no CVAs occurred during delivery. A poor prognosis was noted in only one patient who experienced ventricular hemorrhage at 30 weeks of pregnancy. In this case, bilateral ventricular drainage was performed after Caesarian section, but the patient entered a state of akinetic mutism. The remaining patients had a good prognosis. On the other hand, 23 patients were reported to have become symptomatic and were first diagnosed with moyamoya disease following the occurrence of a CVA during the period of pregnancy and delivery (16 with cerebral hemorrhage, 3 with cerebral ischemia, and 4 with other events). Cerebral hemorrhage occurred at gestation periods ranging from 15 to 37 weeks, with an average of 28.1 weeks. One patient who underwent spontaneous vaginal delivery experienced a cerebral hemorrhage in early postpartum. While no hemorrhagic attacks were noted during delivery, ischemic episodes occurred at periods ranging from 4 months to 40 weeks of gestation. The outcomes for the patients who presented with hemorrhagic or ischemic attacks were three deaths, six with poor recovery, two with akinetic mutism, and ten with good recovery. With one exception, all maternal deaths and cases of poor prognosis were the result of cerebral hemorrhage.

In sum, the prognosis for pregnant patients known to have moyamoya disease is generally good, whereas that for women newly diagnosed with this disease is poor.

Nationwide Survey in Japan on Management of Pregnancy and Delivery in Women with Moyamoya Disease

Although the review by Komiyama et al. is quite valuable, it does not provide a full understanding of the state of pregnancy and delivery in women with moyamoya disease. In 2008, the author and his colleagues conducted a nationwide survey on the management of pregnancy and delivery in women with moyamoya disease [7]. This survey targeted the experiences of 280 centers for maternal, fetal, and neonatal medicine in Japan during the preceding 5 years. The survey cited 64 deliveries comprising 59 cases of previously diagnosed moyamoya disease and 5 cases of moyamoya disease newly diagnosed as a result of perinatal CVA.

The results of this survey indicated that the incidence of perinatal CVA was low in pregnant women previously diagnosed with moyamoya disease. Only one case of cerebral hemorrhage during pregnancy was reported in which the maternal prognosis was poor (modified Rankin scale score 4). Although Caesarian section was mainly employed for women previously diagnosed with moyamoya disease (76%), no attacks during delivery were observed in either the Caesarian sections or vaginal deliveries. Therefore, no evidence exists that vaginal delivery should be avoided. Extracranial–intracranial (EC–IC) bypass surgery had been performed on 58% of the patients before pregnancy, and the experience of previous EC–IC bypasses had no significant influence on the selection of delivery method.

On the other hand, it was proved that serious cerebrovascular events (three cases of cerebral hemorrhage and two cases of cerebral ischemia) occurred in patients who had not been diagnosed with moyamoya disease before pregnancy and that one patient with intracerebral hemorrhage died despite an emergent neurosurgical operation and Caesarian section. No hemorrhagic attack during delivery was described in the review by Komiyama et al., but in this survey, one patient with intracranial hemorrhage during natural labor was reported. The modified Rankin scale scores of these all patients at discharge were 6 (death), 2, 1, 0, and 0.

Management of Pregnancy and Delivery in Women with Moyamoya Disease

It has been confirmed that most pregnant patients known to have moyamoya disease can deliver safely. This could be attributable to the adequate management provided by obstetricians. It is also possible that previous EC–IC bypass surgery has a favorable influence on the course of a pregnancy, although whether bypass surgery reduces the rate of hemorrhagic events in moyamoya disease remains unclear [8–10]. However, serious cerebrovascular events occur in patients whose moyamoya disease was undiagnosed before their pregnancy, indicating that the risk of pregnancy and delivery in women with moyamoya disease should not be underestimated. Patients known to have moyamoya disease should be made aware of the risks of pregnancy. Moreover, it should be emphasized that a poor prognosis is mostly likely to result from cerebral hemorrhage and not cerebral ischemia.

It is essential that obstetricians and neurosurgeons cooperate closely in managing pregnant patients with moyamoya disease. To avoid catastrophic intracranial hemorrhage, blood pressure should be strictly controlled throughout the gestation period and during puerperium. In cases of PIH or eclampsia, prompt treatment including emergent Caesarian section is needed. When the clinical course is favorable, however, insistence on a Caesarean section for patients known to have moyamoya disease appears to be unnecessary. Vaginal delivery with forceps under epidural anesthesia can be used to reduce stress on the cardiovascular system, as can avoidance of hyperventilation during delivery [6, 11].

Clearly, all physicians have an obligation to provide accurate information and appropriate management of patients with moyamoya disease.

In conclusion, we expect the rapid formulation of guidelines on management of pregnancy and delivery in women with moyamoya disease.

References

1. Handa H, Yonekawa Y (1985) The occlusion of the circle of Willis: 1,500 case files including 200 long follow-up cases [in Japanese]. No Socchu 7:477–480
2. Jennett WB, Cross JN (1967) Influence of pregnancy and oral contraception on the incidence of strokes in women of childbearing age. Lancet 1:1019–1023
3. Wiebers DO (1985) Ischemic cerebrovascular complications of pregnancy. Arch Neurol 42:1106–1113
4. Kittner SJ, Stern BJ, Feeser BR et al (1996) Pregnancy and the risk of stroke. N Engl J Med 335:768–774
5. Sameshima H (1999) Ninshin,bunbenji no nousyukketu (cerebral hemorrhage during pregnancy and delivery) [in Japanese]. Perinat Med 29:205–209
6. Komiyama M, Yasui, T, Kitano S et al (1998) Moyamoya disease and pregnancy: case report and review of the literature. Neurosurgery 43:360–368
7. Takahashi JC, Ikeda T, Iihara K et al (2009) A nationwide survey on the management of pregnancy and delivery in association with moyamoya disease [in Japanese]. Jpn J Neurosurg (Tokyo) 18:367–375
8. Kawaguchi S, Okuno S, Sakaki T (2000) Effect of direct arterial bypass on the prevention of future stroke in patients with the hemorrhagic variety of moyamoya disease. J Neurosurg 93:397–401

9. Miyamoto S (2004) Study design for a prospective randomized trial of extracranial-intracranial bypass surgery for adults with moyamoya disease and hemorrhagic onset – the Japan Adult Moyamoya Trial Group. Neurol Med Chir (Tokyo) 44:218–219
10. Yoshida Y, Yoshimoto T, Shirane R et al (1999) Clinical course, surgical management, and long-term outcome of moyamoya patients with rebleeding after an episode of intracerebral hemorrhage: an extensive follow-up study. Stroke 30:2272–2276
11. Ikeda T, Neki R, Suga S et al (2009) Intrapartum epidural analgesia for patients with moyamoya disease. Jpn J Neurosurg (Tokyo) 18:376–382

Asymptomatic Moyamoya Disease

Satoshi Kuroda

Introduction

Moyamoya disease is an uncommon cerebrovascular disorder that is characterized by progressive stenosis of the supraclinoid internal carotid arteries and its main branches within the circle of Willis. This occlusion results in the formation of a fine vascular network (the moyamoya vessels) at the base of the brain. Moyamoya vessels are the dilated perforating arteries and function as collateral pathways. Recent investigations have rapidly developed our knowledge on basic and clinical aspects in moyamoya disease, including its etiology, pathophysiology, surgical results, and long-term prognosis. Thus, recent epidemiological and genetic studies have suggested the involvement of some genetic factors in its pathogenesis. The potential contribution of infections has also been pointed out, although specific pathogens have not been identified. Pediatric patients with moyamoya disease often develop transient ischemic attacks (TIA) or cerebral infarction, while adult patients also suffer intracranial bleeding. Surgical revascularization such as superficial temporal artery to middle cerebral artery (STA–MCA) anastomosis and indirect bypass improves their cerebral hemodynamics and prevents further ischemic attacks. An on-going multicenter randomized clinical trial is being performed to examine whether surgical revascularization including STA–MCA anastomosis reduces hemodynamic stress on the dilated moyamoya vessels and contributes to prevent further intracranial bleeding [1].

Despite increasing knowledge on basic and clinical aspects of moyamoya disease, there are few data on the epidemiology, radiological findings, and prognosis of asymptomatic moyamoya disease. Asymptomatic moyamoya disease has been believed to be quite rare for a long time. However, the recent development of noninvasive diagnostic modality such as MR imaging (MRI) and angiography (MRA) has revealed that the incidence of asymptomatic moyamoya disease may be higher than previously thought. The author believes that the accumulation of their clinical data would be essential to issue the guideline for the diagnosis and management for asymptomatic patients with moyamoya disease and to improve their long-term prognosis. In this chapter, therefore, the author reviews recent knowledge on asymptomatic moyamoya disease and discusses future perspectives.

S. Kuroda (✉)
Department of Neurosurgery, Hokkaido University Graduate School of Medicine,
North 15 West 7, Kita-ku, Sapporo 060-8638, Japan
e-mail: skuroda@med.hokudai.ac.jp

B.-K. Cho and T. Tominaga (eds.), *Moyamoya Disease Update*,
DOI 10.1007/978-4-431-99703-0_46, © Springer 2010

Definition

"Asymptomatic" patients with moyamoya disease have been defined as those who have experienced neither ischemic nor hemorrhagic episodes since their birth. In fact, according to previous reports, clues to the diagnosis of asymptomatic moyamoya disease included tension-type headache, dizziness, head trauma, and so on. Some patients were incidentally diagnosed on MRI and MRA performed for a brain health check-up. Other diagnoses were made on MRI and MRA performed for screening, because a member of their family had had moyamoya disease diagnosed [2, 3].

Epidemiology

As aforementioned, even in Japan, the epidemiology of asymptomatic moyamoya disease is still obscure. Previously, asymptomatic cases of moyamoya disease have been only sporadically reported [4, 5]. Screening of family members with moyamoya disease has also identified small numbers of asymptomatic patients [6–8]. Therefore, the incidence of asymptomatic moyamoya disease had been considered to be very low. However, Nanba et al. (2003) recently reviewed their single-center experiences and precisely reported the clinical features of 10 asymptomatic patients with moyamoya disease [3]. Yamada et al. (2005) also reported the results of a nation-wide questionnaire conducted in 1994 and identified 33 asymptomatic patients (1.5%) out of a total of 2,193 [9]. Very recently, Kuroda et al. (2007) conducted the first multicenter, nation-wide survey focused on asymptomatic patients with moyamoya disease in Japan between 2003 and 2006, with 40 patients enrolled from 12 participating hospitals [2]. Baba et al. (2008) performed an all-inclusive survey of moyamoya disease in Hokkaido, one of major islands in Japan with a population of 5.63 million [10]. They found that asymptomatic patients comprised 17.8% of 267 newly registered patients with moyamoya disease between 2002 and 2006 (Fig. 1). Therefore, the prevalence of asymptomatic moyamoya disease may be much higher than previously considered.

According to these recent reports, most of asymptomatic patients with moyamoya disease are adults. A nationwide survey in Japan reported that their mean age at diagnosis was 41.4 ± 12.6 years, ranging from 13 to 67 years [2]. The female to male ratio and mean age of the patients in these studies were similar to those of moyamoya disease as a whole [11].

Radiological Findings

The information on radiological findings in asymptomatic moyamoya disease is limited. Nanba et al. (2003) reported that silent cerebral infarction was identified in three (30%) of ten asymptomatic patients with moyamoya disease [3]. Kuroda et al. (2007) found cerebral infarction in 16 (20.8%) of a total of 77 involved hemispheres [2]. Asymptomatic moyamoya disease may be closely related to the development of silent cerebral infarction, because a population-based consecutive autopsy study in Japan has revealed that the incidence of silent cerebral infarction is 4.4% in the 40- to 59-year-old population [12]. In these studies, no intracranial bleeding was noted at initial diagnosis.

In a multicenter, nationwide survey in Japan, 37 of 40 asymptomatic patients had typical "bilateral" moyamoya disease and the other 3 had "unilateral" moyamoya disease. The disease

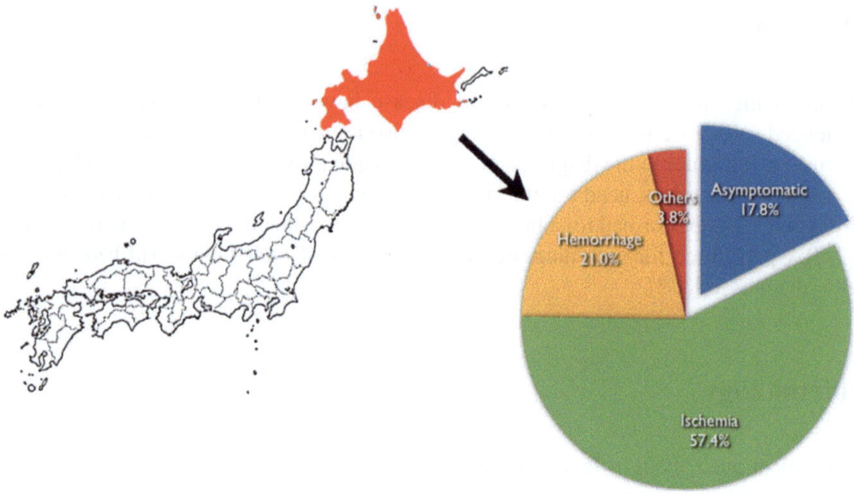

Fig. 1 Recent all-inclusive survey in Hokkaido (*left*, red island) revealed that about 18% of newly registered patients with moyamoya disease were asymptomatic [10]

stage on cerebral angiography widely varied. However, correlation analysis revealed that older patients had a significantly more advanced disease stage [2]. This fact correlates with recent findings that occlusive arterial lesions in adult moyamoya disease are not steady and often progress in both anterior and posterior circulation, in both bilateral and unilateral types, and in both symptomatic and asymptomatic patients [13]. Therefore, it should be remembered that disease progression may silently occur and can suddenly cause ischemic or hemorrhagic stroke even in asymptomatic patients (see below).

It is unknown when moyamoya disease shifts from an asymptomatic to a symptomatic disorder. Kuroda et al. (2008) reported that about 40% of the involved hemispheres had a moderate or severe reduction of cerebral perfusion reserve in asymptomatic moyamoya disease. Thus, 24 (34.3%) of 77 hemispheres had normal cerebral blood flow but reduced reactivity to acetazolamide on single photon emission computed tomography. Seven (10%) had reduced cerebral blood flow and its reactivity to acetazolamide [2]. These parameters would be important to consider their long-term prognosis (Fig. 2).

Outcome

The natural course of asymptomatic moyamoya disease is still unclear. Kuroda et al. (2008) reported that 7 of 34 non-surgically treated patients experienced TIA ($n=3$), ischemic stroke ($n=1$), or intracranial bleeding ($n=3$) during 43.7 months of follow-up periods. Therefore, the annual risk for any stroke was 3.2%. Disturbed cerebral hemodynamics was significantly linked to ischemic episodes. Disease progression was associated with ischemic events or silent infarction in 4 of 5 patients. Furthermore, silent radiological changes were identified in another 3 patients [2]. These findings strongly suggest the importance to repeat MRI and MRA at regular intervals when asymptomatic patients are conservatively followed up in order to detect silent radiological changes such as disease progression, cerebral infarction and microbleeds before stroke occurs.

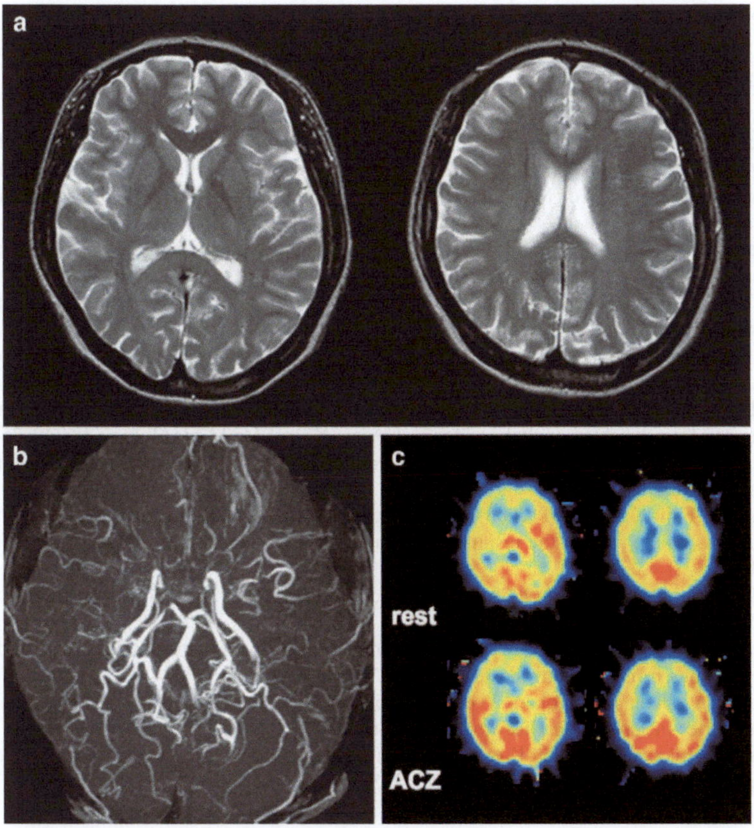

Fig. 2 Representative radiological findings of a 43-year-old female with asymptomatic moyamoya disease. No parenchymal lesion was noted on MRI (**a**). However, MRA revealed that she had bilateral moyamoya disease (**b**). Blood flow study demonstrated the reduction of both cerebral blood flow and its reactivity to acetazolamide (ACZ) in the bilateral frontal lobes (**c**)

On the other hand, none of 6 patients who underwent surgical revascularization had any cerebrovascular event during follow-up periods, except for surgical morbidity [2]. Therefore, surgical revascularization may be indicated, at least, in patients who have disturbed cerebral hemodynamics if surgical morbidity is enough low.

Conclusions

A recent multicenter, nationwide survey in Japan shed light on asymptomatic moyamoya disease. We should now clearly recognize that asymptomatic moyamoya disease is not a "silent" disorder and might potentially cause ischemic or hemorrhagic stroke. However, the clinical information to clarify the whole picture of asymptomatic moyamoya disease is still limited. Further investigations are essential to clarify how we should manage each asymptomatic patient with moyamoya disease.

References

1. Kuroda S, Houkin K (2008) Moyamoya disease: current concepts and future perspectives. Lancet Neurol 7:1056–1066
2. Kuroda S, Hashimoto N, Yoshimoto T et al (2007) Radiological findings, clinical course, and outcome in asymptomatic moyamoya disease: results of multicenter survey in Japan. Stroke 38:1430–1435
3. Nanba R, Kuroda S, Takeda M et al (2003) [Clinical features and outcomes of 10 asymptomatic adult patients with moyamoya disease]. No Shinkei Geka 31:1291–1295
4. Akasaki T, Kagiyama S, Omae, T et al (1998) Asymptomatic moyamoya disease associated with coronary and renal artery stenoses – a case report. Jpn Circ J 62:136–138
5. Aoki T, Saiki M, Ishizaki R et al (2004) [A case report of the adult patient with asymptomatic moyamoya disease]. Pract Curr Neurosurg 14:597–602
6. Houkin K, Aoki T, Takahashi A et al (1994) Diagnosis of moyamoya disease with magnetic resonance angiography. Stroke 25:2159–2164
7. Kaneko Y, Imamoto N, Mannoji H et al (1998) Familial occurrence of moyamoya disease in the mother and four daughters including identical twins. Neurol Med Chir (Tokyo) 38:349–354
8. Yamauchi T, Houkin K, Tada M et al (1997) Familial occurrence of moyamoya disease. Clin Neurol Neurosurg 99:S162–S167
9. Yamada M, Fujii K, Fukui M (2005) [Clinical features and outcomes in patients with asymptomatic moyamoya disease – from the results of nation-wide questionnaire survey]. No Shinkei Geka 33: 337–342
10. Baba T, Houkin K, Kuroda S (2008) Novel epidemiological features of moyamoya disease. J Neurol Neurosurg Psychiatry 79:900–904
11. Wakai K, Tamakoshi A, Ikezaki K et al (1997) Epidemiological features of moyamoya disease in Japan: findings from a nationwide survey. Clin Neurol Neurosurg 99:S1–S5
12. Shinkawa A, Ueda K, Kiyohara Y et al (1995) Silent cerebral infarction in a community-based autopsy series in Japan. The Hisayama Study. Stroke 26:380–385
13. Kuroda S, Ishikawa T, Houkin K et al (2005) Incidence and clinical features of disease progression in adult moyamoya disease. Stroke 36:2148–2153

Hyperthyroidism in Moyamoya Disease

So-Hyang Im

Introduction

Hyperthyroidism is a clinical condition caused by the effects of excessive circulating thyroid hormones on various tissues of the body [1]. The various actions of thyroid hormone on many organ systems produce a broad spectrum of clinical signs and symptoms in patients with hyperthyroidism. An increased body's metabolism is characteristic in hyperthyroidism [2]. For this reason, patients often feel hotter than those around them and can slowly lose body weight even though they may be eating more food. When hyperthyroidism is severe, patients can suffer shortness of breath, chest pain, and muscle weakness [2]. Although there are several different causes of hyperthyroidism, most of the symptoms that patients experience are the same regardless of the cause [3]. Hyperthyroidism, thyroid storm, and Graves disease are conditions of excess thyroid hormone. Thyroid storm is a rare and potentially fatal complication of hyperthyroidism [4]. It typically occurs in patients with untreated or partially treated thyrotoxicosis who experience a precipitating event such as surgery, infection, or trauma [2]. Patients typically appear markedly hypermetabolic with high fevers, tachycardia, nausea and vomiting, tremulousness, agitation, and psychosis [5]. Graves disease (diffuse toxic goiter), the most common underlying cause of hyperthyroidism, is an autoimmune disease in which autoantibodies against the thyroid-stimulating hormone receptors inappropriately stimulate thyroid gland with ensuing excessive production and release of thyroid hormones [6]. The resultant hyperthyroid state produces multiorgan physiological derangements. Graves disease is associated with various autoimmune diseases such as pernicious anemia, vitiligo, type 1 diabetes mellitus, autoimmune adrenal insufficiency, systemic sclerosis, myasthenia gravis, Sjögren syndrome, rheumatoid arthritis, and systemic lupus erythematosus [7]. Utku et al. described reversible angiographical findings mimicking moyamoya disease at magnetic resonance (MR) angiography in a woman with a stroke-like episode and encephalopathy diagnosed as Graves disease [8]. In this case, her neurological status improved dramatically after methylprednisolone treatment and plasmapheresis, and the MR angiography abnormalities

S.-H. Im (✉)
Department of Neurosurgery, Thomas Jefferson University Hospital, 909 Walnut Street, Suite 200, Philadelphia, PA 19107, USA
e-mail: shyim@medimail.co.kr

B.-K. Cho and T. Tominaga (eds.), *Moyamoya Disease Update*,
DOI 10.1007/978-4-431-99703-0_47, © Springer 2010

resolved after 3 months. Utku et al. suggested that elimination of thyroid antibodies from circulation by plasmapheresis had a significant role in the reversal of vasculitic changes [8]. Intracranial vascular abnormalities were not confirmed by cerebral angiography in that case. Rarely, Graves disease has been reported to occur in association with moyamoya disease/syndrome. Although moyamoya disease has been described in association with various autoimmune diseases, its concurrence with Graves disease is extremely rare. A total of 24 cases of Graves disease associated with moyamoya disease or moyamoya variant have been described in the literature [9–23]. Although it has been hypothesized that both conditions may share a common autoimmune mechanism, there is no clear pathogenetic relationship between Graves disease and moyamoya disease [13, 24]. In most of these cases, cerebrovascular accidents occurred when patients were thyrotoxic, suggesting that thyroid hormones could have facilitated these accidents, possibly through hemodynamic changes and (or) sympathetic nervous system-mediated vasculopathy [13, 21]. A clear pathoetiological link remains to be elucidated. Hsu et al. reported a case of Graves disease with thyroid storm associated with moyamoya syndrome, which was particularly noteworthy because of a very rapid progression of the cerebrovascular occlusive disease that was ultimately fatal [19]. The authors have reported four cases of moyamoya disease developing in association with Graves thyrotoxicosis [21]. Although possible conclusions may be limited because of the small number of patients in the study (four cases), data from the cases indicated that thyrotoxicosis may trigger cerebral ischemia in moyamoya disease. The transient ischemic symptoms of moyamoya disease disappeared after control of hyperthyroidism, and cerebral infarction developed as hyperthyroidism reappeared in our cases. Our experiences have suggested that the surgical risk for moyamoya disease might be higher in patients with uncontrolled or poorly controlled thyrotoxicosis. Cerebral ischemic injury during perioperative period occurred only in the patient in our series whose thyrotoxicosis was incompletely controlled during the perioperative period. In patients with both moyamoya disease and Graves thyrotoxicosis, the importance of optimal hormonal remission during the perioperative period should be remembered. It is also important to prevent relapse of hyperthyroidism after restoring euthyroid function in patients with moyamoya disease. In one patient in our series, cerebral ischemic symptoms aggravated during the relapse of thyrotoxicosis following the initial clinical and laboratory remission of Graves disease. A possible evolving thyroid dysfunction must be considered when cerebral ischemic symptoms appear during the follow-up period. However, the pathophysiology during hyperthyroidism are yet to be clarified in patients with moyamoya disease. It is necessary to study more patients with concurrent moyamoya disease and Graves thyrotoxicosis to obtain more evidence on the relationship between these two conditions. Physiological effects of thyroid hormone on cerebral metabolism and cerebrovascular hemodynamics should be elucidated by experimental and clinical studies to improve knowledge regarding the underlying pathophysiological or biochemical mechanisms of cerebrovascular accidents in patients with concurrent moyamoya disease.

References

1. McKeown NJ, Tews MC, Gossain VV et al (2005) Hyperthyroidism. Emerg Med Clin North Am 23:669–685
2. Tietgens ST, Leinung MC (1995) Thyroid storm. Med Clin North Am 79:169–184
3. Ringel MD (2001) Management of hypothyroidism and hyperthyroidism in the intensive care unit. Crit Care Clin 17:59–74
4. Waldstein SS, Slodki SJ, Kaganiec GL (1960) A clinical study of thyroid storm. Ann Intern Med 52:626–642

5. Fisher JN (2002) Management of thyrotoxicosis. South Med J 95:493–505
6. Weetman AP (2000) Graves' disease. N Engl J Med 343:1236–1248
7. Cruz AA, Akaishi PM, Vargas MA et al (2007) Association between thyroid autoimmune dysfunction and non-thyroid autoimmune diseases. Ophthal Plast Reconstr Surg 23:104–108
8. Utku U, Asil T, Celik Y et al (2004) Reversible MR angiographic findings in a patient with autoimmune Graves disease. Am J Neuroradiol 25:1541–1543
9. Kushima K, Satoh Y, Ban Y et al (1991) Graves' thyrotoxicosis and Moyamoya disease. Can J Neurol Sci 18:140–142
10. Liu JS, Juo SH, Chen WH et al (1994) A case of Graves' diseases associated with intracranial moyamoya vessels and tubular stenosis of extracranial internal carotid arteries. J Formos Med Assoc 93:806–809
11. Tendler BE, Shoukri K, Malchoff C et al (1997) Concurrence of Graves' disease and dysplastic cerebral blood vessels of the moyamoya variety. Thyroid 7:625–629
12. Wakamoto H, Ishiyama N, Miyazaki H et al (2000) The stenoses at the terminal portion of the internal carotid artery improved after initiation of antithyroid therapy: a case report. No Shinkei Geka 28:379–383 (Abstract)
13. Nakamura K, Yanaka K, Ihara S et al (2003) Multiple intracranial arterial stenoses around the circle of Willis in association with Graves' disease: report of two cases. Neurosurgery 53:1210–1215
14. Kim JY, Kim BS, Kang JH (2001) Dilated cardiomyopathy in thyrotoxicosis and Moyamoya disease. Int J Cardiol 80:101–103
15. Matsumoto K, Nogaki H, Yamamoto K et al (1992) A case of moyamoya disease complicated with Basedow disease. Jpn J Stroke 14:409–413
16. Garcin B, Louissaint T, Hosseini H et al (2008) Reversible chorea in association with Graves' disease and moyamoya syndrome. Mov Disord 23:620–622
17. Ni J, Gao S, Cui LY et al (2006) Intracranial arterial occlusive lesion in patients with Graves' disease. Chin Med Sci J 21:140–144
18. Sasaki T, Nogawa S, Amano T (2006) Co-morbidity of moyamoya disease with Graves' disease. report of three cases and a review of the literature. Intern Med 45:649–653
19. Hsu SW, Chaloupka JC, Fattal D (2006) Rapidly progressive fatal bihemispheric infarction secondary to moyamoya syndrome in association with Graves thyrotoxicosis. Am J Neuroradiol 27:643–647
20. Golomb MR, Biller J, Smith JL et al (2005) A 10-year-old girl with coexistent moyamoya disease and Graves' disease. J Child Neurol 20:620–624
21. Im SH, Oh CW, Kwon OK et al (2005) Moyamoya disease associated with Graves disease: special considerations regarding clinical significance and management. J Neurosurg 102:1013–1017
22. Shen AL, Ryu SJ, Lin SK (2006) Concurrent moyamoya disease and Graves' thyrotoxicosis: case report and literature review. Acta Neurol Taiwan 15:114–119
23. Garcin B, Louissaint T, Hosseini H et al (2008) Reversible chorea in association with Graves' disease and moyamoya syndrome. Mov Disord 23:620–622
24. Squizzato A, Gerdes VE, Brandjes DP et al (2005) Thyroid diseases and cerebrovascular disease. Stroke 36:2302–2310

Enhancer of Revascularization, Gene and Stem Cell Therapies

Koji Tokunaga and Isao Date

Introduction

Various surgical techniques for direct or indirect vasoreconstruction have been developed for moyamoya disease [1–6]. The induction of neovascularization can be achieved in most patients by indirect surgery on the brain surface through vascularized tissues such as the galea, the dura mater, and the temporal muscle [7, 8], although the development of neovascularization after indirect surgery is slower than that induced by direct bypass and not sufficient in some patients. The results of direct bypass are not always excellent in terms of the extent of blood supply and the long-term patency [9]. Adjunctive therapies to enhance neovascularization after indirect surgery may improve the angiographic and clinical results of patients with moyamoya disease.

Recently, research in the field of gene therapy and cell transplantation for cerebral ischemia has advanced tremendously [10]. We have reported basic studies concerning treatments for brain ischemia, including neurotrophic factor-secreting cell line grafting [11], adult-derived neural stem cell grafting [12, 13], gene therapy [14], and protein induction [15]. The application of induced pluripotent stem cells is a promising method for the regeneration of multiple cell types in damaged brains [16]; however, the replacement of lost neurons and reformation of synapses with the surrounding neurons is still difficult. This chapter focuses on gene therapy and stem cell transplantation methods used to enhance neovascularization in ischemic brains to assess the possibility of their future combination with indirect revascularization surgery.

K. Tokunaga (✉) and I. Date
Department of Neurological Surgery, Okayama University Graduate School of Medicine, Dentistry and Pharmaceutical Sciences, 2-5-1 Shikata-cho, Kita-ku, Okayama 700-8558, Japan
e-mail: kojitoku@md.okayama-u.ac.jp

B.-K. Cho and T. Tominaga (eds.), *Moyamoya Disease Update*,
DOI 10.1007/978-4-431-99703-0_48, © Springer 2010

Gene Therapy for Cerebral Ischemia

Many molecules have been implicated as positive regulators of physiological or pathological angiogenesis [17]. Vascular endothelial growth factor (VEGF), which was originally identified as a vascular permeability factor, is one of the key regulators of angiogenesis, and its mRNA expressions is induced by hypoxia [18]. Alternative exon splicing gives rise to several VEGF isoforms with different numbers of amino acids. Among them, $VEGF_{165}$ has optimal characteristics in terms of both its diffusible nature; high affinity for the extracellular matrix; and its ability to bind to VEGFR-1, VEGFR-2, and neuropilin-1, which enhances VEGFR-2 dependent signaling [17, 18]. Regarding the choice of an appropriate formulation or vector in the case of VEGF, continuous and local production of VEGF resulting from gene transfer is considered to be preferable to a single larger dose of recombinant protein from the standpoints of safety and efficacy. The administration of a naked plasmid encoding the 165-amino-acid isoform of human VEGF ($phVEGF_{165}$) for myocardial or limb ischemia resulted in favorable experimental and clinical results without the use of liposomes or viral vectors [19–24].

We reported enhanced brain angiogenesis in a chronic cerebral hypoperfusion model after the administration of $phVEGF_{165}$ in combination with indirect revascularization surgery [14]. We induced a chronic hypoperfusion model by permanent ligation of both common carotid arteries in rats [25]. Seven days later, encephalo-myo-synangiosis (EMS) and 50 μg of $phVEGF_{165}$ administration into the temporal muscle was performed. Histological examinations 14 days after treatment disclosed that the numbers and the areas of capillary vessels in the brain and the temporal muscle were significantly greater in the group treated with the VEGF gene than the control group. Immunohistochemical staining and western blot analysis revealed positive expression of VEGF protein in the $phVEGF_{165}$-treated muscles but no expression in the brain. We concluded that local and indirect application of VEGF into the muscle was able to induce transmuscular anastomosis and might have contributed to the apparent lack of brain edema.

Discussion on the optimum dose of plasmid DNA is essential for the clinical application of this method [19, 24, 26], because high microenvironmental and long-term expression of VEGF may cause hemangioma growth or leaky immature blood vessels [22]. Yasuhara et al. demonstrated that low-dose administration of VEGF exerted enhanced neuroprotective effects on dopaminergic neurons in comparison to high-dose therapy [27]. We performed EMS and administered various doses of $phVEGF_{165}$ (25, 50, 75, 100, 125, 150, 175, and 200 μg) into the temporal muscle of the abovementioned chronic hypoperfusion model rats. Thirty days later, the animals that received 100 μg $phVEGF_{165}$ exhibited a marked increase in the number of capillary vessels in their muscles and brain, although the high-dose group showed less striking effects on angiogenesis (Fig. 1; Katsumata et al., unpublished data).

Other angiogenic cytokines may play a role in enhancing neovascularization in combination with vasoreconstructive surgery. Angiopoietin-1 (Ang 1), which acts in the late phase of vessel formation during vessel remodeling and maturation, suppresses plasma leakage, and VEGF-induced inflammation [28,29]. Coadministration of Ang 1 and VEGF to the ischemic hindlimb models produced higher capillary density and formed thicker vessels than VEGF alone [30, 31].

Hepatocyte growth factor (HGF) stimulates the migration of both endothelial cells and vascular smooth muscle cells (VSMC), whereas, VEGF does not stimulate the migration of VSMC, which is necessary for the appropriate maturation of vessels. Morishita et al. reported that intramuscular injection of a naked HGF plasmid achieved successful improvement of the ischemic limbs of six patients without any evidence of the edema that was seen in a VEGF trial [32]. Yoshimura et al. demonstrated successful angiogenesis on the brain surface using

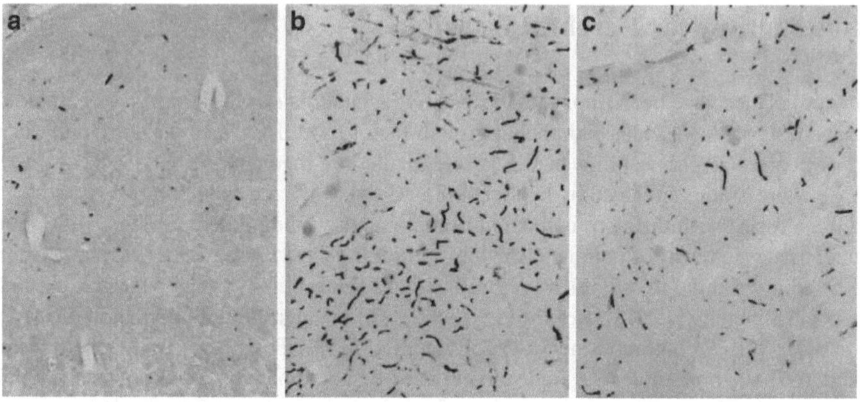

Fig. 1 Light microphotographs of brain tissue after the injection of India ink into a control rat (**a**) and chronic cerebral hypoperfusion model rats in which 100 μg (**b**) and 200 μg (**c**) of phVEGF$_{165}$ had been injected into their temporal muscles. The number and density of capillaries in the brain was largest when 100 μg phVEGF$_{165}$ was administered, whereas a higher dose of phVEGF$_{165}$ demonstrated a less striking effect. Original magnification: ×40

the viral envelope method to transfer the HGF gene or the VEGF gene into the subarachnoid space of a cerebral hypoperfusion model rat [33].

Cell Therapy for Cerebral Ischemia

The clinical efficacy of cell transplantation has already been demonstrated in patients who have suffered from myocardial infarction or limb ischemia. In ischemic stroke, the processes of recovery are more complex. The ultimate goal of cell therapy for cerebral ischemia is not only to secrete neurotrophic and angiogenic factors for neuroprotection and neuroregeneration but also to induce differentiation of the grafted cells into functional neurons or glial cells in damaged brains.

We have reported neurotrophic factor-secreting cell line grafting and adult-derived neural stem cell grafting for the treatment of cerebral ischemia. An encapsulated VEGF-secreting cell line grafted into the striatum of a middle cerebral artery occlusion model rat demonstrated neurotrophic and angiogenic effects on focal cerebral ischemia [11]. We also established glial cell line-derived neurotrophic factor-secreting adult-derived neural stem cells [12]. Transplantation of these cells into the ischemic boundary zone of rats after middle cerebral artery occlusion resulted in a decreased infarct volume, better behavioral assessment, and migration toward the ischemic core of grafted cells that expressed immature neuronal markers [34].

Transplantation of autologous stem cells overcomes the ethical issues, immunological response, and tumor formation that may be encountered during other types of cell transplantation. Although stem cells in humans and rats have the potential to differentiate into neurons [35], replacement of neurons is not necessarily required in cell therapy for moyamoya disease similar to ischemic heart or limb disease. Kim et al. performed an EMS operation 7 days after the induction of chronic cerebral ischemia and injected 1×10^6 bone marrow stromal cells (BMSC) into the temporal muscle [26]. Three weeks later, a greater increase of the capillary/muscle ratio in the temporal muscle was observed in the BMSC transplantation group compared to the control group, although the angiogenesis in the brain was not significantly different between the two groups. The injected BMSC did not directly cause the angiogenesis, but were assumed to provide a favorable environment for angiogenesis through the paracrine effect. They concluded that a large number of BMSC or simultaneous transplantation adjacent to the brain might be required to facilitate angiogenesis in the brain.

We transplanted cultured mesenchymal stem cells (MSCs) into chronic cerebral ischemic model rats. First, an oxidized cellulose sheet containing 1×10^6 MSC was placed on the surface of the rat brain, but no successful engraftment of the transplanted MSC or neovascularization in the brain was observed 1 week later. Then, we transplanted MSC into the brain at a depth of 1 mm from the surface. One week later, marked neovascularization in the brain had been induced by angiogenic cytokines. Some of the transplanted cells differentiated into endothelial cells that were positive for von Willebrand factor (Watanabe et al., unpublished data).

Stem cell transplantation has already been applied to the treatment of patients with cerebral ischemia. Bang et al. treated five patients with cerebral infarction in the middle cerebral artery territory by intravenous infusion of culture-expanded autologous MSC. Neurological outcomes were consistently improved in the MSC-treated group compared with the control patients during the 1-year follow-up period. They concluded that the intravenous infusion of autologous MSC is a feasible and safe therapy that may improve functional recovery from ischemic stroke [36].

Taguchi et al. administered human umbilical cord blood-derived $CD34^+$ cells containing endothelial progenitor cells and secreting numerous angiogenic factors to immunocompromised mice that had been subjected to stroke 48 h earlier. They demonstrated that the $CD34^+$ cells directly or indirectly promoted an environment conducive to neovascularization of the ischemic brain and thereby enabled neuronal regeneration [37].

Although it remains uncertain which type of cells are the most appropriate for treatment of cerebral ischemia, a variety of cell types have shown sufficient potential to be subjected to clinical trials to test their efficacy for the treatment of cerebral ischemia in the near future.

Conclusion

We summarized the basic and clinical studies regarding gene therapy and stem cell transplantation intended to enhance neovascularization after cerebral ischemia. Various types of genes and stem cells can be used in vasoconstructive surgery for cerebral ischemia including moyamoya disease.

References

1. Karasawa J, Kikuchi H, Furuse S et al (1977) A surgical treatment of "moyamoya" disease "encephalo-myo synangiosis". Neurol Med Chir (Tokyo) 17:29–37
2. Matsushima Y, Fukai N, Tanaka K et al (1981) A new surgical treatment of moyamoya disease in children: a preliminary report. Surg Neurol 15:313–320
3. Kinugasa K, Mandai S, Tokunaga K et al (1994) Ribbon enchephalo-duro-arterio-myo-synangiosis for moyamoya disease. Surg Neurol 41:455–461

4. Kinugasa K, Mandai S, Kamata I et al (1993) Surgical treatment of moyamoya disease: operative technique for encephalo-duro-arterio-myo-synangiosis, its follow-up, clinical results, and angiograms. Neurosurgery 32:527–531
5. Karasawa J, Kikuchi H, Furuse S et al (1978) Treatment of moyamoya disease with STA-MCA anastomosis. J Neurosurg 49:679–688
6. Tokunaga K, Kinugasa K, Mandai S et al (1994) Ribbon encephalo-duro-arterio-myo-synangiosis (ribbon EDAMS) for patients with moyamoya disease. Nerv Syst Child 19:131–137
7. Kawaguchi T, Fujita S, Hosoda K et al (1996) Multiple burr-hole operation for adult moyamoya disease. J Neurosurg 84:468–476
8. Isono M, Ishii K, Kobayashi H et al (2002) Effects of indirect bypass surgery for occlusive cerebrovascular diseases in adults. J Clin Neurosci 9:644–647
9. Houkin K, Kuroda S, Ishikawa T et al (2000) Neovascularization (angiogenesis) after revascularization in moyamoya disease. Which technique is most useful for moyamoya disease? Acta Neurochir (Wien) 142:269–276
10. Date I, Yasuhara T (2009) Neurological disorders and neural regeneration, with special reference to Parkinson's disease and cerebral ischemia. J Artif Organs 12:11–16
11. Yano A, Shingo T, Takeuchi A et al (2005) Encapsulated vascular endothelial growth factor-secreting cell grafts have neuroprotective and angiogenic effects on focal cerebral ischemia. J Neurosurg 103:104–114
12. Muraoka K, Shingo T, Yasuhara T et al (2008) Comparison of the therapeutic potential of adult and embryonic neural precursor cells in a rat model of Parkinson disease. J Neurosurg 108:149–159
13. Muraoka K, Shingo T, Yasuhara T et al (2006) The high integration and differentiation potential of autologous neural stem cell transplantation compared with allogeneic transplantation in adult rat hippocampus. Exp Neurol 199:311–327
14. Kusaka N, Sugiu K, Tokunaga K et al (2005) Enhanced brain angiogenesis in chronic cerebral hypoperfusion after administration of plasmid human vascular endothelial growth factor in combination with indirect vasoreconstructive surgery. J Neurosurg 103:882–890
15. Ogawa T, Ono S, Ichikawa T et al (2007) Novel protein transduction method by using 11R: an effective new drug delivery system for the treatment of cerebrovascular diseases. Stroke 38:1354–1361
16. Takahashi K, Tanabe K, Ohnuki M et al (2007) Induction of pluripotent stem cells from adult human fibroblasts by defined factors. Cell 131:861–872
17. Ferrara N, Gerber HP, LeCouter J (2003) The biology of VEGF and its receptors. Nat Med 9:669–676
18. Harrigan MR (2003) Angiogenic factors in the central nervous system. Neurosurgery 53:639–660; discussion 660–631
19. Baumgartner I, Pieczek A, Manor O et al (1998) Constitutive expression of phVEGF165 after intramuscular gene transfer promotes collateral vessel development in patients with critical limb ischemia. Circulation 97:1114–1123
20. Isner JM, Pieczek A, Schainfeld R et al (1996) Clinical evidence of angiogenesis after arterial gene transfer of phVEGF165 in patient with ischaemic limb. Lancet 348:370–374
21. Losordo DW, Vale PR, Symes JF et al (1998) Gene therapy for myocardial angiogenesis: initial clinical results with direct myocardial injection of phVEGF165 as sole therapy for myocardial ischemia. Circulation 98:2800–2804
22. Ozawa CR, Banfi A, Glazer NL et al (2004) Microenvironmental VEGF concentration, not total dose, determines a threshold between normal and aberrant angiogenesis. J Clin Invest 113:516–527
23. Takeshita S, Weir L, Chen D et al (1996) Therapeutic angiogenesis following arterial gene transfer of vascular endothelial growth factor in a rabbit model of hindlimb ischemia. Biochem Biophys Res Commun 227:628–635
24. Tsurumi Y, Kearney M, Chen D et al (1997) Treatment of acute limb ischemia by intramuscular injection of vascular endothelial growth factor gene. Circulation 96:II-382–388
25. Tanaka K, Wada N, Hori K et al (1998) Chronic cerebral hypoperfusion disrupts discriminative behavior in acquired-learning rats. J Neurosci Methods 84:63–68
26. Kim HJ, Jang SY, Park JI et al (2004) Vascular endothelial growth factor-induced angiogenic gene therapy in patients with peripheral artery disease. Exp Mol Med 36:336–344
27. Yasuhara T, Shingo T, Muraoka K et al (2005) The differences between high and low-dose administration of VEGF to dopaminergic neurons of in vitro and in vivo Parkinson's disease model. Brain Res 1038:1–10

28. Kim I, Moon SO, Park SK et al (2001) Angiopoietin-1 reduces VEGF-stimulated leukocyte adhesion to endothelial cells by reducing ICAM-1, VCAM-1, and E-selectin expression. Circ Res 89:477–479
29. Thurston G, Rudge JS, Ioffe E et al. (2000) Angiopoietin-1 protects the adult vasculature against plasma leakage. Nat Med 6:460–463
30. Chae JK, Kim I, Lim ST et al (2000) Coadministration of angiopoietin-1 and vascular endothelial growth factor enhances collateral vascularization. Arterioscler Thromb Vasc Biol 20:2573–2578
31. Shyu KG, Chang H, Isner JM (2003) Synergistic effect of angiopoietin-1 and vascular endothelial growth factor on neoangiogenesis in hypercholesterolemic rabbit model with acute hindlimb ischemia. Life Sci 73:563–579
32. Morishita R, Aoki M, Hashiya N et al (2004) Safety evaluation of clinical gene therapy using hepatocyte growth factor to treat peripheral arterial disease. Hypertension 44:203–209
33. Yoshimura S, Morishita R, Hayashi K et al (2002) Gene transfer of hepatocyte growth factor to subarachnoid space in cerebral hypoperfusion model. Hypertension 39:1028–1034
34. Kameda M, Shingo T, Takahashi K et al (2007) Adult neural stem and progenitor cells modified to secrete GDNF can protect, migrate and integrate after intracerebral transplantation in rats with transient forebrain ischemia. Eur J Neurosci 26:1462–1478
35. Woodbury D, Schwarz EJ, Prockop DJ et al (2000) Adult rat and human bone marrow stromal cells differentiate into neurons. J Neurosci Res 61:364–370
36. Bang OY, Lee JS, Lee PH et al (2005) Autologous mesenchymal stem cell transplantation in stroke patients. Ann Neurol 57:874–882
37. Taguchi A, Soma T, Tanaka H et al (2004) Administration of CD34+ cells after stroke enhances neurogenesis via angiogenesis in a mouse model. J Clin Invest 114:330–338

Part XIV
Special Consideration III

Moyamoya Disease in North America

Raphael Guzman, Nadia Khan, and Gary K. Steinberg

Introduction

Moyamoya disease (MMD) was first described in the Japanese medical literature in 1957 by Takeuchi and Shimizu [1]. The term "moyamoya" (Japanese for "puff of smoke"), was coined by Suzuki and Takaku in 1969 to describe the diagnostic appearance of angiogenesis on catheter angiogram [2]. Since its initial discovery, the features of the disease have become clearer; however, its etiology remains unknown. MMD is a chronic cerebrovascular disease characterized by stenosis or occlusion of the bilateral terminal internal carotid arteries resulting in the characteristic development of an abnormal vascular network in the areas of the arterial occlusions [3]. It is hypothesized that, in the setting of arterial stenosis or occlusion, hypoxic regions of the brain induce deep collateral flow through dilated and tortuous perforating arteries. It has been shown that this native revascularization strategy is orchestrated by the expression of various angiogenic signaling cascades [4, 5]. Despite intense research, the etiology of MMD remains unclear [6]. Familial MMD has been noted in as many as 15% of patients, indicating an autosomal dominant inheritance pattern with incomplete penetrance. Genetic analyses in familial MMD and genome-wide association studies represent promising strategies for elucidating the pathophysiology of this condition. A recent study described that carriers of a mutation in the vascular smooth muscle cell-specific isoform of alpha-actin can present with a diversity of vascular diseases, including premature onset of coronary artery disease and thoracic artery aneurysm and dissection, as well as MMD [7].

While recent literature shows an increase in the number of diagnosed moyamoya cases in non-Asian populations, the exact incidence has not been determined [8]. A survey in the western United States found an annual incidence of 0.086/100,000 persons [9]. The numbers are much lower than those reported for the Asian population, with newest data reporting an incidence of 0.54/100,000/year and a prevalence of 6/100,000 [10]. Amongst the Asian population, the disease often affects children more than adults, with each age group presenting

R. Guzman, N. Khan and G.K. Steinberg (✉)
Department of Neurosurgery, Stanford Stroke Center and Stanford Institute for Neuro-Innovation and Translational Neurosciences, Stanford University School of Medicine,
300 Pasteur Drive, R200, Stanford, CA, 94305-5327, USA
e-mail: gsteinberg@stanford.edu

B.-K. Cho and T. Tominaga (eds.), *Moyamoya Disease Update*,
DOI 10.1007/978-4-431-99703-0_49, © Springer 2010

unique clinical features [11]. While some studies have reported similar presentation characteristics in North America [12], others have shown distinct differences from Asian populations [13–15]. This chapter reviews clinical findings in the North American literature on moyamoya disease and discusses it in comparison to the Asian literature.

Epidemiologic Features

Moyamoya is a rare disease with only limited population-based epidemiological data in North America. In a previous study, analysis of a hospital discharge database combined California and Washington State and reported an incidence of 0.086/100,000 persons/year [9]. In a subgroup analysis, they found an incidence of 0.28/100,000 persons/year for Asian-Americans which would indicate that the incidence is maintained after immigration into the US [9]. The ethnicity adjusted incidence ratio shows a 4.5-times higher incidence for Asian-Americans, 2.1-times higher incidence for African-Americans, and 0.5-times higher incidence for Hispanics as compared to Caucasians [9]. A physician survey performed in Hawaii showed a higher percentage of Asians and Pacific Islanders (56%) compared to the remaining USA (3%) [16]. In this study, the authors found a significantly higher prevalence in patients of Japanese descent as compared to Caucasians [16]. The literature describes a much higher incidence in the Asian population of 0.54/100,000 persons/year and a prevalence of 6/100,000 [10] and up to an incidence of 0.94/100,000 and a prevalence of 10.5/100,000 [17]. There is, however, no nationwide survey available for MMD in North America and therefore conclusions about demographical data should be made with caution. The available data might only be representative for the western United States and Hawaii especially if the ethnicity factor truly accounts for differences in the disease incidence. California has the highest percentage of Asian population and is projected to have the biggest gain in the nation over the next 15 years (source, US Census Bureau). For instance, the ethnic distribution in our series of 329 MMD patients was 59% Caucasian, 32% Asian, 5% African-American, and 4% Hispanic [18], which was comparable to the epidemiological data published for California and Washington State [9]. This was, however, different from previously published North American series in which the majority of patients were Caucasian and African-American [12, 14, 15]. Therefore, most of the current studies represent local demographics reflecting local referral patterns. Additionally, the disease is most likely underdiagnosed in North America. While there were fewer than 200 reported cases in 1992, this number has increased more than five-fold in 2009.

MMD has a higher prevalence in female patients. In our series with 329 patients, the female/male ratio was 2.7:1 [18]. This was comparable to other North American series [12, 14], but higher than reported in the Asian literature with ratios between 1.2 and 1.8:1 [10, 11, 17]. An interesting observation was that in our age group of 0–9 years there was an almost equal distribution between females and males, which later in life was found to be 2.7:1 [18]. Scott et al. in their pediatric series of 143 patients had a female/male ratio of 1.6:1 [19].

There is a well-described bimodal age distribution in patients with MMD. Typically, a pediatric peak age at 5 years and an adult peak age in the mid-40s is described [17]. We found a first peak at 10.1 years and a second peak at 39.5 years [18] which was comparable with other North American series [12, 15]. The mean adult age reported in Uchino's study for the western United States was slightly higher at 55–59 years [9]. These numbers are comparable to larger survey studies in Japan comprising more than 3,000 patients [10, 17, 20, 50].

Disease Presentation

Originally, MMD was described to be a bilateral disease. With the advent of modern radiological modalities, more patients are diagnosed at potentially earlier stages of disease with unilateral manifestation [21–23]. In a recent study, we identified 28/157 patients (17.8%) with unilateral disease [22]. Angiographic progression from unilateral to bilateral disease was seen in 7 patients (38.9%) at a mean follow-up of 12.7±2.4 months. The best predictor for disease progression was the presence of equivocal or mild stenotic changes of the contralateral anterior cerebral artery, middle cerebral artery, or internal carotid artery ($p<0.01$). In the group with equivocal or mild contralateral disease, 5 of 7 patients (71%) progressed, whereas only 1 of 12 patients (8%) with no initial contralateral disease progressed to bilateral MMD [22]. Similar observations are described in the Japanese literature where 36.4% of patients with unilateral disease progressed to bilateral vascular involvement [24]. Interestingly, in the subgroup of patients with neurofibromatosis and associated MMD, 37.5% had a unilateral manifestation which was a significant difference compared to the other syndromic patients or the entire cohort ($p<0.05$) [18].

In our series, 17% of adult patients presented with hemorrhage, while 66% presented with ischemic stroke and 63% with TIAs [25]. Other North American series describe similar findings with ischemia as the most prevalent presenting symptom (70% [12] and 74% [14]) followed by hemorrhagic presentation (15% [12] and 17% [14]) (Table 1). The literature suggests a difference in presenting symptoms between Caucasian and Asian patient populations, with Asian adult patients having a higher incidence of hemorrhage [3, 12, 14, 15]. However, in a large recent Japanese survey study with 267 patients, hemorrhage was the presenting symptom in 21.3% and ischemic stroke in 56.9% [17]. A large study comparing 296 Korean with 731 Japanese MMD patients found a significantly higher incidence of hemorrhage in Korean (42.2%) as compared to Japanese (19.1%) patients, with a lower incidence of presenting ischemic strokes for both groups (27.3 and 14.9%, respectively) [26]. Based on these findings, one would expect to see differences in presenting symptoms between the different ethnicities within North American series. We separately analyzed the presenting symptoms in our adult Asian (69 patients) and Caucasian (137 patients) populations. There was, however, no statistically significant difference in the incidence of ischemic stroke (67 vs 65%) and TIA (61 vs 67%). The rate of hemorrhagic presentation was higher in American-Asian as compared to Caucasian (24 vs 16%), but did not reach statistical significance ($p=0.08$). There was a statistically nonsignificant higher incidence of stroke and lower incidence of hemorrhage in African-American patients. The incidence of hemorrhagic presentation in pediatric patients is known to be rare. In a large series of 143 pediatric MMD patients examined by Scott et al. [19], only 2.8% presented with intracranial hemorrhage. The same was found in our 96 pediatric patients with 2.1% presenting with intracerebral hemorrhages [25] (Table 1). Headache has been described as a symptom associated with a hemorrhagic presentation of MMD [27] or as an independent presenting symptom [28, 29] in children [29] and adult [27, 30] patients. When it is not associated with a hemorrhage, studies have suggested a relation to hypoperfusion and TIAs [31]. The ischemic penumbra can cause spreading cortical depression which has been associated with migraine [31] and has also been described in MMD [28]. A different theory by Seol et al. [29] speculates that the dilation of meningeal and leptomeningeal collateral vessels stimulate dural nociceptors. A significant number of our patients presented with a long history of mild to severe headaches (50% in adult and 44% in pediatric patients) [25]. In the Asian literature, headaches as a presenting symptom have been reported in up to 49% of patients [27, 29, 32].

Neuropsychological changes caused by MMD are rarely described. We found that the highest rate of impairment was for measures of executive functioning and cognitive

Table 1 Demographics, clinical presentation and revascularization procedures in Moyamoya disease.

Author	Year	No. of patients	Ethnicity	Female (%)	Mean age adult/Peds	Ischemic presentation	Hemorrhagic presentation	Treatment
Numaguchi et al. [50]	1997	98	55% Caucasian 8% Asian	71	2 peaks	Most patients	14%	–
Graham et al. [16]	1997	21	10% Caucasian 80% Asian	62	37.3	69	19%	EDAS/STA-MCA
Chiu et al. [14]	1998	35	63% Caucasian	71	32	74	17%	EDAS
Yilmaz et al. [15]	2001	20	90% Caucasian	60	35/8	78	14% of adults	EDAS/STA-MCA
Scott et al. [19]	2004	143	89% Caucasian 11% Asian	62	7.1	67.8	2.8%	EDAS
Uchino et al. [9]	2005	289	Caucasian and Asian	68	55–59/5–9	26	15%	–
Hallemeier et al. [12]	2006	34	68% Caucasian 3% Asian	74	42	71	21%	EDAS
Mesiwala et al. [38]	2008	39	69% Caucasian 31% Asian	77	34	85	13%	STA-MCA/EDAS
Guzman et al. [18]	2009	329	59% Caucasian 32% Asian	70	39.5/10.1	57	14.6% of adults 2.1% of peds	STA-MCA/EDAS

impairment. In a consecutive series of 36 adult patients who underwent neuropsychological assessment, cognitive impairment was present in 11 (31%) of the patients; it was judged to be moderate to severe in 4 patients (11%) [33].

Natural History

The data on natural history for MMD is controversial, and there are only a limited number of studies that have observed untreated patients prospectively.

Common to both North American and Asian studies is the inevitable disease progression [22, 24, 34]. From a radiological perspective, disease progression in unilateral moyamoya of 36.4% [24] and 38.9% [22] have been described.

From a clinical perspective, North American and Asian data report that when left untreated moyamoya is a devastating disease even in initially asymptomatic patients.

The 5-year cumulative risk for any recurrent ipsilateral stroke among medically treated hemispheres with impaired hemodynamic reserve (increased oxygen extraction fraction on PET) is estimated to be 65% and, if stratified for patients with bilateral disease only, the stroke risk increases to 82% over 5 years [12]. A second North American study found a recurrent stroke risk of 18% in the first year and a 5%/year risk thereafter, for a cumulative 5-year risk of 40% [14]. A long-term study on the natural history of hemorrhagic MMD in 42 patients demonstrated a risk of recurrent hemorrhage of 7.09% [35]. A nationwide survey in Japan focused on asymptomatic MMD patients and found that the risk of stroke in medically treated hemispheres was 3.2%/year [32]. In contrast to these devastating numbers, the cumulative 5-year Kaplan–Meier risk of perioperative or subsequent stroke or death was between 5.5% [18] and 17% [12] in surgically treated hemispheres. Hence, even in asymptomatic MMD patients with an estimated annual stroke risk of 3.2% [32], surgery would already be superior to observation after 2 years.

Treatment

Many studies report successful revascularization results in patients with MMD. In these high risk patients, perioperative ischemia seems to be more common than in other cerebrovascular occlusive diseases [36]. Much debate has centered on the safety and efficacy of various revascularization procedures. No randomized study is available comparing direct and indirect revascularization methods, and a review of the literature failed to demonstrate a superiority or a lower surgical morbidity rate for either method [37]. Generally, in adults, direct revascularization, and in children, indirect revascularization are considered the preferred surgical treatments [18, 19, 38]. Nevertheless, several North American reports have used mainly indirect methods in adult patients as well [12, 14] (Table 1). Our philosophy has been to attempt direct revascularization in all patients. Direct revascularization procedures are thought to provide immediate increase of blood flow to the ischemic brain. In our series including 557 revascularization procedures, 95.1% were direct in adults and 76.2% in the pediatric group [18]. Similar approaches were chosen by other North American groups applying direct techniques in 90.8% of their adult population [38].

Surgical outcome data from North American series demonstrate neurological complications in 3.5–13% per surgical hemisphere [12, 14, 18, 19, 38]. Similar findings were described in the Japanese literature where predominantly direct revascularization procedures are used [36, 39]. A large patient volume, a highly specialized team, intraoperative electrophysiological monitoring [40], intra- and postoperative rigorous blood pressure control, and possibly the use of intraoperative mild hypothermia [41] are contributory factors for successful outcomes after revascularization surgery.

Prior studies have attempted to determine risk factors that would predict surgical morbidity. Although not statistically significant in uni- and multivariate analyses, preoperative TIA, stroke, and hemorrhage were associated with a higher risk for postoperative complications. In a large study of 368 revascularization surgeries, Sakamoto et al. found that a high frequency of preoperative TIA (>1–4/months; OR 4.8, $p=0.01$) and indirect revascularization (OR 5.8, $p=0.01$) were predictors of perioperative stroke risk [36]. Frequent TIAs are a sign of cerebral hemodynamic instability and put the patient at higher risk of perioperative stroke if additional events such as hypercapnia or hypotension occur during the surgical procedure [42]. An additional strong predictor of adverse surgical events was the presence of a syndrome associated with moyamoya. This had been previously described for Down's syndrome with associated moyamoya where a perioperative stroke rate of 12.5% was found [43].

Outcome

The main goal of revascularization surgery in MMD patients remains prevention of future ischemic and hemorrhagic strokes and potentially to limit disease progression. Most North American studies agree that surgical treatment will reduce the risk of recurrent stroke and TIA. We found a 5-year cumulative risk of stroke or death of 5.5% [18]. Hallemeier et al. described a reduction in the 5-year cumulative stroke or death risk from 65% in medically to 17% in surgically treated hemispheres [12]. One study failed to demonstrate a benefit of surgical over medical treatment in the 5-year risk of recurrent stroke [14] mainly because of a relatively high initial surgical morbidity.

There is an ongoing debate in the literature over treatment of MMD and prevention of recurring hemorrhage [44–48]. Rebleeding rates of 18% [45] and 14.3% [49] have been described at a mean follow-up of 4 and 6 years mean follow-up, respectively, after revascularization surgery. Even though this would compare favorably to a risk of recurrent hemorrhage estimated to be 7%/person/year with a mortality of 28.6% [35] if left untreated, it is not a satisfying result. We have observed reduction of moyamoya vessels at the 4–6 months follow-up cerebral angiography, sometimes with almost complete resolution of the moyamoya collaterals [20]. Early reduction of the fragile moyamoya vessels is thought to be responsible for the reduction in rebleeding, and direct bypass surgery is suggested to be the preferred revascularization technique.

In our series, 71.2% of patients experienced a significant improvement in quality of life, the strongest predictor being the preoperative MRS (OR 26, $p<0.0001$) [18]. The patients also reported an increased energy level and an improved cognitive function. We had, however, no medical arm to compare outcome data. While most of the groups describe a reduction in stroke risk after treatment, three North American series failed to demonstrate a difference in the functional outcome comparing medical and surgical treatment [12, 14, 15]. Hallemeier et al. [12] found no difference in the modified Rankin, Barthel, or SS-QOL scores between surgically and medically treated patients.

Conclusions

MMD is overall more rare in North America, but if analyzed in the subgroup of Asian-American or Pacific Islanders in Hawaii, findings become more comparable. While the female to male ratio seems to be higher in the North American literature, the age distribution does not seem to be different. The rate of hemorrhagic presentation is lower in North American moyamoya patients, but again the subgroup analysis of Asian-American patients provides more comparable findings to the Asian literature. Overall these findings indicate that there is an ethnicity factor, and that disease characteristics are maintained after immigration into the US.

References

1. Takeuchi K, Shimizu K (1957) Hypogenesis of bilateral internal carotid arteries. No To Shinkei 9:37–43
2. Suzuki J, Takaku A (1969) Cerebrovascular "moyamoya" disease. Disease showing abnormal net-like vessels in base of brain. Arch Neurol 20:288–299
3. Suzuki J, Kodama N (1983) Moyamoya disease – a review. Stroke 14:104–109
4. Lim M, Cheshier S, Steinberg GK (2006) New vessel formation in the central nervous system during tumor growth, vascular malformations, and moyamoya. Curr Neurovasc Res 3:237–245
5. Sakamoto S, Kiura Y, Yamasaki F, et al. (2007) Expression of vascular endothelial growth factor in dura mater of patients with moyamoya disease. Neurosurg Rev
6. Achrol AS, Guzman R, Lee M, et al. (2009) Pathophysiology and genetic factors in moyamoya disease. Neurosurg Focus 26:E4
7. Guo DC, Papke CL, Tran-Fadulu V, et al. (2009) Mutations in smooth muscle alpha-actin (ACTA2) cause coronary artery disease, stroke, and moyamoya disease, along with thoracic aortic disease. Am J Hum Genet 84:617–627
8. Hoffman HJ (1997) Moyamoya disease and syndrome. Clin Neurol Neurosurg 99 Suppl 2:S39–S44
9. Uchino K, Johnston SC, Becker KJ, et al. (2005) Moyamoya disease in Washington State and California. Neurology 65:956–958
10. Kuriyama S, Kusaka Y, Fujimura M, et al. (2008) Prevalence and clinicoepidemiological features of moyamoya disease in Japan: findings from a nationwide epidemiological survey. Stroke 39:42–47
11. Wakai K, Tamakoshi A, Ikezaki K, et al. (1997) Epidemiological features of moyamoya disease in Japan: findings from a nationwide survey. Clin Neurol Neurosurg 99:S1–S5
12. Hallemeier CL, Rich KM, Grubb RL, Jr., et al. (2006) Clinical features and outcome in North American adults with moyamoya phenomenon. Stroke 37:1490–1496
13. Bruno A, Adams HP, Jr., Biller J, et al. (1988) Cerebral infarction due to moyamoya disease in young adults. Stroke 19:826–833
14. Chiu D, Shedden P, Bratina P, et al. (1998) Clinical features of moyamoya disease in the United States. Stroke 29:1347–1351
15. Yilmaz EY, Pritz MB, Bruno A, et al. (2001) Moyamoya: Indiana University Medical Center experience. Arch Neurol 58:1274–1278
16. Graham JF, Matoba A (1997) A survey of moyamoya disease in Hawaii. Clin Neurol Neurosurg 99:S31–S35
17. Baba T, Houkin K, Kuroda S (2008) Novel epidemiological features of moyamoya disease. J Neurol Neurosurg Psychiatry 79:900–904
18. Guzman R, Lee M, Achrol A, Bell-Stephens T, Kelly ME, Do HM, Marks MP, Steinberg GK (2009) Clinical outcome after 450 revascularization procedures for moyamoya disease. J Neurosurg 111:927–935
19. Scott RM, Smith JL, Robertson RL, et al. (2004) Long-term outcome in children with moyamoya syndrome after cranial revascularization by pial synangiosis. J Neurosurg 100:142–149
20. Wang MY, Steinberg GK (1996) Rapid and near-complete resolution of moyamoya vessels in a patient with moyamoya disease treated with superficial temporal artery-middle cerebral artery bypass. Pediatr Neurosurg 24:145–150
21. Hirotsune N, Meguro T, Kawada S, et al. (1997) Long-term follow-up study of patients with unilateral moyamoya disease. Clin Neurol Neurosurg 99:S175–S178
22. Kelly ME, Bell-Stephens TE, Marks MP, et al. (2006) Progression of unilateral moyamoya disease: a clinical series. Cerebrovasc Dis 22:109–115
23. Nagata S, Matsushima T, Morioka T, et al. (2006) Unilaterally symptomatic moyamoya disease in children: long-term follow-up of 20 patients. Neurosurgery 59:830–836; discussion 836–837
24. Kuroda S, Ishikawa T, Houkin K, et al. (2005) Incidence and clinical features of disease progression in adult moyamoya disease. Stroke 36:2148–2153

25. Guzman RLM, Bell-Stephens T, Pickthorn B, et al. (2007) Long term clinical outcome in children who underwent revascularization surgery for moyamoya disease. Abstract, Annual meeting of the CNS
26. Ikezaki K, Han DH, Kawano T, et al. (1997) Epidemiological survey of moyamoya disease in Korea. Clin Neurol Neurosurg 99:S6–S10
27. Hung C-C, Tu Y-K, Su C-F, et al. (1997) Epidemiological study of moyamoya disease in Taiwan. Clin Neurol Neurosurg 99:S23–S25
28. Park-Matsumoto YC, Tazawa T, Shimizu J (1999) Migraine with aura-like headache associated with moyamoya disease. Acta Neurol Scand 100:119–121
29. Seol HJ, Wang KC, Kim SK, et al. (2005) Headache in pediatric moyamoya disease: review of 204 consecutive cases. J Neurosurg 103:439–442
30. Iwama T, Yoshimura S (2008) Present status of moyamoya disease in Japan. Acta Neurochir Suppl 103:115–118
31. Olesen J, Friberg L, Olsen TS, et al. (1993) Ischaemia-induced (symptomatic) migraine attacks may be more frequent than migraine-induced ischaemic insults. Brain 116(Pt 1):187–202
32. Kuroda S, Hashimoto N, Yoshimoto T, et al. (2007) Radiological findings, clinical course, and outcome in asymptomatic moyamoya disease: results of multicenter survey in Japan. Stroke 38:1430–1435
33. Karzmark P, Zeifert PD, Tan S, et al. (2008) Effect of moyamoya disease on neuropsychological functioning in adults. Neurosurgery 62:1048–1051; discussion 1051–1042
34. Imaizumi T, Hayashi K, Saito K, et al. (1998) Long-term outcomes of pediatric moyamoya disease monitored to adulthood. Pediatr Neurol 18:321–325
35. Kobayashi E, Saeki N, Oishi H, et al. (2000) Long-term natural history of hemorrhagic moyamoya disease in 42 patients. J Neurosurg 93:976–980
36. Sakamoto H, Kitano S, Yasui T, et al. (1997) Direct extracranial-intracranial bypass for children with moyamoya disease. Clin Neurol Neurosurg 99:S126–S131
37. Veeravagu A, Guzman R, Patil CG, et al. (2008) Moyamoya disease in pediatric patients: outcomes of neurosurgical interventions. Neurosurg Focus 24:E16
38. Mesiwala AH, Sviri G, Fatemi N, et al. (2008) Long-term outcome of superficial temporal artery-middle cerebral artery bypass for patients with moyamoya disease in the US. Neurosurg Focus 24: E15
39. Fujimura M, Kaneta T, Tominaga T (2008) Efficacy of superficial temporal artery-middle cerebral artery anastomosis with routine postoperative cerebral blood flow measurement during the acute stage in childhood moyamoya disease. Childs Nerv Syst 24:827–832
40. Lopez JR (2009) Neurophysiologic intraoperative monitoring of pediatric cerebrovascular surgery. J Clin Neurophysiol 26:85–94
41. Choi R, Andres RH, Steinberg GK, et al. (2009) Intraoperative hypothermia during vascular neurosurgical procedures. Neurosurg Focus 26:E24
42. Iwama T, Hashimoto N, Yonekawa Y (1996) The relevance of hemodynamic factors to perioperative ischemic complications in childhood moyamoya disease. Neurosurgery 38:1120–1125; discussion 1125–1126
43. Jea A, Smith ER, Robertson R, et al. (2005) Moyamoya syndrome associated with Down syndrome: outcome after surgical revascularization. Pediatrics 116:e694–e701
44. Fujii K, Ikezaki K, Irikura K, et al. (1997) The efficacy of bypass surgery for the patients with hemorrhagic moyamoya disease. Clin Neurol Neurosurg 99:S190–S191
45. Ikezaki K, Inamura T, Kawano T, et al. (1997) Clinical features of probable moyamoya disease in Japan. Clin Neurol Neurosurg 99:S170–S174
46. Kawaguchi S, Okuno S, Sakaki T (2000) Effect of direct arterial bypass on the prevention of future stroke in patients with the hemorrhagic variety of moyamoya disease. J Neurosurg 93:397–401
47. Otawara Y, Ogasawara K, Seki K, et al. (2007) Intracerebral hemorrhage after prophylactic revascularization in a patient with adult moyamoya disease. Surg Neurol 68:335–337; discussion 337
48. Yoshida Y, Yoshimoto T, Shirane R, et al. (1999) Clinical course, surgical management, and long-term outcome of moyamoya patients with rebleeding after an episode of intracerebral hemorrhage: an extensive follow-up study. Stroke 30:2272–2276
49. Houkin K, Kamiyama H, Abe H, et al. (1996) Surgical therapy for adult moyamoya disease. Can surgical revascularization prevent the recurrence of intracerebral hemorrhage? Stroke 27:1342–1346
50. Numaguchi Y, Gonzalez CF, Davis PC, Monajati A, Afshani E, Chang J, et al. (1997) Moyamoya disease in the United States. Clinical Neurology and Neurosurgery 99(Supplement 2):S26–S30

Moyamoya Angiopathy in Europe

Yasuhiro Yonekawa, Javier Fandino, Martina Hug, Markus Wiesli, Masayuki Fujioka, and Nadia Khan

Introduction

This chapter deals with moyamoya angiopathy (MMA) [1, 2], [moyamoya disease (MMD), moyamoya syndrome (MMS), and unilateral MM pathology] in Europe. Although this terminology MMA might give rise to some objections, it is considered to be acceptable from the clinical and practical points of view [2, 3], as the senior author (Y.Y.) has experience of a considerable number of patients with this pathology in Japan and in Europe (Zürich). As knowledge of recent investigation on its pathophysiology and etiology has been outlined elsewhere [2], we focus our attention here on our clinical experience in Zürich and attempt to clarify some differences between MMA in Europe and in Japan.

Y. Yonekawa (✉)
University of Zürich, Rämistrasse 71, 8006, Zürich, Switzerland
Department of Neurosurgery, Kantonsspital Aarau, Tellstrasse, 5001, Aarau, Switzerland
Children's Hospital of Zürich, University Clinic, Steinwiesstrasse 75, 8032, Zürich, Switzerland
Klinik im Park, Zürich, Switzerland
e-mail: yonekawa@bluewin.ch

J. Fandino
Department of Neurosurgery, Kantonsspital Aarau, Tellstrasse, 5001, Aarau, Switzerland

M. Hug
Children's Hospital of Zürich, University Clinic, Steinwiesstrasse 75, 8032, Zürich, Switzerland

M. Fujioka
Department of Neurosurgery, Kantonsspital Aarau, Tellstrasse, 5001, Aarau, Switzerland
University of Zürich, Rämistrasse 71, 8006, Zürich, Switzerland

M. Wiesli
Klinik im Park, Zürich, Switzerland

N. Khan
Department of Neurosurgery and Stanford Stroke Center, Stanford University School of Medicine, 300 Pasteur Drive, R200, Stanford, CA, 94305-5327, USA

B.-K. Cho and T. Tominaga (eds.), *Moyamoya Disease Update*,
DOI 10.1007/978-4-431-99703-0_50, © Springer 2010

Patients and Methods

Diagnosis was made according to the diagnostic criteria proposed by the Research Committee of the Ministry of Welfare and Health (now Ministry of Health and Labor), Japan (RCMWHJ) in 1978 and modernized in 1997 especially as a diagnostic tool using magnetic resonance imaging (MRI) and magnetic resonance angiography (MRA) instead of digital subtraction angiography (DSA) [4, 5]. This series also includes MMS and unilateral pathology as mentioned above. The retrospective consecutive series consists of 67 patients: 43 children (1 month–17 years, mean 6.8 years; female/male 1.36) and 24 adults (21–66 years, mean 39 years; female/male 4.75) during the period 1993–2009, experienced mostly at the university hospital and the children's hospital, Zürich, and partly at Klinik im Park, Zürich, and at the Kantonsspital Aarau. The patients were from Switzerland (27), Germany (15), Holland (11), Denmark (4), Austria (3), Italy (2), Sweden (2), Norway (1), Greece (1), and Qatar (1). Sixty patients were Caucasian except for patients of Middle East origin (4) and Asian origin (3) (Fig. 1). One-third of the patients had basic diseases, such as neurofibromatosis type 1, trisomy 21, hemoglobinopathy, etc., as shown in Table 1, so these patients are to be categorized as MMS.

Four adult patients presented with intracerebral hemorrhage ICH. Almost all other patients presented with ischemia and/or infarction.

Surgical augmentation of cerebral blood flow (CBF) by multiple microvascular extracranial intracranial bypasses [superficial temporal artery–middle cerebral artery (STA–MCA) bypass, superficial temporal artery–anterior cerebral artery (STA–ACA) bypass, or occipital artery–posterior cerebral artery (OA–PCA) bypass] was performed according to the findings of $H_2{}^{15}O$ positron emission tomography (PET) examination on CBF and cerebrovascular reactivity (CVR) identified by Diamox® loading [1, 2, 4].

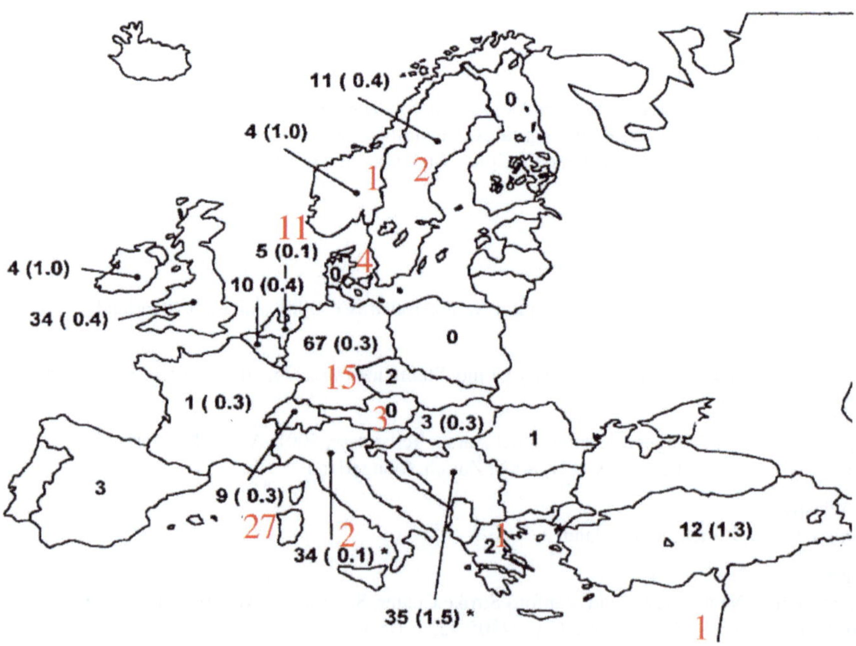

Fig. 1 Distribution of MMA patients in Europe. Numbers of patients obtained at the time of questionnaire in 1996, ( ) indicates patient numbers experienced per year per center [16]. *Numbers* in *red* indicate patient distribution in this series

Table 1 Lists of basic diseases or concomitant diseases in this series of MMA

1. Neurofibromatosis type 1	5 Patients: 1 adult+4 children
2. Hemoglobinopathy	4 Patients: 2 adults+2 children
3. Recurrent severe infection	4 Children: 2 urogenital, 1 laryngitis, 1 gastroenteritis
4. Down syndrome (trisomy 21)	3 Children
5. Pupillary sphincter dysplasia+PFO	2 Children
6. Factor 5 deficiency	2 Children: 1 hypercoagulability, 1 heart valvular disease
7. ADHD syndrome	2 Children
8. Thrombocytopenia+adipositas per magna	1 Adult
9. Hypothalamic glioma	1 Child
10. Grange syndrome	1 Child
11. Protein S deficiency	1 Child
12. Morning glory papille	1 Child
13. ARC resistant coagulopathy	1 Child
14. Glucose-6-dehydrogenase deficiency	1 Child
15. Congenital extremity defect	1 Adult

PFO patent foramen ovale; *ADHD* attention deficit hyperactivity disorder; *ARC* aids related complex

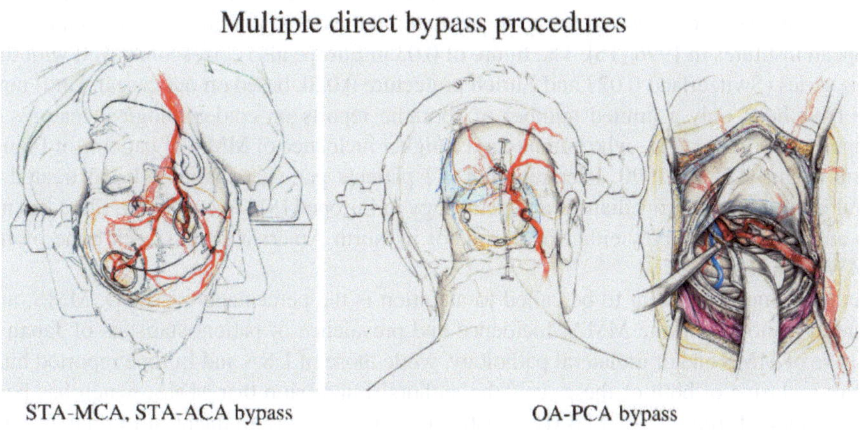

Fig. 2 Artist's drawing of multiple direct bypass procedures [6, 7, 38]

The location of revascularization was determined by findings of the PET scan. In order to find or select an appropriate recipient artery, a craniotomy was centered in the case of STA–MCA bypass ca. 6 cm above the external auditory meatus, in STA–ACA bypass just anterior to the coronal suture at the midline, and in OA–PCA bypass on the superior nuchal line for the subsequent supracerebellar transtentorial approach [6] (Fig. 2). Indirect revascularization with the use of muscle, dura, and arteries was performed only in cases where direct vascularization was impossible or failed due to the small caliber of the donor or recipient arteries (less than 0.5 mm).

Patients were followed up under Aspirin administration usually 3 months postoperatively with an admission of a couple of days for examinations, e.g., assessment of neurological findings, PET scan, DSA, Doppler sonography, etc. Thereafter, they submitted to regular ambulant follow-up with a year base without discontinuation of Aspirin.

Results and Discussion

Results in terms of postoperative improvement of hemodynamics and long-term follow-up have been partly presented [1, 3, 7] and will be presented elsewhere separately, so that some noticeable items or results are dealt with here along with discussion.

After the first report of the disease by Takeuchi and Shimizu in 1957 [8], more than 50 years have passed and its name "moyamoya disease" given by Suzuki [9] now has worldwide acceptance, although "spontaneous occlusion of the circle of Willis" used by Kudo [10] can be considered to be more appropriate for its pathophysiological expression. Since its initial discovery, the clinical features and pathophysiology of the disease have become clearer mostly by systematic survey by the RCMWHJ. Moyamoya vasculature at the base of the brain and transdural anastomosis (vault moya, ethmoidal moya) [11, 12] are considered to become orchestrated by expression of various angiogenetic signaling cascades in accordance with bilateral occlusion of the internal carotid artery (ICA) at the terminal portion [2].

It has been considered that the incidence of MMA in the USA and Europe is lower than in Japan. In 1992, Goto and Yonekawa collected 1,063 patients with MMA from countries other than Japan, and found 625 patients in Asia, 201 in Europe, 176 in North and South America, 52 in Africa, and 9 in Australia, as published in the literature [13]. In Japan, the incidence has been reported to be 0.35 (recently 0.94)/100,000, while it is 0.086 in the USA and around 0.03 in Europe [1, 2, 14–16]. The last figures, of one-tenth incidence in Europe as compared with that of Japan, has been reported from our institute on the basis of a questionnaire-enquiry of European institutes in 1996 [16]. The figure of 0.03 in Europe also corresponds well with that of this series (Switzerland 0.023 and Zürich prefecture 0.020, based on our cases). Until now, there have been only a limited number of sporadic reports on epidemiological features in Europe, e.g., Fodstad et al., who emphasized a higher incidence of MMA of patients of Finno-Uguric origin [17]. In 1990, Isler reported 0.2 patients per year diagnosed and treated at central institutes of neuropediatrics and neurology in Europe [18]. To our regret, there has not been any systematic survey either in Europe or in North America, as has been done by the RCMWHJ in Japan.

Another important point to be called to attention is the percentage of MMD, MMS, and unilateral pathology in the MMA. Incidence and prevalence of patient statistics of Japan is exclusive of MMS and of unilateral pathology, while those of USA and Europe reported hitherto are inclusive of both of these. It is the authors' impression that MMS, which has been always excluded from the RCMWHJ statistics in Japan, is more frequent in Europe as compared to Japan as can be seen in our series (Table 1).

According to the RCMWHJ study, around one-quarter of cases of unilateral MMD in children have been reported to change into bilateral pathology within a few years [19]. Two children and three adults of our series in Europe had unilateral pathology. Adult patients presented in one with headache, and in the other two with intracerebral hematoma (ICH). Four of the five patients did not show any change into the bilateral pathology during the follow-up period.

Age distribution (Fig. 3) is rather similar to that of the Japanese study and this is contrary to reports from other institutions in Europe [20, 21].

Familial incidence has increased in Japan from ca. 10% to ca. 15% [14, 22], although a lower familial incidence of around 6–15% has been reported in patients in the USA [23, 24]. In our series, only one patient showed clear familial incidence. Considering the quite frequent cases of MMS, there must be, however, some more asymptomatic cases which did not undergo active examination concerning this with neuroimaging.

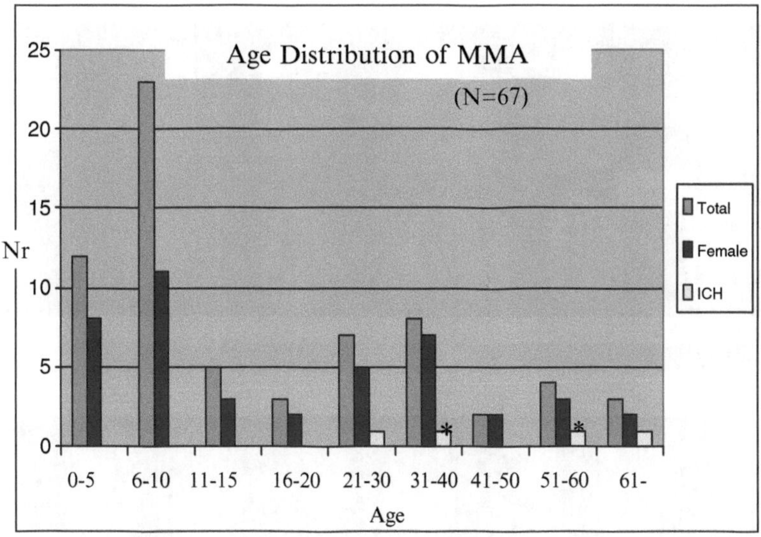

Fig. 3 Age distribution of MMA patients in this series. Two peaks are evident: one higher peak within ten years and the other lower peak around thirties. *indicates the case of unilateral pathology. *ICH* intracerebral hematoma

As for clinical manifestation, it is felt that manifestation with epileptic seizures in children is rather infrequent, and almost all adult patients in our series presented with TIAs or completed stroke. In 24 adult patients, only four presented with ICH (17%) and the rest (83%) with cerebral ischemia partly not necessarily associated with TIAs or infarctions. A sudden drop in performance due to low perfusion has been the only clinical manifestation in two (8%) of our adult patients. This is a considerable contrast to the statistics of Japan, where more than 60% of patients (mostly female) present with ICH [25]. This prevalence in clinical manifestation with ischemia in adult patients has been frequently reported in other European and North American literature [15, 20, 24, 26].

Infarctions are observed at cortico-subcortical regions prevalent in watershed territories or PCA territories in about 40% of ischemic cases, but basal ganglia and thalamus are usually spared [1, 4]. The proximal portion of the posterior cerebral artery (PCA) has been reported to also be involved in up to half of the patients [27], although the posterior circulation has usually been considered not to be affected and to contribute as a main source of collateral circulation to the insufficient anterior circulation. Steno-occlusive lesions were encountered in our series in 11 patients (16%): basilar trunk in two children and PCA in nine patients (six children and three adults).

The other point to draw attention to is that two of four ICHs took place in patients with unilateral pathology, and those in male adults (Fig. 3). ICHs have been reported to be repetitive with an annual rate of rebleeding of 7%, and one-third of the patients go on to have further hemorrhage after a variable interval (days to years) [1, 28]. The Effectiveness of bypass surgery in prevention of rebleeding has to be settled [2]. One of our patients experienced rebleeding after revascularization surgery.

Unruptured aneurysm was encountered in two patients in the series: one (adult) at MCA bifurcation and at the anterior communicating artery, and the other (child) at basilar bifurcation. The former was treated with microsurgical clipping and the latter with endovascular coiling procedure outside our institution. This occurrence of 3% belongs to the lowest figures as compared with usually reported 10% aneurysm combination with MMA [1, 29].

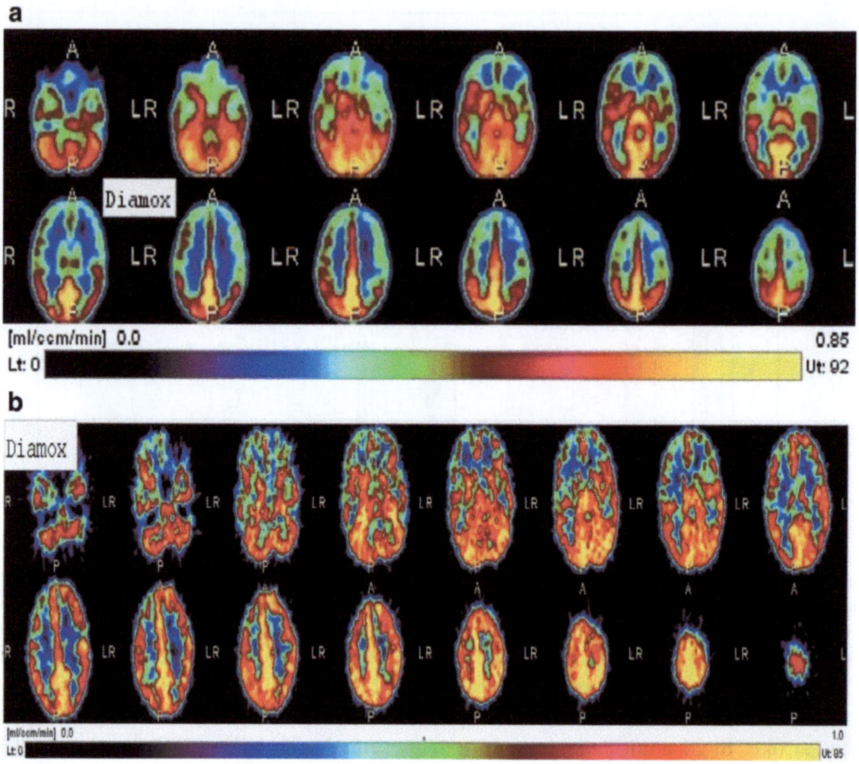

Fig. 4 Hemodynamic improvement identified by PET scan three months after direct bypass revascularization procedures (bilateral STA-MCA bypasses and a STA-ACA bypass on the left side) on a female 4 yrs. patient. Note the remarkable increase of the postoperative CVR on Diamox loading (a: Preoperative b: Postoperative)

Currently, there are no clear data of definite superiority of either of the methods; direct revascularization pioneered by Donaghy and Yasargil, indirect revascularization by Henschen later Matsushima, or their combination [30–33]. The senior author is of the opinion, in terms of predictability above all, that direct revascularization procedure should be performed whenever possible, although being aware of new cortico-subcortical infarction and hyperperfusion syndrome as infrequent postoperative complications [34, 35]. Some additional bypasses turned out to be necessary, as was observed in several patients of ours in the course of follow-up years, due to redistribution or segmentation of perfusion territory presumably due to progression of occlusive process [4, 34].

As in the case of mental retardation in children, adult patients presenting with a remarkable drop of performance due to low perfusion in the ACA territory could profit from the STA–ACA bypass in combination with standard STA–MCA bypass [7, 36, 37]. In the face of rather frequent ischemia in the PCA territory with visual problems, some revascularization procedures such as OA–PCA bypass should be taken into consideration as have been cases in our series [6, 38].

In total, on these 67 patients, direct revascularization procedures were performed 156 times [129 times to the MCA, 25 times to the anterior cerebral artery (ACA), mostly to the middle internal frontal artery, and twice to the PCA], and indirect 25 times (24 times to the

ACA and twice to the PCA), so that 2.75 revascularization procedures were performed on average per patient.

One adult patient died of perioperative ischemic edema (on the contralateral side of bypass). Among others, three other patients had perioperative ischemic complication but showed good recovery. One ICH complicated several hours after surgery remote from the site of a STA–MCA bypass near the wall of temporal horn. This patient underwent immediate surgical removal. There must have been some vascular anomaly, which bled soon after the bypass construction. The bypass continued to be patent. Three children had postoperative subdural effusions. Two of them underwent subduroperitoneal shunt and the remainder simple evacuation.

Other patients profited from augmentation of CBF by multiple bypass surgery (Fig. 4).

It should be emphasized again that ischemic complication can easily take place under compromised hemodynamic situation of these MMA patients with diminished reserve in any intervention, even at the time of diagnostic angiography or PET scan with Diamox loading, so that every preventive measure should be taken, as has been reported elsewhere [39, 40].

Conclusion

MMA is a rare disease of unknown etiology. As compared with Japan and other Asian countries, the disease in Europe seems to have somewhat different features: lower incidence, prevalence with ischemia and not ICH in adult patients, and prevalence of MMS in MMA. Multiple direct revascularization procedures with the use of STA–MCA bypass, STA–ACA bypass, and OA–PCA bypass depending on findings of PET scan were recommended from our experience of 67 patients since 1993.

Acknowledgments The authors are indebted to Ms. R. Frick for secretarial work and Mr. P. Roth for artistic drawings. They are also grateful for the excellent cooperative work to: Prof. E. Boltshauser, Prof. A. Buck, Prof. A. Valavanis and Prof. B. Schuknecht.

References

1. Yonekawa Y, Khan N (2003) Moyamoya disease. In: Barnett HJM, Bogousslavsky J, Meldrum H (eds) Ischemic stroke: advances in neurology, vol 92. Lippincott Williams & Wilkins, Philadelphia, pp 113–118
2. Yonekawa Y, Takagi Y, Khan N (2009) Adult moyamoya disease. In: Winn HR (ed) Youman's neurological surgery, 6th edition. Elsevier (in press)
3. Peerless SJ (1997) Risk factors of moyamoya disease in Canada and the USA. Clin Neurol Neurosurg 99(Suppl 2):45–48
4. Yonekawa Y, Goto Y, Ogata N (1992) Moyamoya disease: diagnosis, treatment, and recent achievement. Part IV. Specific medical disease and stroke. In: Barnett HJM, Mohr JP, Stein BM, Yatsu FM (eds) Stroke, pathophysiology, diagnosis and management. Churchill Livingstone, New York, pp 721–747
5. Fukui M, Members of Research Committee on Spontaneous Occlusion of the Circle of Willis (Moyamoya disease) of the Ministry of Health and Welfare, Japan (1997) Guidelines for the diagnosis and treatment of spontaneous occlusion of the circle of Willis ('Moyamoya' disease). Clin Neurol Neurosurg 99(Suppl 2):S238–S240
6. Yonekawa Y (2009) Brain revascularization by extracranial intracranial arterial bypass. In: Sindou M (ed) Practical handbook of neurosurgery, vol 1. Springer, Wien, pp 355–381

7. Khan N, Schuknecht B, Boltshauser E et al (2003) Moyamoya disease and moyamoya syndrome: experience in Europe: choice of revascularisation procedures. Acta Neurochir (Wien) 145:1061–1071
8. Takeuchi K, Shimuzu K (1957) Hypoplasia of the bilateral internal carotid arteries. No To Shinkei 9:37–43
9. Suzuki J, Takaku (1969) Cerebrovascular "moyamoya" disease: disease showing abnormal net-like vessels in base of brain. Arch Neurol 20:288–299
10. Kudo T (1968) Spontaneous occlusion of the circle of Willis: a disease apparently confined to Japanese. Neurology 18:485–496
11. Kodama N, Fujiwara S, Hone Y et al (1980) Transdural anastomosis in moyamoya disease: vault moyamoya. No Shinkei Geka 8:729–739
12. Suzuki J, Kodama N (1971) Cerebrovascular "moyamoya" disease. Second report. Collateral routes to forebrain via ethmoidal sinus and superior nasal meatus. Angiology 23:233–236
13. Goto Y, Yonekawa Y (1992) Worldwide distribution of moyamoya disease. Neurol Med Chir (Tokyo) 32:883–886
14. Baba T, Houkin K, Kuroda S (2008) Novel epidemiological features of moyamoya disease. J Neurol Neurosurg Psychiatry 79:900–904
15. Uchino K, Johnston SC, Becker KJ et al (2005) Moyamoya disease in Washington State and California. Neurology 65:956–958
16. Yonekawa Y, Ogata N, Kaku Y et al (1997) Moyamoya disease in Europe, past and present status. Clin Neurol Neurosurg 99(Suppl 2):S58–60
17. Fodstad H, Bodosi M, Forsell A et al (1996) Moyamoya disease in Finno-Uguric origin. Br J Neurosurg 10:179–186
18. Isler W (1991) Moyamoya disease in Europe. In: Yonekawa Y (ed) Annual Report of Research Committee on Spontaneous Occlusion of the Circle of Willis (Moyamoya disease) of the Ministry of Welfare and Health, Japan 1990. Tokyo, pp 16–21
19. Kawano T, Fukui M, Hashimoto N et al (1994) Follow-up study of patients with "unilateral" moyamoya disease. Neurol Med Chir (Tokyo) 34:744–747
20. Kraemer M, Heienbrok W, Berlit P (2008) Moyamoya disease in Europeans. Stroke 39:3193–3200
21. Czabanka M, Vajkoczy P, Schmiedek P et al (2009) Age-dependent revascularization patterns in the treatment of moyamoya disease in a European patient population. Neurosurg Focus 26(4):E9
22. Fukuyama Y, Sugawara N, Osawa M (1991) A genetic study of idiopathic spontaneous occlusion of the circle of Willis. In: Yonekawa Y (ed) Annual Report of Research Committee on Spontaneous Occlusion of the Circle of Willis (Moyamoya disease) of the Ministry of Welfare and Health, 1990. Tokyo, pp 139–144
23. Scott RM, Smith ER (2009) Moyamoya disease and moyamoya syndrome. N Engl J Med 360:1226–1237
24. Hallemeier CL, Rich KM, Grubb RL et al (2006) Clinical features and outcome in North American adults with moyamoya phenomenon. Stroke 37:1490–1946
25. Handa H, Yonekawa Y (1985) Analysis of filing data bank of 1500 cases of spontaneous occlusion of the circle of Willis and study of 200 cases for more than 5 years. Stroke (Tokyo) 7:477–480
26. Chiu D, Shedden P, Bratina P et al (1998) Clinical features of moyamoya disease in the United States. Stroke 29:1347–1351
27. Miyamoto S, Kikuchi H, Karasawa J et al (1984) Study of the posterior circulation in moyamoya disease. Clinical and neuroradiological evaluation. J Neurosurg 61:1032–1037
28. Kawaguchi S, Sakaki T, Kakizaki T et al (1996) Clinical features of the haemorrhage type moyamoya disease based on 31 cases. Acta Neurochir (Wien) 138:1200–1210
29. Kawaguchi S, Sakaki T, Morimoto T et al (1996) Characteristics of intracranial aneurysms associated with moyamoya disease. A review of 111 cases. Acta Neurochir (Wien) 138:1287–1294
30. Donaghy RM, Yasargil G (1968) Extracranial blood flow diversions in microvascular surgery. The 36th Annual Meeting of the American Association of Neurological Surgeons, Chicago, Iiinois
31. Yasargil MG (1969) Microsurgery applied to neurosurgery. Thieme, Stuttgart
32. Henschen C (1950) Operative revascularization des zirkulatorisch geschädigten Gehirns durch Auflage gestielten Muskellappen (Encephalo-myo-synangiose). Langenbecks Arch Klein Chir 264:392–401
33. Matsushima Y, Fukai N, Tanaka K et al (1981) A new surgical treatment of moyamoya disease in children: a preliminary report. Surg Neurol 15(4):313–320

34. Yonekawa Y, Handa H, Moritake K et al (1985) Revascualrization in children with moyamoya disease: low-density area and regional cerebral blood flow after operation. In: Handa H, Kikuchi H, Yonekawa Y (eds) Microsurgical anastomosis for cerebral ischemia. Igaku-shoin, Tokyo, pp 272–274
35. Fujimura M, Kaneta T, Mugikura S et al (2007) Temporary neurologic deterioration due to cerebral hyperperfusion after superficial temporal artery-middle cerebral artery anastomosis in patients with adult-onset moyamoya disease. Surg Neurol 67:273–282
36. Iwama T, Hashimoto N, Miyake H et al (1998) Direct revascularization to the anterior cerebral artery territory in patients with moyamoya disease. Report of five cases. Neurosurgery 42:1157–1161
37. Tanaka K, Yonekawa Y, Satou K et al(1992) STA–ACA anastomosis with interposed vein graft. A case report. No Shinkei Geka (Tokyo) 20:171–176
38. Yonekawa Y, Imhof HG, Taub E et al (2001) Supracerebellar transtentorial approach for posterior temporomedial structures. J Neurosurg 94:339–345
39. Muroi C, Yonekawa Y, Khan N et al (2003) Case report. Metabolic changes after H215O-positron emission tomography with acetazolamide in a patient with moyamoya disease: case report and review of previous cases. J Neurosurg Anesthiol 15:131–139
40. Iwama T, Hashimoto N, Yonekawa Y (1996) The relevance of hemodynamic factors in perioperative complications in childhood moyamoya disease. Clinical studies. Neurosurgery 38:1120–1126

Moyamoya Disease in China

Jianmin Liu, Wenyuan Zhao, and Weimin Wang

Introduction

Moyamoya disease (MMD) was considered to be rare in China. With the tremendous improvement of medical care over the past 30 years, especially with the current universal availability of magnetic resonance imaging (MRI) and digital subtraction angiography (DSA), more MMD has been diagnosed. Data concerning its pathophysiological features, clinical presentation, and treatment have been reviewed. The ethnical difference between Chinese and Japanese or Korean seemed not be so large as previously believed [1].

Pathophysiological Features

Li [2] performed microscopical and elctronmicroscopical studies in 13 MMD cases documented by angiography. Segments of superficial temporal artery and middle meningeal artery (MMA) were sampled and the histological findings were compared with corresponding manifestation in angiography. Intimal thickening and internal elastic laminal disruption were found in superficial temporal artery (STA) and MMA no matter whether the angiographical manifestation in the corresponding segment was normal or abnormal. These findings challenge the conception that MMD was confined to the internal carotid artery (ICA) system.

Leptospirosis was reported to be an important cause of MMD in China. However, the prevalence of epidemic diseases is continuously changing and, thus, leptospirosis is no longer the major concern in China. Nowadays, most of the reported cases had no leptospirosis-related history. Wegener Granulomatosis was also reported in patients with MMD [3], but this was sporadic and, on the whole, no specific cause had been found for MMD in Chinese up to this time.

J.M. Liu (✉) and W.Y. Zhao
Department of Neurosurgery, Changhai Hospital, 168 Changhai Road, 200433, Shanghai, China
e-mail: liu118@vip.163.com

W.M. Wang
Department of Neurosurgery, Guangzhou General Hospital of Guangzhou Military Area Command, 510010, Guangzhou, China

B.-K. Cho and T. Tominaga (eds.), *Moyamoya Disease Update*,
DOI 10.1007/978-4-431-99703-0_51, © Springer 2010

Allergic injuries and certain cytokines may play a role in the development of MMD. An experimenta l rabbit model of MMD was established with normal horse serum injected into the neck regions on both sides of the common carotid arteries [4]. The concentrations of basic fibroblast growth factor (bFGF) in the cerebrospinal fluid of patients with MMD were measured using an enzyme-linked immunoadsorbent assay method [5]. The bFGF's average concentration in patients with MMD was significantly higher than that in the control group, which implies that bFGF may possibly lead to the constriction and obstruction of ICA and the formation of new blood vessels. Jin [6] measured the serum hepatocyte growth factor (HGF) concentrations in 30 patients with MMD, 60 healthy control subjects, and 8 non-MMD control patients with cerebral ischemia. Meanwhile, they detected the expression of HGF and its receptor c-Met by immunohistochemical technique in six branches of STAs and six branches of MMAs obtained from 12 patients with MMD, in comparison with the branches of STAs taken from two control patients with other diseases. The serum HGF concentrations in patients with MMD tended to be somewhat higher than those in patients with cerebral ischemic non-MMD, although the difference was not statistically significant. The sections of STAs and MMAs taken from the patients with MMD showed dense and strong HGF and c-Met immunoreactivity in smooth muscle cells and endothelial cells of the arterial walls, whereas the control sections had only scattered or faint immunoreactivity. The elevated serum HGF concentrations and the high expression of HGF and c-Met in the arterial walls of the STAs and MMAs in patients with MMD suggest that HGF may be a factor in the development of MMD. Xin [7] evaluated the concentration of vascular endothelial growth factor (VEGF) and transforming growth factor β1 (TGFβ1) in the serum of MMD patients and healthy controls. The average concentrations of VEGF and TGFβ1 in the serum of patients with MMD were significantly higher than that in the control group. Therefore, VEGF and TGFβ1 may also be considered MMD-related cytokines.

Clinical Presentation

There have been few systemically epidemic investigations on MMD in China. Our data mainly relied on sporadic clinical reports. Currently, we have less than 400 cases with MMD reported, although the actual number of diagnosed or treated MMD should be far higher. Certain clinical features of MMD in Chinese may be different from those in the people of other countries [8–10] .The age distribution among Chinese patients showed two peaks that were similar to Japanese and Korean patients. The first peak was within the first decade and the second was between 21 and 40 years. However, there was a male prevalence over female and the incidence of adult MMD was higher than that of children in Chinese. Duan [8] analyzed 54 cases with MMD that was strictly diagnosed according to MMD criteria [11]. The male to female ratio was about 1.16:1 and the child to adult ratio was 1:3.5.

Transient ischemic attacks such as hemiparesis, monoparesis, and sensory impairment are common in children. Intracranial hemorrhage is not common in the pediatric group. In contrast, adult patients usually presented with intracranial hemorrhage, such as intraventricular, subarachnoid, or intracerebral. In 2006, a study reviewed 4,564 cases of spontaneous SAH presented to 33 medical centers in China (sponsored by Huasan hospital, unpublished). A total of 3,728 cases had full cerebral vessel angiography and 527 of them were nonaneurysmal SAH, among which 42 (8%) were MMD. Intraventricular hemorrhage was prone to occur in females and the prognosis was usually benign. In Duan's series of a total of 72 patients, 22% had symptoms related with ischemia, among which 44.44% were cerebral infarction and 27.78% were TIA [8].

Only 20.37% of the patients presented with intracranial hemorrhage and 81.8% of them were female. The incidence of cerebral infarction may be higher in Chinese patient but transient ischemic attack and seizure may be lower than in Japanese. However, we should be cautious in interpreting these differences. Firstly, there is no strict discrimination between MMD and moyamoya syndrome in some papers. Many reported cases had incomplete etiological examinations. Therefore, "moyamoya" often refers to the distinctive findings on cerebral arteriography, independent of the cause. Secondly, bias may exist concerning the age of onset and preponderance of hemorrhagic to ischemic presentation. Neurological pediatrics is not popular in the mainland of China and MMD in children can easily be ignored by the parents and physicians. Ischemic symptoms may less likely arouse a thorough etiological examination than hemorrhagic cases.

CT or MRI is routinely performed as preliminary screening work-up for MMD, while single photon emission CT or CT perfusion is used for evaluating the cerebral hemodynamic, but the Acetazolamide loading test [12] is only performed in a few institutes in China.

Although MRI, MRA, and CTA were used for diagnosis by some institutes, DSA was performed for the definitive diagnosis and hemodynamic evaluation in most of the reported cases in China. Tang [13] reviewed the angiogram of 19 MMD cases, among which 12 revealed posterior cerebral artery involvement and 5 demonstrated basilar artery stenosis. Such a high incidence of posterior circulation involvement was not common; however, there was no etiological study in the paper and patient bias may exist.

Treatment

There is a trend towards performing surgical operations on either ischemic or hemorrhagic MMD patients although there are few data verifying efficacy in preventing recurrent hemorrhage among Chinese. Medical therapy is mainly adopted as postoperative management. Direct bypass or indirect revascularization was practised by different institutes. While direct bypass immediately increased the cerebral blood flow, indirect revascularization procedures include encephalo-duro-arterio-synangiosis, encephalo-myo-arterio-synangiosis, dural inversion, and multiple burr holes without vessel synangiosis can establish collateral circulation within 3–6 months. The efficacy of indirect revascularization was well documented and the establishing of a new blood supply was seen in 58–100% of patients confirmed by ECT, CT perfusion, and angiography [8,14]. It is worth mentioning that in a series of 27 adults MMD treated with the multiple burr holes operation in Changhai hospital (unpublished), 3 months follow-up angiogram after operation was available in 17 cases with all cases showed abundant collateral blood flow from an extra-carotid artery, mainly from MMA. It is satisfying to achieve this result in adult patients. Combined operation procedures which include direct bypass integrating with indirect revascularization or EDAS integrating with multiple burr holes are being practised in some institutes. However, the benefit of such combined procedures still requires further evaluation.

References

1. Matsushima Y, Qian L, Aoyagi M (1997) Comparison of moyamoya disease in Japan and moyamoya disease (or syndrome) in the People's Republic of China. Clin Neurol Neurosurg 99 Suppl 2:s19–s22
2. Li B, Wang ZC, Zhao JZ et al (1990) Extracarotid angiography and ultrastructure study in moyamoya. Chin J Neurosurg 6(3):173–175

3. Wang Y, Zeng W, Xue XP et al (2003) Wegener granulomatosis accompanied with cerebral infarction and moyamoya. Case report. Chin J Rbeumatol 7(10):647
4. Zhang HO, Rao ML, Zhang SQ et al (2001) An experimental study on the pathogenic role of immune complex to moyamoya disease. Chin J Neuroimmunol Neuro 13(2):121–123
5. Zhang Y, Meng GL, Zhao JZ et al (2003) The role of basic fibroblast growth factors in the pathogenesis of moyamoya disease. Chin J Nerv Ment Dis 29(1):39–41
6. Jin H, Zou LP, Duan L et a1 (2007) The roles of HGF in the pathogenesis of moyamoya disease. J Apoplexy Nerv Dis 24(2):150–153
7. Xin Y, Zhao JZ et al (2005) Changes of the serum level of vascular endothelial growth factor and transforming growth factor β1 in patients with moyamoya disease. Beijin Med 27(6):321–323
8. Duan L, Sun WJ, Wang FY et al (2005) Analysis of clinical features in Chinese patients with moyamoya disease. Chin J Clin Neurosurg 10(4):269–272
9. Sien TC, Yang HL, Chung YH et al (1988) Moyamoya disease in Taiwan. Stroke 19:53–59
10. Wang ZC (1994) Cerebral vascular diseases and surgical treatment. Beijing: Beijing publishing company 180–195
11. Fukui M (1997) Guidelines for the diagnosis and treatment of spontaneous occlusion of the circle of Willis ('moyamoya' disease). Clin Neurol Neurosurg 99 Suppl 2:S238–S240
12. Gao QY, Li N, Li YM et al (2004) Evaluation of cerebral hemodynamic in moyamoya disease using acetazolamide (Diamox)99mTc-HMPAO SPECT. J Chin Med Univ 33(1):80–82
13. Tang WJ, Fan WJ, Huang XL (1999) DSA analysis of moyamoya disease. J Prac Radio 15(12):720–723
14. Yang MQ, Ni M, Wang S et al (2007) Clinical analysis of the hemorrhagic type moyamoya disease. J Cap Med Univ 28(4):528–531

Part XV
Future Perspectives

Future Perspectives in Moyamoya Disease

Byung-Kyu Cho

Introduction

It has been half a century since K. Takeuchi and K. Shimizu first reported a new entity in vascular disease in 1957, moyamoya disease (MMD) [1]. This disease is a relatively rare vascular disease and has a high prevalence in children and Asian ethnics; thus, it has not been of great interest to physicians and researchers in non-Asian countries. The Research Committee on Spontaneous Occlusion of the Circle of Willis (Moyamoya Disease) of the Ministry of Health and Welfare in Japan launched a project in 1977 to investigate the disease, and continues to study its pathogenesis, epidemiology, and treatment. Most of the reported literature about MMD is from Japan. The annual report of the Committee has accumulated many clinical as well as research data, and studies are ongoing. The incidence of reports on MMD is increasing in Western countries. It is important to understand the current status of MMD management with its unsolved problems. No standardized surgical method of choice has yet been established. One reason for this is the absence of standardized evaluation measures and protocols. Here, current evaluation measures for pre- and post-operative outcomes are reviewed, and novel therapeutic research trials are presented as potential future perspectives on this disease.

Outcome Evaluation

Clinical Outcome Measurements

Clinical outcomes in patients with MMD are graded according to symptoms and neurologic deficits. Matsushima et al. [2] graded outcomes into four grades: Grade I (Excellent: neurological deficits recovered completely and transient ischemic attacks (TIAs), disappeared), Grade II (Good: minor neurological deficits improved to a certain degree or reduced in severity;

B.-K. Cho (✉)
Division of Pediatric Neurosurgery, Pediatric Clinical Neuroscience Center,
Seoul National University Children's Hospital, Seoul National University College of Medicine,
101 Daehangno, Jongno-gu, Seoul, 110-744, Republic of Korea
e-mail: bkcho@snu.ac.kr

B.-K. Cho and T. Tominaga (eds.), *Moyamoya Disease Update*,
DOI 10.1007/978-4-431-99703-0_52, © Springer 2010

the occurrence of TIAs was markedly reduced after surgery), Grade III (Fair: preoperative neurological symptoms partially improved), and Grade IV (Poor: neurologic deficits were unchanged, worsened, or new after surgery). Matsushima later simplified this system into three clinical outcome grades [3]: Grade A (symptoms completely disappeared), Grade B (symptoms improved, but remained to some extent), and Grade C (symptoms unchanged). This latter grading system has been widely used.

A somewhat different grading of four clinical outcomes has also been used in patients with MMD. These include: Excellent – preoperative symptoms (such as TIAs or seizures) disappeared, without neurologic deficits; Good – symptoms disappeared but neurologic deficits remained; Fair – symptoms persisted, albeit less frequently; and Poor – symptoms remained unchanged or worsened. These four gradings can be simplified into two categories: Favorable – excellent and good grades; and Unfavorable – fair and poor grades. This grading focuses on the importance of the disappearance of TIAs [4].

Another three gradings of revascularization (RV) in patients with MMD have been introduced. These include: Improved disease – complete disappearance of TIAs and neurologic improvement; Stable disease – absence of new neurologic deficits during follow-up with persistence of manifest preoperative deficits, TIAs decreased; and Progressive disease – worsening of observed symptoms. Observed neurologic symptoms included hemiparesis, sensory deficits, aphasia, and TIAs. Diffuse neurologic symptoms, such as cognitive deficits or persistent headaches, were not included [5].

The degree of reduction in TIAs and neurologic deficits is mainly measured for clinical outcomes. However, the grading of these measurements differs in each institution; thus, direct comparison of clinical outcome data is not accurate. Furthermore, the time frame of evaluation of clinical outcomes differs between studies. For example, the outcome report based on the duration of follow-up differs in each report. To compare different studies accurately, outcome data would need to be reported within defined periods of observation; for example, after 6 months, 1 year, or 2 years.

Angiographic Evaluation of Revascularization

The most widely used grading system of postoperative angiographic RV is Matsushima's three-grade method: Grade A – Good (collateral formation supplied for more than two-thirds of middle cerebral artery, MCA, distribution); Grade B – Fair (between one-third and two-thirds of MCA distribution); and Grade C – Poor (slight or no collateral formation). This method was basically devised for indirect RV procedures and for RV of the MCA territory. This classification is very simple and practical; however, it presents some difficulties in classifying borderline RV [3].

A more detailed evaluation system for RV is angiographic scoring according to the degree of dilatation of the dural artery and the donor artery, degrees of RV, and decrease in moyamoya vessels. This method involves 23 grades (14 scores) [6]. Unfortunately, this integrative method of evaluation has not been widely applied, probably because it is a little complex and time consuming.

An analysis of RV, used mainly for direct RV procedures, is to classify the degree of RV according to the number of MCA branches that are filled and the flow direction; that is, GI (anastomosed MCA filled only), GII (two or more MCA branches filled), and GIII (ante- and retro-grade filling of the entire MCA system) [5, 7]. In fact, we often confirm antegrade as well as retrograde flow through the anastomosed superficial temporal artery (STA)–MCA at the end of anastomosis surgery.

RV of anterior cerebral artery (ACA) territory can be classified into three grades, in the same way as the grading of MCA territory by Matsushima, that is: Good – RV of more than two-thirds of the ACA distribution; Fair – RV of one-third to two-thirds of the ACA distribution; and Poor – slight or no RV [4].

The dynamic 2-D cine phase-contrast magnetic resonance imaging (MRI) technique can be used to measure blood volume flow (BVF) of the STA–MCA bypass. In a previous study, angiographic RV grade was correlated with BVF as follows: Grade I (poor) – BVF values of 48 ml/min or lower; Grade II (moderate) – BVF between Grades I and III, mean 73.6 ± 16.7 ml/min (48.3–111); and Grade III (good) – mean 97.2 ± 26.6 ml/min (49.2–177.6). However, only BVF values higher than 111 ml/min (15% of all samples) were specific for extensive angiographic bypass [7].

Another magnetic resonance angiography method introduced scoring of each internal carotid artery (ICA) (0–3), MCA (0–3), ACA (0–2), and posterior cerebral artery (0–2) according to the severity of the steno-occlusive change, and in total 0 to 10 scores were assigned to each hemisphere. Good correlation of this technique with the conventional angiographic stages of Suzuki and Kodama was confirmed [8].

Power Doppler through the temporal-bone window is another method that was introduced to assess angiographic RV after encephalomyosynangiosis (EMS). This method involves grading RV as: Grade 1 – absent (0 vessel); Grade 2 – moderate (one–four vessels); and Grade 3 – extensive (>four vessels) [9, 20].

Different measures are used in different institutions; therefore, comparison of outcome data between institutions or procedures is inaccurate.

Hemodynamic Evaluation

Single-photon emission computed tomography (SPECT) has been most commonly used to assess the regional cerebral blood flow (rCBF), and vascular reactivity to vasodilating agents (vascular perfusion reserve). Diamox-challenge SPECT is most useful to confirm the hemodynamic compromise (decreased vascular reserve) of the ischemic brain. The *N*-isopropyl[^{123}I]-*p*-iodoamphetamine (IMP)-SPECT redistribution pattern (types I, II, III, and IV) has been analyzed to differentiate ischemic and nonischemic regions [10]. However, this study had poor resolution, and only the lobar level of evaluation was possible, making absolute quantitation of CBF difficult. Positron emission tomography (PET) is another powerful technique used to measure rCBF, regional cerebral blood volume (rCBV), regional oxygen extraction fraction (rOEF), regional transit time (rTT), and regional cerebral metabolic rate for oxygen ($rCMRO_2$). This technique is increasingly being used in many centers; however, there are not a lot of data on MMD, particularly for preoperative and postoperative long-term follow-up studies. Decreased rCBF and increased rOEF are important parameters for surgical indication of MMD [11]; however, PET requires technical improvement to obtain better resolution of cerebral hemodynamics.

Perfusion MRI and perfusion computed tomography are rapidly increasing the technical aspects of neuroimaging studies as well as evaluation of the perfusion status of the ischemic brain. Currently, regional cerebral perfusion, rCBV, regional transit time to peak (rTTP), and regional mean transit time are good parameters with which to evaluate hemodynamic function. However, the resolution of imaging is almost the same in SPECT and PET techniques. The advancement of flow-imaging techniques is continuing and will provide higher resolution images and more accurate, useful information of cerebral hemodynamics in the near future.

Evaluation of Cognitive Function

Intelligence quotient and/or development quotient are often measured to evaluate the integrative higher cortical function; however, more quantitative data that analyzes language, learning, memory, calculation, attention, concentration, and visuospatial/ visuoconstructional/ visuo-perceptual abilities are necessary to evaluate the effect of RV surgery on cognitive function. Analysis of the full cognitive function of patients with MMD is not usually available in the literature.

Functional Status and Quality of Life Measurements

The Lansky Play-Performance Scale score for children, and the Karnofsky Performance Scale score, the modified Rankin Scale score, and activities of daily living measures for adults are commonly used to assess follow-up functional neurologic status of patients with MMD. Information about quality of life measures is very limited in the literature.

A standardized evaluation of patients with MMD for presurgical baseline studies and postsurgical follow-ups is essential to accurately analyze and compare the outcomes of each surgical procedure. For this purpose, the establishment of an international cooperative network for standardized protocols of MMD evaluation is mandatory.

Treatment Aspects

Treatment aspects of MMD and their perspectives can be considered in three categories: first, the efficacy of current surgical methods; second, the experimental treatment of ischemic injury; and third, the prevention of MMD.

Current Surgical Methods

Various surgical methods have been introduced using many types of donor tissues individually or in combination, particularly in indirect RV procedures; e.g., STAs, dura (middle meningeal artery), muscles (deep temporal artery), galea, and periosteum. However, it remains unknown which tissue is the most effective to use in surgery. The reasons for this are the small number of patients, the various combinations and modifications of indirect procedures used, and the absence of a standardized evaluation protocol for MMD/MMS, as mentioned in the previous section. The direct RV procedure has a standardized protocol; that is, STA–MCA direct anastomosis. However, many different methods are used for indirect procedures, with various modifications according to donor tissue used. The more donor tissues that are used in wide ischemic areas, the more RV of the ischemic brain may be expected. However, verification of the efficacy of this complex, extensive, and indirect procedure of using more than one type of donor tissue is needed; e.g., whether the encephalo-duro-myo-arterio-periosteal synangiosis (EDMAPS) and STA–MCA bypass conducted by the Hokkaido group [12] has better long-term outcomes than less complex, multiple, combined indirect procedures. The clinical indications of this approach are also an issue. A review of the literature revealed that more complex combined procedures result in significantly better angiographic RV than the indirect RV procedure (as a pooled procedure); however, there was no significant difference in clinical symptomatic outcomes between the pooled indirect RV procedure and the direct and/or combined RV procedures in pediatric MMD [13, 14]. More refined evaluation measures are necessary to differentiate between the efficacies of each surgical procedure.

Experimental Treatment of Ischemic Injury

Strategies for treating ischemic stroke include: (1) neuroprotection, preventing injured neurons from undergoing apoptosis in the acute phase of cerebral ischemia; and (2) stem cell therapy, the repair of disrupted neuronal networks with newly born neurons in the chronic phase of cerebral ischemia [15].

Recently, numerous agents including cytokines and trophic factors have been confirmed to have neuroprotective effects in an animal model of cerebral ischemia, for example angiopoietin 1, glial cell-line-derived neurotrophic factor, brain-derived neurotrophic factor, insulin-like growth factor 1 (IGF-1), retinoic acid, cyclin-dependent kinase-5, systemic lipopolysaccharide, interleukin-10, neurogenin-1, and niacin.

Many of these agents have been transfected into various stem cells via viral vectors, and then transplanted or injected into the ischemic animal model to determine therapeutic effects and mechanisms of action. The most commonly used stem cells are human mesenchymal stem cells (hMSCs), human neuronal stem cells (hNSCs), bone marrow stem cells, hematopoietic stem cells, and human embryonic stem cells.

Human MSCs transfected with angiopoietin-1 and the *VEGF* gene (Ang-VEGF-hMSC) by intravenous injection into a rat MCA-occlusion model showed structural–functional recovery of the animals [15, 16]. Continuous IGF-1 overexpression through an adeno-associated virus transduction system through stereotactic injection promoted long-lasting functional recovery after cerebral infarction in a mouse model of chronic stage infarction [17]. Inhibition of hypoxia-inducible factor-1α (HIF-1α), a proapoptotic factor, with small interfering RNA (siRNA), reduced the infarction volume, decreased mortality, improved neurological deficits, and reduced Evans blue extravasation in a rat model of focal ischemic [18]. Brain transplantation of hNSCs overexpressing Akt1 in an animal model of intracerebral hematoma resulted in functional recovery, survival, and differentiation of grafted hNSCs [19].

Details of gene and stem cell therapy are discussed in the chapter by Tokunaga and Date, in this volume.

These studies indicate that the use of angiogenic, antiapoptotic, siRNA, cytokine, and trophic factors through gene transduction systems for the treatment of the ischemic injured brain may be used in clinical practice in the near future.

Prevention of Disease

Prevention of MMD requires the basic approach of controlling its etiology. Currently, knowledge of familial MMD has been accumulated to clarify genetic defects. In addition, genetic studies of sporadic MMD are necessary to determine the basic genetic abnormalities. Familial MMD is discussed in the chapter "Familial Moyamoya Disease" by Suzuki in this volume.

If relevant genes are identified, the development of novel gene therapy and the early detection of MMD through a screening test will be possible.

References

1. Takeuchi K, Shimizu K (1957) Hypogenesis of bilateral internal carotid artery. No To Shinkei 9:37–43
2. Matsushima T, Fujiwara S, Nagata S et al (1989) Surgical treatment for pediatric patients with moyamoya disease by indirect revascularization procedures (EDAS, EMS, EMAS). Acta Neurochir 98:135–140
3. Matsushima T, Inoue T, Suzuki SO (1992) Surgical treatment of moyamoya disease in pediatric patients-comparison the results of indirect and direct revascularization procedures. Neurosurgery 31:401–405
4. Kim SK, Wang KC, Kim IO et al (2002) Combined encephaloduroarteriosynangiosis and bifrontal encephalogaleo(periosteal)synangiosis in pediatric moyamoya disease. Neurosurgery 50:88–96
5. Czabanka M, Vajkoczy P, Schmiedek P (2009) Age-dependent revascularization patterns in the treatment of moyamoya disease in European patient population. Neurosurg Focus 26(4):E9
6. Matsushima Y, Aoyagi M, Niimi Y et al (1990) Symptoms and their pattern of progression in childhood moyamoya disease. Brain Dev 12(6):784–789
7. Horn P, Vajkoczy P, Schmiedek P et al (2004) Evaluation of extracranial-intracranial arterial bypass function with magnetic resonance angiography. Neuroradiology 46:723–729
8. Houkin K, Nakayama N, Kuroda S et al (2005) Novel magnetic resonance angiography stage grading for moyamoya disease. Cerebrovasc Dis 20:347–354
9. Perren F, Meairs S, Schmiedek P et al (2005) Power Doppler evaluation of revascularization in childhood moyamoya. Neurology 64:558–560
10. Sato H, Sato N, Tamaki N et al (1990) Chronic low-perfusion state in children with moyamoya disease following revascularization. Childs Nerv Syst 6(3):166–171
11. Ikezaki K, Matsushima T, Kuwabara Y et al (1994) Cerebral circulation and oxygen metabolism in childhood moyamoya disease: a perioperative positron emission tomography study. J Neurosurg 81:843–850
12. Kuroda S, Houkin K (2008) Moyamoya disease: current concepts and future prospective. Lancet Neurol 7:1056–1066
13. Guzman R, Lee M, Achrol A et al (2009) Clinical outcome after 450 revascularization procedures for moymoy disease. J Neurosurg. doi: 10.3171/2009.4.JNS081649
14. Veeravagu A, Guzman R, Path CG et al (2008) Moyamoya disease in pediatric patients: outcomes of neurosurgical interventions. Neurosurg Focus 24(2):1–9
15. Yamashita T, Deguchi K, Nagotani S et al (2009) Gene and stem cell therapy in ischemic stroke. Cell Transplant Apr 29 Pii:CT-2061 [Epub ahead of print]
16. Toyama K, Honmou O, Harada K et al (2009) Therapeutic benefits of angiogenetic gene-modified human mesenchymal stem cells after cerebral ischemia. Exp Neurol 216(1):47–55
17. Zhu W, Fan Y, Hao Q et al (2009) Postischemic IGF-1 gene transfer promotes neurovascular regeneration after experimental stroke. J Cereb Blood Flow Metab 29(9):1528–1537
18. Chen C, Hu Q, Yan J et al (2009) Early inhibition of HIF-1alpha with small interfering RNA reduce ischemic-reperfused brain injury in rats. Neurobiol Dis 33(3):509–517
19. Lee HJ, Kim MK, Kim HJ et al (2009) Human neural stem cells genetically modified to overexpress Akt1 provide neuroprotection and functional improvement in mouse stroke model. PLoS One 4(5):e5586
20. Perren F, Horn P, Vajkoczy P et al (2005) Power Doppler imaging in detection of surgically induced indirect neoangiogenesis in adult moyamoya disease. J Neurosurg 103:869–872

Index

MIX
Papier aus verantwortungsvollen Quellen
Paper from responsible sources
FSC® C105338

If you have any concerns about our products,
you can contact us on
ProductSafety@springernature.com

In case Publisher is established outside the EU,
the EU authorized representative is:
Springer Nature Customer Service Center GmbH
Europaplatz 3, 69115 Heidelberg, Germany

Printed by Libri Plureos GmbH
in Hamburg, Germany